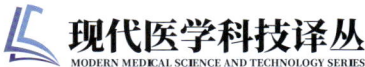

# 现代医学科技译丛
MODERN MEDICAL SCIENCE AND TECHNOLOGY SERIES

# 肺移植
# 胸外科临床问题

Lung Transplantation, An Issue of Thoracic Surgery Clinics

[美] 弗吉尼亚·R.利特尔（Virginia R. Litle）
**顾问主编**

[美] 贾斯琳·库克雷亚（Jasleen Kukreja）
[美] 艾达·维纳多（Aida Venado）
**主编**

陈静瑜　张兰军
**主审**

周建平
**主译**

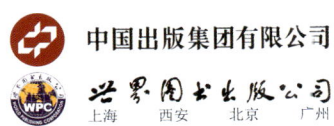

中国出版集团有限公司
世界图书出版公司
上海　西安　北京　广州

图书在版编目（CIP）数据

肺移植：胸外科临床问题 /（美）贾斯琳·库克雷亚,（美）艾达·维纳多主编；周建平译. -- 上海：上海世界图书出版公司, 2025.7. -- ISBN 978-7-5232-1938-6

Ⅰ. R655.3

中国国家版本馆CIP数据核字第2025T89N24号

| | |
|---|---|
| 书　　名 | 肺移植：胸外科临床问题<br>Feiyizhi: Xiongwaike Linchuang Wenti |
| 主　　编 | [美] 贾斯琳·库克雷亚　　[美] 艾达·维纳多 |
| 主　　译 | 周建平 |
| 策　　划 | 曹高腾 |
| 责任编辑 | 芮晴舟 |
| 出版发行 | 上海世界图书出版公司 |
| 地　　址 | 上海市广中路88号9-10楼 |
| 邮　　编 | 200083 |
| 网　　址 | http://www.wpcsh.com |
| 经　　销 | 新华书店 |
| 印　　刷 | 运河（唐山）印务有限公司 |
| 开　　本 | 787 mm × 1092 mm　1/16 |
| 印　　张 | 15.25 |
| 字　　数 | 300千字 |
| 版　　次 | 2025年7月第1版　2025年7月第1次印刷 |
| 版权登记 | 图字09-2025-0409号 |
| 书　　号 | ISBN 978-7-5232-1938-6 / R·775 |
| 定　　价 | 128.00元 |

版权所有　翻印必究
如发现印装质量问题，请与印刷厂联系
（质检科电话：022-59658568）

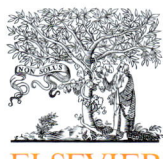

Elsevier (Singapore) Pte Ltd.
3 Killiney Road,
#08-01 Winsland House I,
Singapore 239519
Tel: (65) 6349-0200; Fax: (65) 6733-1817

Lung Transplantation, An Issue of Thoracic Surgery Clinics.

Copyright © 2022 Elsevier Inc. All rights are reserved, including those for text and data mining, AI training, and similar technologies.

Publisher's note: Elsevier takes a neutral position with respect to territorial disputes or jurisdictional claims in its published content, including in maps and institutional affiliations.

ISBN-13: 978-0-323-89768-6

This translation of Lung Transplantation, An Issue of Thoracic Surgery Clinics by Jasleen Kukreja, Aida Venado was undertaken by World Publishing Shanghai Corporation Limited and is published by arrangement with Elsevier (Singapore) Pte Ltd.

Lung Transplantation, An Issue of Thoracic Surgery Clinics by Jasleen Kukreja, Aida Venado由世界图书出版上海有限公司进行翻译，并根据世界图书出版上海有限公司与爱思唯尔（新加坡）私人有限公司的协议约定出版。

《肺移植：胸外科临床问题》（周建平 主译）
ISBN 978-7-5232-1938-6

Copyright © 2025 by Elsevier (Singapore) Pte Ltd. and World Publishing Shanghai Corporation Limited.

All rights reserved. No part of this publication may be reproduced or transmitted in any form or by any means, electronic or mechanical, including photocopying, recording, or any information storage and retrieval system, without permission in writing from Elsevier (Singapore) Pte Ltd and World Publishing Shanghai Corporation Limited.

声明

本译本由世界图书出版上海有限公司独立完成。相关从业及研究人员必须凭借其自身经验和知识对文中描述的信息数据、方法策略、搭配组合、实验操作进行评估和使用。由于医学科学发展迅速，临床诊断和给药剂量尤其需要经过独立验证。在法律允许的最大范围内，爱思唯尔、译文的原文作者、原文编辑及原文内容提供者均不对译文或因产品责任、疏忽或其他操作造成的人身及/或财产伤害及/或损失承担责任，亦不对由于使用文中提到的方法、产品、说明或思想而导致的人身及/或财产伤害及/或损失承担责任。

Printed in China by World Publishing Shanghai Corporation Limited under special arrangement with Elsevier (Singapore) Pte Ltd. This edition is authorized for sale in the People's Republic of China only, excluding Hong Kong SAR, Macau SAR and Taiwan. Unauthorized export of this edition is a violation of the contract.

译者团队风采

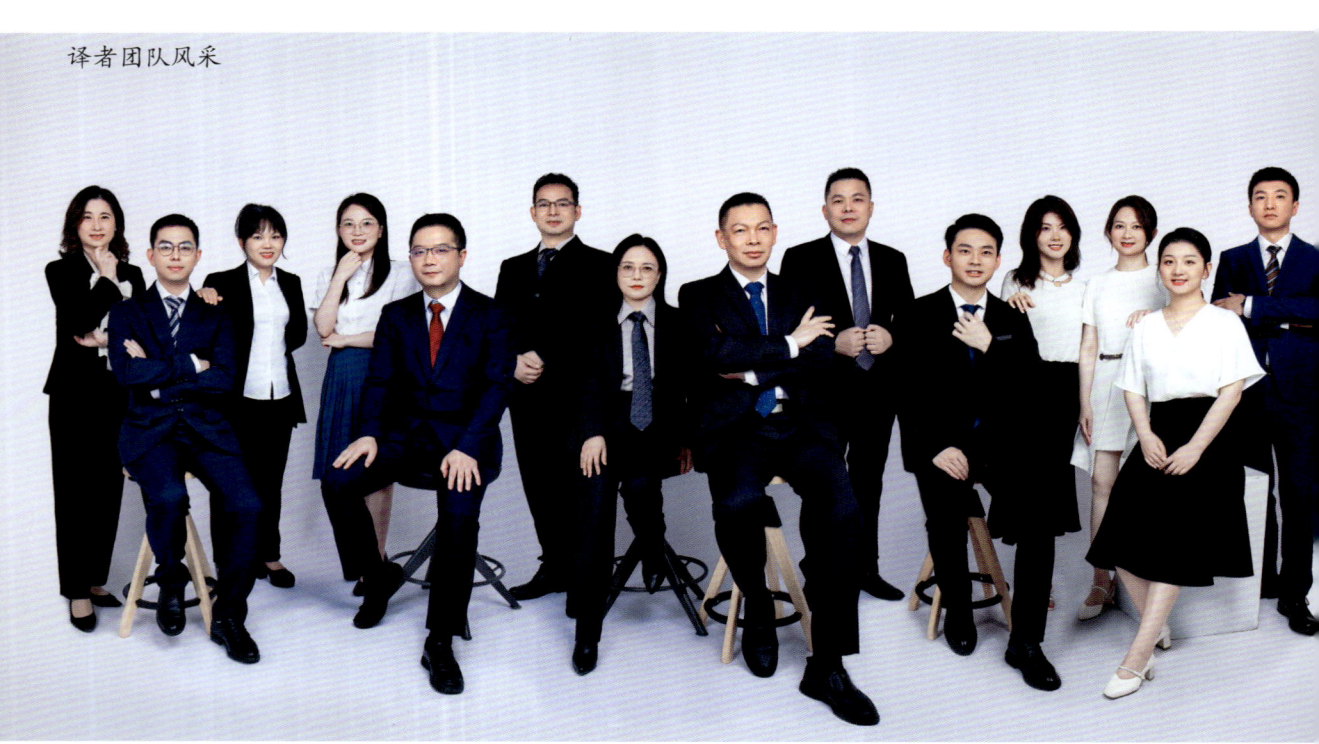

# 译者名单

## 主 审

陈静瑜　浙江大学医学院附属第二医院
张兰军　中山大学附属肿瘤医院

## 主 译

周建平　东莞市人民医院（南方医科大学第十附属医院）

## 副主译

郭素峡　东莞市人民医院（南方医科大学第十附属医院）
方年新　东莞市人民医院（南方医科大学第十附属医院）
付春来　东莞市人民医院（南方医科大学第十附属医院）

## 译 者（按姓氏笔画排序）

单位：东莞市人民医院（南方医科大学第十附属医院）

朱小冬　孙　昊　孙树楷　扶志敏　李　聪
杨燕华　陈晓渝　周　伟　周永巧　袁金权
梁瑞茵　谢哲凡　谢锐文　廖敏琪　黎昱江

# 主审简介

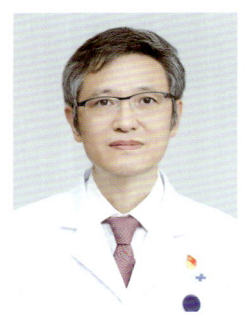

**陈静瑜** 南京医科大学二级教授、博士生导师，南京医科大学附属无锡市人民医院副院长、江苏省肺移植中心主任。浙江大学医学院附属第二医院副院长、肺移植中心主任。

中国人体器官捐献与移植委员会委员，中华医学会器官移植学分会常务委员、肺移植组组长，国家卫健委肺移植数据管理单位负责人，国家肺移植质控中心主任。主持国家重点研发项目、"十一五"国家科技攻关项目。第十一届、十二届、十三届全国人大代表。

从事胸部疾病的诊断、治疗及胸部癌症的综合治疗近40年。2021年以来，专攻肺移植临床研究及基础研究，所带领肺移植中心成为全球前三的肺移植中心。个人肺移植手术量超1500例，近3年每年主刀肺移植手术量超200例。同时建立了中国肺移植质控体系，发表了10多个指南、规范、标准。扶持国家23个省近40家医院开展了肺移植，推动了肺移植在全国的普及。完成多项创新性的肺移植手术。全球首创劈裂式异位双肺叶移植、漏斗胸纠正同期双肺移植，完成全球首例产妇心脏修补肺移植。

发表有关肺移植的"中华级"论文130多篇，*Cell* 等SCI论文50多篇，主持编写专著3部。

先后荣获全国五一劳动奖章、全国先进工作者，国务院特殊津贴获得者，国家卫生健康突出贡献中青年专家。荣获华夏建设科学技术一等奖、中华医学科技奖二等奖、江苏省科技奖三等奖、教育部科技奖一等奖。2020年荣获"中国医师奖"称号。

# 主审简介

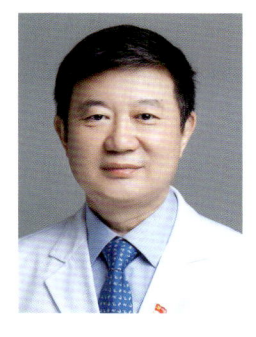

**张兰军** 教授，博士及博士后导师，主任医师。中山大学附属肿瘤医院胸科主任、肺癌首席专家。

中华医学会胸心血管外科学分会委员兼肺癌外科学组副组长，国际肺癌研究协会（IASLC）Active Member，全国控烟与肺癌防治协作组副组长，中国医师协会整合医学会胸外科分会副主任委员，中国抗癌协会科普专业委员会常务委员，国家癌症中心肺癌质控专家委员会委员，中国抗癌协会肺癌专业委员会委员，中国抗癌协会食管癌专业委员会委员，中国医疗保健国际交流促进会理事兼胸外科分会、肺癌防控分会副主任委员，中国医药教育协会肺癌医学教育委员会副主任委员，中国医药教育协会胸部肿瘤微创诊疗专业委员会副主任委员，中国医药教育协会胸外科专业委员会副主任委员，中国临床肿瘤学会（CSCO）非小细胞肺癌专业委员会常务委员，海峡两岸医药卫生交流协会胸外科专业委员会副主任委员，中国胸外科肺癌联盟（CLCU）南方联盟主席，广东生物医学工程学会理事兼胸心外科分会主任委员，广东临床医学学会资深专家委员会副主任委员，广东临床医学学会精准医疗学会副主任委员。第三届"国之名医·优秀风范"获得者（2019年），"羊城好医生"及"岭南名医"获得者，广东省委医疗保健专家。

# 主译简介

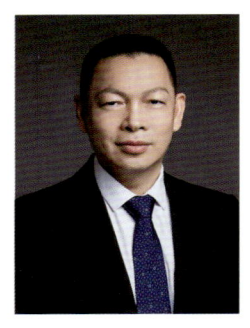

**周建平** 广东医科大学兼职教授,硕士生导师,心胸外科主任医师。东莞市人民医院(南方医科大学第十附属医院)副院长。

海峡两岸医药卫生交流协会胸外科分会常务委员,广东省医学会胸外科学分会常务委员,广东省医师协会胸外科分会常务委员,广东省生物医学工程学会心胸外科分会副主任委员。

东莞地区最早从事心胸外科专业的医生之一,擅长胸外科创伤和胸部肿瘤诊断与治疗,建立和发展了地区微创胸外科技术,牵头建立地区肺部肿瘤 MDT,对于胸外科疑难重症治疗、肺部肿瘤综合治疗、复合伤治疗有丰富经验。在 *Lung Cancer* 等国内外杂志发表学术论文 30 余篇,管理类论文 4 篇;主编、参编论著 3 部。担任《中国卫生产业》杂志编委。获得全国卫生系统先进个人、岭南名医、东莞名医、东莞特色人才荣誉称号。

# 原著贡献者

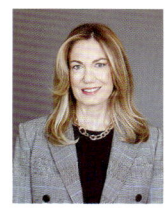

顾问主编

弗吉尼亚·R. 利特尔（Virginia R. Litle），医学博士

美国犹他州默里市山间医疗保健系统，胸外科及心血管外科主任

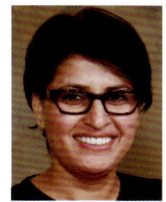

主　编

贾斯琳·库克雷亚（Jasleen Kukreja），医学博士、公共卫生硕士

美国加利福尼亚州旧金山市，加利福尼亚大学旧金山分校，心胸外科及肺移植外科主任，外科教授

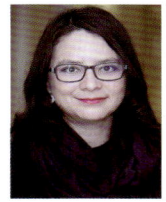

主　编

艾达·维纳多（Aida Venado），医学博士、应用统计硕士

美国加利福尼亚州旧金山市，加利福尼亚大学旧金山分校，呼吸与危重症医学科、过敏与睡眠医学科，肺移植外科医生，医学助理教授

## 作　者

**Aadil Ali**，博士

加拿大安大略省多伦多市，多伦多综合医院，多伦多大学健康网络，外科系，胸外科分部，多伦多肺移植项目

**Selim M. Arcasoy**，医学博士、公共卫生硕士

美国纽约州纽约市，哥伦比亚大学欧文医学中心，肺移植项目

**Ashwini Arjuna**，医学博士

美国亚利桑那州凤凰城，克雷顿大学医学院凤凰城分校，圣约瑟夫医疗中心，诺顿胸科研究所，医学临床助理教授

**Amit Bery**，医学博士

美国密苏里州圣路易斯市，华盛顿大学医学院，医学系，肺病与重症监护医学科

**Ankit Bharat**，医学博士

美国伊利诺伊州芝加哥市，西北大学范伯格医学院，胸外科分部，外科教授

**Ross M. Bremner**，医学博士、哲学博士
美国亚利桑那州凤凰城，克雷顿大学医学院凤凰城分校，圣约瑟夫医疗中心，诺顿胸科研究所

**Marek Brzezinski**，医学博士、哲学博士
美国加利福尼亚州旧金山市，加利福尼亚大学旧金山分校，旧金山退伍军人医疗中心麻醉科，麻醉与围手术期护理系

**Marie M. Budev**，骨科博士、公共卫生硕士、美国胸科医师学会会员
美国俄亥俄州克利夫兰市，克利夫兰医学中心，呼吸研究所，勒纳医学院，教授

**Laurens J. Ceulemans**，医学博士、哲学博士
比利时勒芬市，鲁汶大学，勒芬大学医院，胸外科系，加斯图斯贝格分院，慢性疾病与代谢科

**Marcelo Cypel**，医学博士、理学硕士、美国外科学院院士
加拿大皇家外科医师学会院士，加拿大安大略省多伦多市，多伦多综合医院，多伦多大学健康网络，外科系，胸外科分部，多伦多肺移植项目

**Eduardo Fontena**，医学博士
巴西里约热内卢，圣路易斯医疗集团，科帕多尔医院，肺移植研究项目

**Matthew Galen Hartwig**，医学博士、卫生科学硕士
美国北卡罗来纳州达勒姆市，杜克大学医学中心，杜克大学医学院，外科系，心血管与胸外科分部，终身职外科副教授

**Hilary J. Goldberg**，医学博士、公共卫生硕士
美国马萨诸塞州波士顿市，哈佛医学院，布莱根妇女医院

**Harpreet Singh Grewal**，医学博士
美国纽约州纽约市，肺移植项目部，哥伦比亚大学欧文医学中心

**John R. Greenland**，医学博士、哲学博士
美国加利福尼亚州旧金山市，旧金山退伍军人医疗保健系统，主治医师；加利福尼亚大学旧金山分校，肺病、重症监护、过敏与睡眠医学科分部，医学副教授

**Ramsey R. Hachem**，医学博士
美国密苏里州圣路易斯市，圣路易斯华盛顿大学，肺病与重症监护医学科

**Konrad Hoetzenecker**，医学博士
奥地利维也纳，维也纳医科大学，胸外科系，外科教授

**Daniel Kreisel**，医学博士、哲学博士
美国密苏里州圣路易斯市，华盛顿大学医学院，病理学与免疫学系，外科系

**Erika D. Lease**，医学博士、美国胸科医师学会
美国华盛顿州西雅图市，华盛顿大学，医学系肺病、重症监护与睡眠医学科分部，副教授

**Deborah J. Levine,医学博士**
美国得克萨斯州圣安东尼奥市,得克萨斯大学健康科学中心圣安东尼奥分校,肺病与重症监护医学科

**Bronwyn Levvey,注册护士**
澳大利亚维多利亚州墨尔本市,阿尔弗雷德医院与莫纳什大学,肺移植服务中心

**Gabriel Loor,医学博士**
美国得克萨斯州休斯顿市,得克萨斯心脏研究所,心胸移植与循环支持分部,贝勒医学院,外科系及贝勒肺研究所

**Tiago N. Machuca,医学博士、哲学博士**
美国佛罗里达州盖恩斯维尔市,佛罗里达大学胸外科分部,成人 Ecmo 项目主任;佛罗里达大学肺移植项目外科主任;胸外科分部主任

**Luciana Mascia,医学博士**
意大利博洛尼亚市,博洛尼亚大学,生物医学与神经运动科学系,麻醉、重症监护与疼痛医学住院医师项目主任,麻醉与重症监护副教授

**Aladdein Mattar,医学博士**
美国得克萨斯州休斯顿市,贝勒医学院,贝勒肺研究所,外科系

**Anna Teresa Mazzeo,医学博士**
意大利墨西拿市,墨西拿大学,成人与儿科病理学系,麻醉与重症监护副教授

**Eriberto Michel,医学博士**
美国马萨诸塞州波士顿市,麻省总医院,外科系,心脏外科分部

**Domagoj Mladinov,医学博士、哲学博士**
美国阿拉巴马州伯明翰市,阿拉巴马大学伯明翰分校,麻醉学与围手术期医学系

**Arne Neyrinck,医学博士、哲学博士**
比利时勒芬市,鲁汶大学,心血管科学系;加斯图斯贝格分院,勒芬大学医院,麻醉学系

**Joseph M. Pilewski,医学博士**
美国宾夕法尼亚州匹兹堡市,匹兹堡大学医学系,肺病、过敏与重症监护医学科分部

**Juan C. Salgado,医学博士**
美国宾夕法尼亚州费城市,宾夕法尼亚大学,佩雷尔曼医学院,医学系,肺病、过敏与重症监护医学科分部,医学副教授

**Marcos N. Samano,医学博士、哲学博士**
巴西圣保罗市,以色列阿尔伯特·爱因斯坦医院,肺移植项目,圣保罗大学,胸外科分部

**David M. Sayah**，医学博士、哲学博士
美国加利福尼亚州洛杉矶市，加利福尼亚大学洛杉矶分校，大卫·格芬医学院，医学系，肺病、重症监护、过敏与睡眠医学科分部

**Lara Schaheen**，医学博士
美国亚利桑那州凤凰城，克雷顿大学医学院凤凰城分校，圣约瑟夫医疗中心，诺顿胸科研究所

**Abbas Shahmohammadi**，医学博士
美国佛罗里达州盖恩斯维尔市，佛罗里达大学，医学系，肺病、重症监护与睡眠医学科分部，肺移植与 ECMO 项目

**Gregory I. Snell**，医学学士、医学博士
澳大利亚维多利亚州墨尔本市，阿尔弗雷德医院与莫纳什大学，肺移植服务中心

**Stephan A. Soder**，医学博士
巴西南里奥格兰德州阿雷格里港，阿雷格里港圣卡萨慈善兄弟会医院，胸外科分部与肺移植项目

**Wiebke Sommer**，医学博士
德国海德堡市，海德堡大学，心脏外科系

**Tany Thaniyavarn**，医学博士
美国马萨诸塞州波士顿市，哈佛医学院，布莱根妇女医院

**Tommaso Tonetti**，医学博士
意大利博洛尼亚市，圣奥索拉教学医院，麻醉与重症监护医学科；博洛尼亚大学，医学与外科学系

**Binh N. Trinh**，医学博士、哲学博士
美国加利福尼亚州旧金山市，加利福尼亚大学旧金山分校，心胸外科分部

**Dirk Van Raemdonck**，医学博士、哲学博士
比利时勒芬市，鲁汶大学，慢性疾病与代谢科；加斯图斯贝格分院，勒芬大学医院，胸外科系

**Rajat Walia**，医学博士
美国亚利桑那州凤凰城，克雷顿大学医学院凤凰城分校，圣约瑟夫医疗中心，诺顿胸科研究所，医学教授

# 主审序言(一)

肺移植手术至今仍是治疗肺纤维化、肺动脉高压等终末期肺疾病的唯一有效手段,可以延长患者生命并极大改善其生活质量。全球超过半个世纪的肺移植实践表明,肺移植学科的蓬勃发展,与外科技术进步、多学科协作模式建立、新型抗感染药物和免疫抑制剂研发的成功密不可分。时至今日,肺移植领域形成了完善的关于肺移植供体维护、受者选择、围手术期管理和随访的指南和程序,使得肺移植术后的并发症和死亡率不断降低,惠及更多濒死的患者。

中国的肺移植技术走过了近半个世纪的风雨历程,2002年9月28日,我在无锡市人民医院完成了第一例肺移植,自此我国的肺移植工作展开了新的篇章。20年来,我国的肺移植数量已经超过4900例,且目前已有60家医疗机构取得肺移植资质,特别是儿童肺移植的发展令人瞩目。参与肺移植工作的医疗同行越来越多,共同为提升肺移植的数量和质量做出了巨大的贡献。我们看到,肺移植的成功是社会和政府共同努力的结果,其关乎人民群众的生命健康,也涉及生命伦理和社会公平,是国家医学发展和社会文明进步的重要标志,同时也是医院综合实力的体现,需要上下一心,共同努力,才能完成这一伟大使命。

周建平主任医师带领东莞市人民医院一批优秀的中青年医疗专家,涵盖胸外科、心外科、重症监护室、心内科及一批科研骨干,以及护理专家共同翻译了这部《肺移植:胸外科临床问题》。本书详细介绍了等待肺移植患者的管理、肺移植术中患者的监测及术后的院内院外管理,以及围手术期生命支持及术后各种并发症的处理,并重点阐述了肺移植术后的专科护理。通读下来,该书内容丰富,图文并茂,是临床工作者不可或缺的参考资料。

医术之美以及救治患者之精神高尚,在以肺移植为代表的器官移植领域,得到了充分的诠释。我国的肺移植技术既学自于西方,在未来也当贡献于东西方肺移植的发展与进步。希望本书能为每一位愿意投身肺移植事业的学者提供指引和参考,以对提高我国肺移植患者的管理水平发挥重要的作用。相信广大从事肺移植的医务工作者必以极大的仁心和专业素养对待每一位肺移植患者,让肺移植事业之树常青。

浙江大学医学院附属第二医院副院长

# 主审序言（二）

肺移植作为胸外科诊疗领域的关键部分，对晚期肺部疾病治疗意义非凡。加利福尼亚大学旧金山分校的专家们精心汇集相关课题，全面总结了肺移植外科治疗现状、待供体患者的管理、失代偿患者的治疗及紧急移植手术、供体的统筹管理及分配、最先进的移植手术方法、麻醉进展等内容，同时涵盖了多种急慢性疾病。虽全球肺移植手术量有所增长，但仍难以满足需求，供体来源等挑战犹存，排斥与感染问题亟待攻克。周建平教授及其团队在充分尊重原著的基础上，结合专业中文的表达方式，精准地翻译了《肺移植：胸外科临床问题》这部著作，凝聚了多方心血。望读者及致力于肺移植工作的学者们能借此深入领略肺移植的奥秘，激发对这一复杂亚学科的探索热情，为我国肺移植的发展贡献力量。在此，特向所有参与者致谢，愿大家在阅读中能够有所收获并积极分享。

中山大学附属肿瘤医院
胸科主任、肺癌首席专家

# 主译前言

作为一名胸外科医生，不断挑战自我是成长的动力，目前外科领域最高和最有挑战性的技术之一就是器官移植。2007年5月1日前，东莞市人民医院也曾开展了器官移植工作，我亲自参与了供体的获取、心脏移植手术等实际工作。从此，器官移植成为我向往突破的一项技术。与此同时，我也时刻关注器官移植尤其是肺移植相关的前沿技术及其法律法规要求。自2007年5月1日实施《人体器官移植条例》以来，国家在供体来源、供体管理、医院资格认定、医师培训和认定等方面日趋成熟，许多医院因此停止了器官移植工作，东莞市人民医院也包含在内。经过多年的探索，我们国家在器官捐献和移植工作方面取得了非常大的成果，也制定了多部法律法规。2023年国务院令第767号《人体器官捐献和移植条例》和《人体器官移植技术临床应用管理规范（2020年版）》等重要法律文件和技术管理规范的发布，进一步完善了我国器官移植法治体系。

2021年5月，我进入南开大学攻读医院管理硕士学位，接触了更先进的国际前沿医院管理理念，改变了我对器官移植的看法。器官移植不仅仅只是一项技术，而是集法规、伦理、管理及技术于一体的综合项目，使我心中对肺移植的向往增加了更多内涵。为追随国家高质量发展的脚步，我屡次建议将器官移植作为我院医疗新技术发展的重点工作。目前，器官移植已成为我院"十四五"规划和高水平医院建设的重点工作之一。

在此过程中，我有幸认识了我国肺移植第一人陈静瑜教授。在与陈静瑜教授的交流中，使我对肺移植工作的艰难历程以及国家对此项工作的高度关注有了更进一步的了解，同时地方政府的支持和社会共同参与也是肺移植快速发展的动力。纵观我国肺移植的发展，自2002年9月无锡市人民医院陈静瑜教授开展了我国第一例肺移植手术以来，2022年全国进行肺移植710例，到2023年前10个月我国肺移植手术已经达到789例。开展肺移植工作是医院从上至下整合资源、建立发展规划的过程，是新质生产力的重要体现。

2024年年初，我萌生了为肺移植工作尽绵薄之力的想法，也算是自己职业生涯的一次飞跃。在请教了中山大学附属肿瘤医院张兰军教授并获得了他的肯定后，我备受鼓舞。

2024年3月，一批来自我院的优秀中青年专家，配合医院器官移植的建设需要，共同翻译了这部《肺移植：胸外科临床问题》。本书详细介绍了等待肺移植患者的管理、术中麻醉、监测，肺移植术后患者的院内和院外管理，并专门讲述了肺移植术后的专科护理，是一部为肺移植的临床工作提供专业支持的工具书。翻译本书的初衷是让参与者对标国际最新理念，初步了解肺移植的指南，掌握适应证和禁忌证、手术时机、术前检查、术后康复护理和药物应用，以及如何进行多学科联动协助等内容，为推动医院肺移植工作打下基础，也为我国的肺移植工作尽绵薄之力。

东莞市人民医院副院长
（南方医科大学第十附属医院）

# 原著序言

## 肺移植：前进道路上的两大挑战——感染与排斥

我们很高兴能为您带来《肺移植：胸外科临床问题》这部书。本书由加利福尼亚大学旧金山分校胸外科医生 Jasleen Kukreja 博士（医学博士、公共卫生硕士）和移植肺病学家 Aida Venado 博士（医学博士、应用统计硕士）作为特邀编辑，汇集了一系列关于肺移植的最新课题。通过与该领域专家的共同努力，本书编辑为晚期肺部疾病的外科治疗提供了一份综述，涵盖肺纤维化、慢性阻塞性肺疾病等慢性问题以及急性呼吸窘迫综合征等急性病症。每年大约有 2500 例美国患者接受肺移植手术，全球范围内接受肺移植的患者超过 4000 例，但这还远远不够。据 Sayah 和 Pilewski 称，在被列入移植名单后的 1 年内仅有 70% 的患者接受了移植手术。增加供体来源的方法包括更多地识别心脏停搏后的供体（心脏死亡供者）和维持体外肺灌注，以扩大供体肺的可移植标准并减少小型肺移植项目手术的地域差异。心脏死亡供者涉及相关的伦理、法律和专业挑战；不过，移植界正在努力解决这些问题，以增加心脏停搏后捐献（心脏死亡供者）的来源。随着器官保存和围术期重症监护管理的改善，65 岁以上患者的移植手术数量增加了 400%，并取得了较好的结果，推动了肺移植的进展。可用于临床试验的肺移植面临的挑战包括需要新的免疫抑制方案，使首年的移植物急性细胞性排斥反应发生率控制在 0~50%，术后 30 天内死亡率控制在 0~3%。另外，感染并发症的发病率与死亡率也是肺移植术后的一大挑战，在接受肺移植术后 1 年内，有 35% 的患者死于感染。虽然在改善供体器官来源方面取得了很大进展，但一些持续性的移植后挑战仍然存在。

感谢所有撰稿人以及特邀编辑 Kukreja 博士和 Venado 博士。祝您阅读愉快并与专业人员分享本书的内容，以激发他们对胸外科这一知识领域和临床复杂微观世界的热情和兴趣。希望您会喜欢这部书！

Virginia R. Litle，医学博士
心血管外科胸外科科室主任
胸外科医疗主任

电子邮箱：virginia.litle@imail.org
Twitter: @vlitlemd (V.R. Litle)

# 原著前言

## 肺移植：协作推动进步

照顾一个肺移植的患者需要一个团队共同的努力。在过去的 60 年中，随着移植外科技术、供体器官保存以及恢复、免疫抑制和医疗管理的进步，肺移植术后的结局有了显著的改善。目前，肺移植后的总体中位生存期为 6.7 年。事实上，在一些中心，中位生存期已接近 10 年，有少数肺移植受者存活时间接近 30 年。这一瞩目的成就成为可能，离不开外科医生、呼吸病学家、麻醉师、护士、药剂师、免疫学家、呼吸治疗师、物理治疗师、营养师和社会工作者之间的多学科协作。虽然取得了这一成功，但随着时间的推移，保留移植肺功能和实现长期存活仍然是一个挑战。首先，肺移植术后的早期并发症，如原发性移植物功能不全和急性细胞性排斥反应，可导致慢性肺同种异体移植物功能障碍（CLAD），反过来又限制了器官和受体的长期存活。截至 2022 年，有半数受者在移植后 5 年内发生 CLAD。其次，慢性免疫抑制的并发症，如感染、慢性肾脏疾病、心血管疾病和恶性肿瘤等，也会导致肺移植后的预期寿命缩短。此外，突发的病毒大流行事件也可能对受者和医疗系统造成威胁。因此，创新和协作仍然是未来肺移植取得长期成功的关键。作为一名移植外科医生和一名肺科医生，我们怀着这种精神，编著了这部《肺移植：胸外科临床问题》。

为了在全球范围内提供更加可靠的肺移植治疗视角，我们尽可能地邀请了来自世界各地的专家合作撰写每个章节。同样，我们以"医学和外科"为主题，以吸引更多的读者，并为读者提供"一站式"体验（即通过一个单一的资源可以全面地了解肺移植的最新技术）。

我们从各位同仁对"肺移植"问题的贡献中获益良多，并相信这将同样帮助其他人朝着我们共同的目标前进，以改善全世界肺移植患者的预后。

Jasleen Kukreja，医学博士，公共卫生硕士
心胸外科

Aida Venado，医学博士，应用统计硕士
呼吸与危重症医学科、过敏与睡眠医学科
加利福尼亚大学旧金山分校

电子邮箱：
Jasleen.Kukreja@ucsf.edu (J. Kukreja)
Aida.Venado@ucsf.edu (A. Venado)

# 目　录

**第 1 章　等待名单上的肺移植候选者的门诊药物管理** ········· 1
    1.1 引言 ········· 1
    1.2 药物管理 ········· 2
    1.3 讨论 ········· 9

**第 2 章　急性失代偿肺移植候选者的住院管理** ········· 15
    2.1 引言 ········· 15
    2.2 疾病严重程度对肺移植后预后的影响 ········· 17
    2.3 急性失代偿肺移植候选者的医疗管理 ········· 19
    2.4 移植前桥接 ········· 22
    2.5 急性失代偿期间的康复 ········· 26
    2.6 除名触发因素 ········· 27
    2.7 总结 ········· 28

**第 3 章　急性呼吸窘迫综合征的肺移植** ········· 34
    3.1 引言 ········· 34
    3.2 总结 ········· 40

**第 4 章　潜在肺捐献者的管理** ········· 45
    4.1 引言 ········· 45
    4.2 通气管理和血气交换 ········· 46
    4.3 液体管理 ········· 48
    4.4 死亡原因及其影响 ········· 50
    4.5 支气管镜检查 ········· 50
    4.6 胸部放射成像 ········· 51
    4.7 微生物培养结果与抗生素 ········· 51
    4.8 输血对供肺管理的影响 ········· 51

4.9 2019 冠状病毒病（COVID-19）筛查指南 ········· 52
4.10 总结 ········· 54
4.11 未来发展方向 ········· 54

## 第 5 章　肺移植心脏死亡后的捐献 ········· 58

5.1 引言 ········· 58
5.2 DCD 的捐献类别 ········· 59
5.3 DCD 供体的评估 ········· 59
5.4 可耐受的热缺血 ········· 60
5.5 WLST（包括 cDCD 中的安慰治疗） ········· 61
5.6 DCD 肺恢复手术 ········· 62
5.7 死后肺移植前的质量评估 ········· 64
5.8 DCD LTx 的结局 ········· 66
5.9 DCD LTx 的障碍 ········· 69
5.10 总结 ········· 70

## 第 6 章　建立集中化供体器官获取和分配中心 ········· 76

6.1 引言 ········· 76
6.2 器官获取模式的比较 ········· 77
6.3 对外科医生倦怠的影响 ········· 79
6.4 体外肺灌注复苏设施 ········· 80
6.5 讨论 ········· 81
6.6 总结 ········· 82

## 第 7 章　肺移植手术麻醉管理——2021 年新进展 ········· 87

7.1 引言 ········· 87
7.2 术中同种异体移植物和肺外终末器官保护的关键概念 ········· 88
7.3 术中关键时段维持血流动力学稳定 ········· 88
7.4 肺移植过程中机械辅助循环支持的关键概念 ········· 91
7.5 总结 ········· 96

## 第 8 章　肺移植受者术后的早期管理 ········· 102

- 8.1 引言 ········· 102
- 8.2 患者选择 ········· 103
- 8.3 术中管理 ········· 103
- 8.4 血流动力学术后管理 ········· 104
- 8.5 镇静和疼痛管理 ········· 105
- 8.6 移植物功能的管理 ········· 106
- 8.7 免疫抑制 ········· 107
- 8.8 感染管理 ········· 108
- 8.9 其他医疗并发症的管理 ········· 110
- 8.10 总结 ········· 111

## 第 9 章　肺移植的手术并发症 ········· 118

- 9.1 引言 ········· 118
- 9.2 伤口并发症 ········· 118
- 9.3 原发性移植物功能不全 ········· 120
- 9.4 气道缺血 ········· 121
- 9.5 血管并发症 ········· 123
- 9.6 出血并发症 ········· 125
- 9.7 胸膜腔并发症 ········· 127
- 9.8 匹配供者和受者尺寸大小的挑战 ········· 129
- 9.9 再移植 ········· 130
- 9.10 总结 ········· 131

## 第 10 章　肺移植受者的感染性并发症 ········· 136

- 10.1 引言 ········· 136
- 10.2 抗菌药物预防 ········· 136
- 10.3 供体来源的感染 ········· 139
- 10.4 细菌感染的管理 ········· 140
- 10.5 随时间变化的感染风险 ········· 140

10.6 病毒感染的管理 ·········· 141

10.7 真菌感染的管理 ·········· 143

10.8 人型支原体和解脲支原体感染 ·········· 146

10.9 总结 ·········· 146

## 第 11 章　同种异体肺移植排斥反应 ·········· 151

11.1 引言 ·········· 151

11.2 急性细胞性排斥反应 ·········· 152

11.3 抗体介导的排斥反应（AMR） ·········· 155

11.4 总结 ·········· 159

## 第 12 章　慢性移植肺功能障碍 ·········· 164

12.1 慢性移植肺功能障碍定义 ·········· 164

12.2 CLAD 的病理生理学 ·········· 166

12.3 CLAD 的治疗 ·········· 169

12.4 争议 ·········· 174

12.5 总结 ·········· 174

## 第 13 章　非同种异体肺移植的并发症 ·········· 181

13.1 引言 ·········· 181

13.2 糖尿病 ·········· 182

13.3 高血压 ·········· 184

13.4 高脂血症 ·········· 186

13.5 急性肾损伤 ·········· 187

13.6 慢性肾病 ·········· 189

13.7 恶性肿瘤 ·········· 190

13.8 总结 ·········· 196

## 第 14 章　肺再移植 ·········· 203

14.1 背景 ·········· 203

14.2 肺再移植的指征 ·········· 204

14.3 肺再移植患者的评估和选择 ……………………………………… 207
14.4 肺再移植的免疫学方面 …………………………………………… 207
14.5 手术技术 …………………………………………………………… 209
14.6 术后管理和其他重要考虑因素 …………………………………… 212
14.7 长期结果 …………………………………………………………… 212
14.8 总结 ………………………………………………………………… 213

# 第 1 章 等待名单上的肺移植候选者的门诊药物管理

David M. Sayah, Joseph M. Pilewski 著

郭素峡 译

周建平 校

【关键词】
- 肺移植
- 糖皮质激素
- 皮质类固醇
- 抗纤维化药物
- 尼达尼布
- 吡非尼酮
- mTOR 抑制剂
- 西罗莫司

【要点】
- 许多用于常规治疗肺部疾病的药物可能会影响肺移植受者的围移植期过程。
- 对等待名单上的肺移植候选者成功的医疗管理必须考虑到移植前药物对术中和术后结果的影响，如伤口愈合、出血和感染。
- 在移植后影响方面值得注意的药物类别包括糖皮质激素、抗纤维化药物、哺乳动物雷帕霉素靶蛋白（mTOR）抑制剂、囊性纤维化跨膜传导调节因子（CFTR）调节剂、针对肺动脉高压（PAH）的靶向治疗和抗凝药物。

## 1.1 引 言

肺移植（lung transplantation，LTx）是一种越来越常用的终末期肺疾病的疗法，在美国每年完成肺移植的患者超过 2500 例，全球则超过 4000 例[1,2]。2019 年，仅在美国的肺移植等待名单上就有超过 3000 例，其中绝大多数是门诊患者[2]。尽管这些患者从等待到接受移植的中位时间为 2~3 个月，但个体之间的等待时间有着显著的差异[2]。这种差异是由许多因素导致的，包括患者基础肺部疾病的诊断、疾病严重程度［由肺源分配评分（lung allocation score，LAS）确定］、血型、身高以及器官可用性的地域差异。结果只有 60% 的候选者在列名后 6 个月内接受了移植，而 1 年内移植的比例仅为 70%[2]。因此，对处于肺移植等待名单上的这些终末期肺疾病患者进行持续的门诊医疗护理是成

功移植的关键组成部分。

移植前医疗护理的首要目标是保障患者的健康状态，在许多情况下，更是确保患者在等待肺移植过程中的存活。患有终末期肺疾病的患者容易发生衰弱和出现其他医疗并发症。预测并预防可能使患者暂时或永久失去移植资格的并发症是移植前护理的基础。

然而，一些在其他情况下为常规治疗的手段可能会在围术期产生不良的挑战或并发症。因此，与不等待肺移植的类似肺部疾病患者相比，医疗决策不仅须考虑疾病和特定患者的最佳治疗方法，还须考虑这些治疗对肺移植术后即刻的影响。

更为复杂的是，特定患者收到合适的捐献者供体并进行肺移植的时间是不可预测的。必须考虑到这种不可预测性，以避免危及患者的术后结果。或者如果患者因为某种药物或其他治疗导致的围术期风险对移植项目来说是不可接受的，那么就可能危及其接受特定供体的资格。因此，对这些药物的风险和益处进行全面评估时，必须考虑它们在管理患者当前疾病状态的潜在效用，以及影响肺移植术后结果的风险。

在这篇综述中，我们的目标是总结关于肺移植候选者在移植等待名单上的最佳医疗管理的可用数据和共识意见。由于这个主题涉及范围广泛，我们将重点关注肺移植前患者群体中常见的具体用药方案及典型临床情况。

## 1.2 药物管理

### 1.2.1 糖皮质激素

糖皮质激素被广泛用于治疗多种可能最终需要肺移植的肺部疾病，包括慢性阻塞性肺疾病（chronic obstructive pulmonary disease，COPD）、肺结节病、结缔组织病相关间质性肺病（connective tissue disease associated interstitial lung disease，CTD-ILD）、变应性支气管肺曲菌病（allergic bronchopulmonary aspergillosis，ABPA）等。这些药物具有多种抗炎和免疫抑制作用，在治疗广泛的肺部疾病中非常有用[3]。遗憾的是，它们也会引起广泛的不良反应，尤其是长期使用时，许多副作用（如伤口愈合受损）可能会对肺移植术后造成不利影响[4,5]。

虽然糖皮质激素目前是肺移植后维持免疫抑制治疗的主要方式[1]，但关于肺移植前长期系统性糖皮质激素治疗仍存在显著担忧。早期临床前研究表明，糖皮质激素暴露会增加支气管吻合口裂开风险[6,7]。事实上，早期的肺移植专家意见认为，慢性糖皮质激素治疗是肺移植的禁忌证[8]。

随着人类肺移植的临床经验的积累和外科技术的改进，后续回顾性、观察性研究表明，移植前长期"低剂量"糖皮质激素治疗［定义存在差异如：泼尼松 ≤ 20 mg/d[9]，或泼尼松龙 ≤ 0.3 mg/（kg·d）[10]，或泼尼松 ≤ 0.42 mg/（kg·m²）[11] 等］不会对移植后的结果产生负面影响。

相反，McAnally 及其同事报告称，每天长期服用超过 0.42 mg/（kg·m²）泼尼松的患者早期移植后死亡率增加，这种影响是由移植后早期感染和吻合口并发症的增加导致的[11]。他们的患者群体平均身体质量指数（Body Mass Index，BMI）为 22.5 kg/m²，该阈值对应的泼尼松平均剂量刚好低于每天 10 mg。使用相同的移植前高剂量与低剂量糖皮质激素的定义，Sugimoto 及其同事报告了他们对一小组在异基因造血干细胞移植后接受活体叶肺移植的患者的经验[12]。他们也发现了高剂量组的生存率下降。

国际心肺移植学会（International Society for Heart and Lung Transplantation，ISHLT）注册数据库的一项分析发现，接受者移植前使用糖皮质激素与移植后 1 年内死亡风险增加相关[13]。值得注意的是，这种效应似乎仅限于患有 COPD 的接受者，而非特发性间质性肺炎（idiopathic interstitial pneumonia，IIP）的患者。然而，一项利用移植受者科学登记数据库（Scientific Registry of Transplant Recipients，SRTR）的研究并未确定移植前使用糖皮质激素为气道裂开的风险因素[14]，因此，尚不确定移植前使用糖皮质激素可能对移植后生存产生不利影响的潜在机制。

鉴于对移植前糖皮质激素治疗的问题存在模糊性，因此领域内尚未就肺移植候选者使用该类药物的最大剂量（如果有的话）达成共识。实际上，虽然早期的国际指南曾明确建议在肺移植前最小化糖皮质激素剂量[15]，但后续修订版指南并未讨论这一主题[16-18]。

## 1.2.2 抗纤维化药物

吡非尼酮（Pirfenidone）和尼达尼布（Nintedanib）都是抗纤维化药物，2014 年获得美国食品药品监督管理局（the US Food and Drug Administration，FDA）批准使用。此前有研究表明，它们在减缓特发性肺纤维化（idiopathic pulmonary fibrosis，IPF）患者肺功能下降的速度方面有效[19,20]。尼达尼布随后在治疗硬皮病相关的间质性肺病（interstitial lung disease，ILD）以及一组多样化的进展性慢性纤维化 ILD 中显示出了类似的效果[21,22]。使用抗纤维化疗法治疗 IPF 已迅速被采用，最近的一项美国注册研究发现，超过 70% 的患者在注册登记时正在接受其中一种疗法[23]。

由于吡非尼酮和尼达尼布都会抑制成纤维细胞的功能和增殖，理论上认为这些药物可能会影响伤口愈合并导致肺移植术后并发症[24]。此外，尼达尼布抑制血管内皮生长因子，可能会增加围术期出血的风险[25]。

尽管对继续在积极等待肺移植的患者中使用抗纤维化疗法的安全性存在假设性的、机制上的担忧，但多项观察性研究发现没有证据表明这些药物会增加术后并发症的风险。在最早的一项研究中，Leuschner 及同事在 30 例接受抗纤维化治疗的 IPF 患者（23 例使用吡非尼酮，7 例使用尼达尼布）与 32 例未接受抗纤维化治疗的对照患者中发现，两组患者在使用血液制品、伤口愈合和吻合口并发症，以及移植后死亡率方面没有差异[26]。尽管接受抗纤维化治疗的患者年龄显著较大，但这些发现依然成立。迄今为止最大的研究调查了在 226 例接受肺移植的肺纤维化患者中，40 例直到移植时刻接受抗纤维化治疗的患者的结果（29 例使用吡非尼酮，11 例使用尼达尼布）[27]。尽管抗纤维化治疗组的气道裂开发生率（7.5%）较对照组（2.2%）呈现升高趋势，但这一差异未达到统计学显著性，且实际发生事件的绝对数量较少。两组 30 天生存率没有显著差异，而抗纤维化组 1 年生存率高于对照组（93% *vs.* 88%）。若干较小的研究，对吡非尼酮、尼达尼布或两者均进行了调查，发现在伤口愈合或其他外科并发症上差异均没有统计学意义[28-31]。

鉴于抗纤维化治疗与肺移植术后并发症之间没有一致的关联性。因此，该领域的共识是患者可以安全地继续使用这些药物，直至移植时刻[18]。

Veit 及其同事调查了 17 例既往接受过吡非尼酮治疗的 IPF 患者与 26 例未接受抗纤维化治疗的患者在单肺移植后的结果。与其他研究一致，两组在失血量、伤口愈合和吻合口并发症方面没有差异[32]。然而，值得注意的是，吡非尼酮组在原发性移植物功能不全（primary graft dysfunction，PGD）的严重程度、机械通气持续时间以及 ICU 停留时间上均有所减少，这表明吡非尼酮对这组患者可能具有潜在的有益效果。最后，一项近期的回顾性分析表明，在移植时使用尼达尼布或吡非尼酮与原发性移植物功能不全的改善和吻合口并发症更少相关，而并发症并未增加[33]。是否有更多、更大规模的研究显示类似的发现，以及尼达尼布与吡非尼酮相比效果是否相似，仍有待确定。

### 1.2.3 雷帕霉素靶蛋白抑制剂

西罗莫司及其衍生物依维莫司是强大的免疫抑制剂，其通过抑制哺乳动物雷帕霉素靶蛋白（mammalian target of rapamycin，mTOR）发挥作用[34,35]。除了免疫抑制效果外，这些药物还能干扰多种细胞类型的增殖（包括成纤维细胞），并具有抗肿瘤效果，在某些恶性肿瘤的治疗中很有用[36]。

由于兼具免疫抑制和潜在的抗纤维化效果，mTOR 抑制剂被认为是肺移植后免疫抑制的有前景的药物。然而，早期关于在肺移植后立即使用包含西罗莫司的免疫抑制方案的经验报告发现灾难性且通常是致命的支气管吻合口裂开的发生率很高[37,38]。这促使 FDA 特别警告避免在肺移植后使用西罗莫司进行初始免疫抑制[39]。

虽然在治疗终末期肺疾病时，并不经常使用 mTOR 抑制剂，但一个值得注意的例外是淋巴管平滑肌瘤病（lymphangioleiomyomatosis，LAM），这是一种罕见的进展性的囊性肺疾病，可能会导致呼吸衰竭，并且是肺移植的明确适应证。西罗莫司的治疗可以稳定 LAM 患者的肺功能，改善症状，并提高生活质量[40]。

西罗莫司在肺移植术后早期可能导致气道裂开的潜在风险，引发了关于继续西罗莫司治疗对等待肺移植的 LAM 患者安全性，以及是否应在列入移植名单前停用西罗莫司的争议。关于在服用 mTOR 抑制剂期间进行肺移植的患者的研究十分有限[41]。在一项关于 3 例继续使用西罗莫司治疗直至移植的 LAM 患者的研究中，没有出现支气管裂开的病例[42]。另一项研究描述了 7 例使用西罗莫司治疗直至移植的 LAM 患者，其中 1 例在移植后 12 天发展为致命的吻合口裂开[43]。最后，一份报告描述了 2 例在肺移植后接受依维莫司维持免疫抑制治疗的非 LAM 患者，并且继续使用依维莫司直至进行肺再移植的案例[44]。这两例患者均未出现气道裂开。

依维莫司的半衰期比西罗莫司短（30 小时 *vs.* 60 小时）[39,45]。因此，有人建议，由于半衰期较短可能减少气道裂开的风险，依维莫司或许是等待肺移植的 LAM 患者治疗的更安全选择[18,41]。目前尚未具有支持这种方法的研究。

最终，对于等待移植的 LAM 患者，mTOR 抑制剂治疗的最佳方法尚无定论，决策应基于对风险和益处的个体化讨论[18]。在我们的中心，我们通常建议患者在积极列入移植名单前停止使用 mTOR 抑制剂，因为移植的平均等待时间相对较短，使得关于停止治疗导致的 LAM 患者肺功能下降的担忧不那么具有相关性。然而，每个移植中心，以及潜在的每个患者，在这方面都可能有不同的风险/益处计算，因此建议根据各中心或患者的具体情况而定。

### 1.2.4 囊性纤维化跨膜传导调节因子调节剂

囊性纤维化跨膜传导调节因子（cystic fibrosis transmembrane conductance regulator，CFTR）调节剂的开发在呼吸医学领域是一个显著的进展。通过对 CF 突变的遗传、分

## 肺移植：胸外科临床问题

子和细胞生物学特点进行定义，高通量筛选得以识别部分恢复 CFTR 功能的化合物。第一个高效的 CFTR 调节剂 Ivacaftor（Kalydeco，IVA）在 2012 年获得 FDA 批准，用于 G551D CFTR 突变的个体。依伐卡托（IVA）可显著降低汗液氯化物、改善呼吸功能、促进体重增加、减少发作频率，并提高 $FEV_1$ 为 40%~90% 预测值的患者的生活质量[46]。从那时起，IVA 被批准用于其他几种门控突变。到 2020 年初，为约 20% 的 CF 患者提供了使用这种疾病修饰的口服药物的机会。若干研究调查了 IVA 对于晚期肺病患者的影响，并显示出与肺病较轻患者观察到的类似改善[47-50]。

在 2019 年末，第二种高效的 CFTR 调节剂疗法 Elexacaftor/Tezacaftor/Ivacaftor（Trikafta，ETI）被批准用于 F508del CFTR 突变的个体。ETI 同样能够显著改善汗液氯化物、$FEV_1$（绝对预测值提高约 14%）、营养状况、发作频率以及 $FEV_1$ 为 40%~90% 预测值的个体的生活质量[51-53]。由于 F508del 是最常见的 CFTR 突变，现在约 90% 的 CF 患者可以使用有效的疾病修饰疗法。尽管 ETI 在轻至中度 CF 肺病患者中的转化效果已有广泛研究，但对于重度肺病患者的临床影响描述仍较少。

在 2021 年初，一项研究报告了在法国通过早期获取计划接受 ETI 治疗的具有严重肺疾病 CF 患者的 ETI 效果[54]。与先前的研究一致，ETI 在 $FEV_1$ 小于 40% 预测值的个体中耐受良好，并且其肺功能和体重均有显著改善。绝对预测值 $FEV_1$ 平均增加 15%，与三期研究中 $FEV_1$ 刚好小于 40% 预测值的患者子集一致[52]。这项研究为 ETI 对于重度肺病患者的转化效果提供了额外证据，ETI 的使用减少了 50% 的辅助氧疗需求、30% 的无创通气（noninvasive ventilation，NIV）需求和 50% 的肠内管喂养需求。或许对于肺移植项目而言更重要的是，在该人群开始使用 ETI 之前，16 例患者在肺移植等待名单上，37 例正在接受移植评估。尽管受 COVID-19 大流行的某种干扰，但仍有 2 例患者接受了肺移植，1 例死亡，仍在移植的仅有 5 例。鉴于研究的持续时间，这些结果是非同寻常的，其导致在 ETI 可用的国家，转诊进行肺移植的 CF 患者数量显著减少，并且因 CF 进行的肺移植数量也减少。ETI 的效果对何时列入肺移植等待名单的决策也有影响。

最近的长期研究表明，IVA 在 5 年内显著减缓了 CF 肺疾病的进展[55]。这与 IVA[49] 和 ETI[54] 对患有 CF 及严重疾病的个体的短期效果结合起来，表明具有严重 CF 肺疾病的患者的存活时间将显著增加。尽管还需要更多的研究，但到目前为止的经验表明，使用 ETI 的患者迅速进展到呼吸衰竭和死亡的可能性较低。ETI 可能减缓肺疾病的进展，使得使用 ETI 的 CF 患者的进展更像是由于非 CF 疾病（如原发性纤毛运动障碍或免疫缺陷）引起的支气管扩张症患者。患有严重 CF 肺疾病的存活可能发生缓慢，这表明对于这一人群，应谨慎做出列入移植名单的决定，以避免过早的移植可能缩短寿命。

相比之下，对于约 10% 没有 F508del 突变且未使用 IVA 或 ETI 的个体，疾病进展可能接近 $FEV_1$ 小于 30% 预测值时的 6.6 年中位生存期，在临床稳定期间每年有死亡或接受移植的个体多达 10%[56]。对于这一小部分 CF 患者，关于移植列名的决策不需要改变实践。

CFTR 调节剂改善了许多 CF 患者的营养状况，接受移植时体重指数异常低的 CF 患者将会更少。实际上，肥胖成为 CF 中新出现的挑战。此外，随着肺功能下降的减缓，CF 患者在接受移植时年龄更大，可能会出现额外的并发症（如冠心病），而这在 CF 患者中历来很少出现。

与 IVA 和 ETI 相关的肺功能改善、肺部加重频率减少、体重增加和生活质量提高表明，它们应该持续使用到接受移植手术时。这一点尤为重要，因为有报告显示，在患有严重 CF 肺疾病的个体中停用 IVA 会与快速进展相关，可能会导致某些个体死亡[57]。

更困难的决策是是否以及何时在移植后恢复使用高效的 CFTR 调节剂。大多数 CF 患者在移植后的营养状况有所改善，并不需要使用 CFTR 调节剂，而且与唑类药物和钙调磷酸酶抑制剂的药物相互作用，使得移植后使用 IVA 或 ETI 变得复杂并且具有潜在风险。由于受体肺在遗传上是正常的，移植后恢复使用 IVA 或 ETI 的潜在指征是改善营养、药物治疗和外科治疗难以控制的鼻窦疾病，以及在罕见情况下的血糖控制。到目前为止的经验表明，ETI 的开始使用与适度的体重增加相关。早期经验表明，不能耐受 ETI 的肺移植受者多达 1/3，与移植前的不耐受率不到 5% 形成鲜明对比。需要更多的注册数据来更好地定义移植后使用 IVA 或 ETI 的情况。

### 1.2.5 肺血管扩张剂

肺动脉高压（pulmonary arterial hypertension，PAH，第 1 类）是肺移植的一个常见主要适应证，而肺动脉压力升高经常与其他终末期肺疾病（第 3 类肺高压）并发[1,2]。目前，FDA 批准用于治疗第 3 组肺高压的药物仅限于单一药物（吸入用曲前列尼尔），因此大部分数据和建议都是基于 PAH 的。虽然对 PAH 治疗的全面概述超出了本综述的范围，但等待肺移植的 PAH 患者通常都接受针对 PAH 治疗的靶向疗法。因此，在患者等待肺移植期间对这些药物进行管理是移植前护理的一个重要组成部分。

目前有几种不同的疗法可用于 PAH 的治疗。当前的靶向疗法针对以下 3 个途径之一：内皮素 -1（波生坦、马西替坦和安立生坦）、前列腺素（依普前列素、曲前列尼尔、伊洛前列素和司来帕格）以及一氧化氮（西地那非、他达拉非和利奥西呱），患者在考虑移植时通常接受针对多个途径的治疗[58]。尚无高质量研究评估特定药物或这些药物组合在肺移植后结果方面的效果，但在移植前继续使用这些药物没有重大的理论上的问题。重要的是，无论是由于 PAH 还是继发性（第3类）肺高压，肺移植时肺动脉压力升高都是移植后原发性移植物功能不全的一个重要风险因素[59,60]。因此，包括我们在内的大多数中心都采取优化 PAH 靶向药物治疗的方法，在列入移植名单前和期间进行治疗，在移植后立即停止这些药物。

尽管进行了最佳药物治疗，但右心衰竭的发展仍是一个不祥的征兆，可能预示着快速的失代偿和死亡[58,61,62]。因此，对于等待肺移植的 PAH 患者，如果出现右心衰竭恶化的体征或症状，就低门槛地使其住院治疗。这些患者有时可以通过调整利尿剂方案改善，但通常可能需要血管加压药和(或)正性肌力药的支持作为移植的桥梁。在选定的病例中，可能需要进行房间隔造口术或静动脉体外膜肺氧合作为将重度 PAH 患者成功桥接到肺移植的措施[61,63]，尽管在这种危机中对患者的具体处理方法高度依赖于患者和中心的具体情况，并且应该只由在这一领域有显著经验的中心来进行。

### 1.2.6 抗凝药物

活跃的肺移植名单上的患者如果要使用抗凝药物，需要特别注意最小化由于残留抗凝效应导致的出血风险。器官提供的时间是不可预测的，从器官提供到开始肺移植手术的时间也是如此。因此，制定手术前抗凝药物逆转计划非常重要。由于较高的术中和术后输血可能增加原发性移植物功能不全和发展特异性人类白细胞抗原（human leukocyte，HLA）抗体的风险，因此最小化术中出血是高优先级任务。

对于使用华法林的患者，逆转抗凝状态的方法有几种。除了停用华法林外，还可以通过慢速静脉输注剂量为 5 mg 或 10 mg 维生素 K，假设肝功能正常的情况下预期在不少于 6 小时内恢复维生素 K 依赖的凝血因子水平。因此，对于入院到手术时间小于 24 小时的患者，应在手术前重复检查凝血酶原时间和国际标准化比值（international normalized ratio，INR），如果 INR 仍在治疗范围内，应给予快速逆转剂。快速逆转的选择包括新鲜冷冻血浆或 3 因子或 4 因子凝血酶原复合物浓缩物（prothrombin complex concentrate，PCC）。尽管缺乏比较试验，但由于 3 因子 PCC 缺乏第Ⅶ因子，因此 4 因子 PCC 相比 3 因子 PCC 更受青睐。更重要的是，一项将 4 因子 PCC 与新鲜冷冻血浆进行比较的随机试验表明，与血浆相比，4 因子 PCC 止血作用更有效且 INR 降低更快，二者安全性相似，并且 4 因子 PCC 的容量超负荷风险更低[64,65]。因此，4 因子 PCC 是首选的逆转剂。如果 PCC 不可用，应使用血浆来快速逆转华法林引起的抗凝状态。

长期使用直接作用口服抗凝药物（direct-acting oral anticoagulants，DOACs）的肺移植候选者越来越多。直到最近，已获批准的 DOACs 中还没有有效的逆转剂，因此许多甚至所有移植项目都在移植列名时将患者 DOACs 转换为华法林，以便在手术前快速逆转。随着依达赛珠单抗（idarucizumab）的开发和 FDA 批准，使用达比加群的患者可继续使用该 DOACs，并在接受移植时接受依达赛珠单抗治疗。来自心肺移植项目的最近数据表明，依达赛珠单抗逆转是一种合理的方法。在一项单中心回顾性评审中，4 例使用达比加群且预计在手术前没有足够停药时间的患者，在确认供体器官适合移植后，在术前候诊区接受了依达赛珠单抗[66]。这 4 例患者需要 4 个单位或更少的浓缩红细胞，有 0 级或 1 级原发性移植物功能不全（PGD），并且没有院内死亡。然而，术后 4 例中有 3 例在多普勒超声监测中发现有下肢深静脉血栓。总的来说，这些经验以及来自心脏移植项目的经验表明[67]，对于活跃名单上需要抗凝的一些移植候选者来说，使用达比加群并计划使用依达赛珠单抗逆转是华法林的合理替代方案。

## 1.3 讨 论

在过去的十年中，一些新的医学疗法已经可用于治疗晚期肺部疾病，对于肺移植的准备具有重要意义。门诊患者接近肺移植时，需要与转诊医师和长期护理团队进行沟通和协作，以确保医疗方案得到优化，提高在等待名单上的生存率，同时确保患者的医疗方案不会增加移植后出现更糟糕结果的风险。特别需要关注的是皮质类固醇的使用和剂量、现常用于肺纤维化的抗纤维化药物、用于 LAM 患者和潜在其他疾病的 mTOR 抑制剂、用于 CF 患者的 CFTR 调节剂以及抗凝药物。基于仔细的风险/收益分析和准备，通常与移植药师合作，对肺移植候选者在列名前和列名时使用本文评述的药物的医疗管理不会对移植结果产生不利影响。

### 【临床护理要点】

在等待肺移植的患者中：

- 糖皮质激素的最大安全剂量尚不明确，因此慢性剂量应最小化。
- 抗纤维化药物（吡非尼酮和尼达尼布）可能是安全的，可以继续使用。
- mTOR抑制剂（西罗莫司和依维莫司）的数据有限，因此应权衡每位患者风险与收益。依维莫司半衰期较短，可能是首选。
- 停药可能有危险，因此CFTR调节剂应继续使用。
- 应继续PAH治疗，并调整以优化右心功能。
- 在移植手术前需要紧急逆转时，抗凝药物最好使用PCC来逆转华法林，或使用依达赛珠单抗来逆转直接作用口服抗凝药物。

## 声明

D. M. Sayah：没有需要声明的商业或财务利益冲突。没有与此工作相关的资金来源。

J.M. Pilewski：没有商业或财务利益冲突。J.M. Pilewski博士接受了Vertex公司对CFTR调节剂多中心研究的研究资助。

## 参考文献

1. Chambers DC, CherikhWS, Harhay MO, et al. The International Thoracic Organ Transplant Registry of the International Society for Heart and Lung Transplantation: Thirty-sixth adult lung and heart-lung transplantation Report-2019; Focus theme: Donor and recipient size match. J Heart Lung Transpl 2019;38(10):1042–55.
2. Valapour M, Lehr CJ, Skeans MA, et al. OPTN/SRTR 2019 Annual Data Report: Lung. Am J Transplant 2021;21(Suppl 2):441–520.
3. Rhen T, Cidlowski JA. Antiinflammatory action of glucocorticoids–new mechanisms for old drugs. N Engl J Med 2005;353(16):1711–1723.
4. Wang AS, Armstrong EJ, Armstrong AW. Corticosteroids and wound healing: clinical considerations in the perioperative period. Am J Surg 2013;206(3):410–417.
5. Rice JB, White AG, Scarpati LM, et al. Long-term Systemic Corticosteroid Exposure: A Systematic Literature Review. Clin Ther 2017;39(11):2216–2229.

6. Lima O, Cooper JD, Peters WJ, et al. Effects of methylprednisolone and azathioprine on bronchial healing following lung autotransplantation. J Thorac Cardiovasc Surg 1981;82(2):211–215.
7. Goldberg M, Lima O, Morgan E, et al. A comparison between cyclosporin A and methylprednisolone plus azathioprine on bronchial healing following canine lung autotransplantation. J Thorac Cardiovasc Surg 1983;85(6):821–826.
8. Patterson GA, Cooper JD. Status of lung transplantation. Surg Clin North Am 1988;68(3):545–558.
9. Park SJ, Nguyen DQ, Savik K, et al. Pre-transplant corticosteroid use and outcome in lung transplantation. J Heart Lung Transpl 2001;20(3):304–309.
10. Schafers HJ, Wagner TO, Demertzis S, et al. Preoperative corticosteroids. A contraindication to lung transplantation? Chest 1992;102(5):1522–1525.
11. McAnally KJ, Valentine VG, LaPlace SG, et al. Effect of pre-transplantation prednisone on survival after lung transplantation. J Heart Lung Transpl 2006;25(1):67–74.
12. Sugimoto S, Miyoshi K, Kurosaki T, et al. Favorable survival in lung transplant recipients on preoperativelow-dose, as compared to high-dose corticosteroids, after hematopoietic stem cell transplantation. Int J Hematol 2018;107(6):696–702.
13. Yusen RD, Edwards LB, Dipchand AI, et al. The Registry of the International Society for Heart and Lung Transplantation: Thirty-third Adult Lung and Heart-Lung Transplant Report-2016; Focus Theme:Primary Diagnostic Indications for Transplant. J Heart Lung Transpl 2016;35(10):1170–1184.
14. Malas J, Ranganath NK, Phillips KG, et al. Early airway dehiscence: Risk factors and outcomes with the rising incidence of extracorporeal membrane oxygenation as a bridge to lung transplantation. J Card Surg 2019;34(10):933–940.
15. Maurer JR, Frost AE, Estenne M, et al. International guidelines for the selection of lung transplant candidates. The International Society for Heart and Lung Transplantation, the American Thoracic Society, the American Society of Transplant Physicians, the European Respiratory Society. Heart Lung 1998;27(4):223–9.
16. Orens JB, Estenne M, Arcasoy S, et al. International guidelines for the selection of lung transplant candidates: 2006 update–a consensus report from the Pulmonary Scientific Council of the International Society for Heart and Lung Transplantation. J Heart Lung Transpl 2006;25(7):745–755.
17. Weill D, Benden C, Corris PA, et al. A consensus document for the selection of lung transplant candidates: 2014–an update from the Pulmonary Transplantation Council of the International Society for Heart and Lung Transplantation. J Heart Lung Transpl 2015;34(1):1–15.
18. Leard LE, Holm AM, Valapour M, et al. Consensus document for the selection of lung transplant candidates: An update from the International Society for Heart and Lung Transplantation. J Heart Lung Transpl 2021;40(11):1349–1379.
19. Richeldi L, du Bois RM, Raghu G, et al. Efficacy and safety of nintedanib in idiopathic pulmonary fibrosis. N Engl J Med 2014;370(22):2071–2082.
20. King TE Jr, Bradford WZ, Castro-Bernardini S, et al. A phase 3 trial of pirfenidone in patients with idiopathic pulmonary fibrosis. N Engl J Med 2014;370(22):2083–2092.
21. Wells AU, Flaherty KR, Brown KK, et al. Nintedanib in patients with progressive fibrosing interstitial lung diseases-subgroup analyses by interstitial lung disease diagnosis in the INBUILD trial: a randomised, double-

blind, placebo-controlled, parallelgroup trial. Lancet Respir Med 2020;8(5):453–460.
22. Distler O, Highland KB, Gahlemann M, et al. Nintedanib for Systemic Sclerosis-Associated Interstitial Lung Disease. N Engl J Med 2019;380(26):2518–2528.
23. Salisbury ML, Conoscenti CS, Culver DA, et al. Antifibrotic Drug Use in Patients with Idiopathic Pulmonary Fibrosis. Data from the IPF-PRO Registry. Ann Am Thorac Soc 2020;17(11):1413–1423.
24. Lehtonen ST, Veijola A, Karvonen H, et al. Pirfenidone and nintedanib modulate properties of fibroblasts and myofibroblasts in idiopathic pulmonary fibrosis. Respir Res 2016;17:14.
25. Wollin L, Wex E, Pautsch A, et al. Mode of action of nintedanib in the treatment of idiopathic pulmonary fibrosis. Eur Respir J 2015;45(5):1434–1445.
26. Leuschner G, Stocker F, Veit T, et al. Outcome of lung transplantation in idiopathic pulmonary fibrosis with previous anti-fibrotic therapy. J Heart Lung Transpl 2017;37(2):268–274.
27. Mackintosh JA, Munsif M, Ranzenbacher L, et al. Risk of anastomotic dehiscence in patients with pulmonary fibrosis transplanted while receiving anti-fibrotics: Experience of the Australian Lung Transplant Collaborative. J Heart Lung Transpl 2019;38(5):553–559.
28. Mortensen A, Cherrier L, Walia R. Effect of pirfenidone on wound healing in lung transplant patients. Multidiscip Respir Med 2018;13:16.
29. Delanote I, Wuyts WA, Yserbyt J, et al. Safety and efficacy of bridging to lung transplantation with antifibrotic drugs in idiopathic pulmonary fibrosis: a case series. BMC Pulm Med 2016;16(1):156.
30. Tanaka S, Miyoshi K, Higo H, et al. Lung transplant candidates with idiopathic pulmonary fibrosis and long-term pirfenidone therapy: Treatment feasibility influences waitlist survival. Respir Investig 2019;57(2):165–171.
31. Lambers C, Boehm PM, Lee S, et al. Effect of antifibrotics on short-term outcome after bilateral lung transplantation: a multicentre analysis. Eur Respir J 2018;51(6).
32. Veit T, Leuschner G, Sisic A, et al. Pirfenidone exerts beneficial effects in patients with IPF undergoing single lung transplantation. Am J Transplant 2019;19(8):2358–2365.
33. Combs MP, Fitzgerald LJ, Wakeam E, et al. Pretransplant antifibrotic therapy is associated with resolution of primary graft dysfunction. Ann Amer Thorac Soc 2022;19(2):335–338.
34. Kahan BD. Sirolimus: a comprehensive review. Expert Opin Pharmacother 2001;2(11):1903–17.
35. Nashan B. Review of the proliferation inhibitor everolimus. Expert Opin Investig Drugs 2002;11(12):1845–1857.
36. Hua H, Kong Q, Zhang H, et al. Targeting mTOR for cancer therapy. J Hematol Oncol 2019;12(1):71.
37. King-Biggs MB, Dunitz JM, Park SJ, et al. Airway anastomotic dehiscence associated with use of sirolimus immediately after lung transplantation. Transplantation 2003;75(9):1437–1443.
38. Groetzner J, Kur F, Spelsberg F, et al. Airway anastomosis complications in de novo lung transplantation with sirolimus-based immunosuppression. J Heart Lung Transpl 2004;23(5):632–638.
39. Pfizer Inc. Rapamune (sirolimus) [package insert]. U.S. Food and Drug Administration website. 2021. Available at: https://www. accessdata. fda. gov/spl/data/411b5f71-515a-431e-ae12-5db5ea5a06fd/411b5f71-515a-431e-ae12-5db5ea5a06fd. xml. Accessed August 28, 2021.
40. McCormack FX, Inoue Y, Moss J, et al. Efficacy andsafety of sirolimus in lymphangioleiomyomatosis. N

# 第1章　等待名单上的肺移植候选者的门诊药物管理

Engl J Med 2011;364(17):1595–1606.

41. El-Chemaly S, Goldberg HJ, Glanville AR. Should mammalian target of rapamycin inhibitors be stopped in women with lymphangioleiomyomatosis awaiting lung transplantation? Expert Rev Respir Med 2014;8(6):657–660.

42. Baldi BG, Samano MN, Campos SV, et al. Experience of Lung Transplantation in Patients with Lymphangioleiomyomatosis at a Brazilian Reference Centre. Lung 2017;195(6):699–705.

43. Zhang J, Liu D, Yue B, et al. A Retrospective Study of Lung Transplantation in Patients With Lymphangioleiomyomatosis: Challenges and Outcomes. Front Med (Lausanne) 2021;8:584826.

44. Costa AN, Baldi BG, de Oliveira Braga Teixeira RH, et al. Can patients maintain their use of everolimus until lung transplantation? Transplantation 2015;99(6):e42–43.

45. Novartis Inc. Zortress (everolimus) [package insert]. U. S. Food and Drug Administration website. 2018. Available at: https://www. accessdata. fda. gov/drugsatfda_docs/label/2018/021560s021lbl. pdf. Accessed December 20th, 2021.

46. Ramsey BW, Davies J, McElvaney NG, et al. A CFTR potentiator in patients with cystic fibrosis and the G551D mutation. N Engl J Med 2011;365(18):1663–1672.

47. Barry PJ, Plant BJ, Nair A, et al. Effects of ivacaftor in patients with cystic fibrosis who carry the G551D mutation and have severe lung disease. Chest 2014;146(1):152–158.

48. Polenakovik HM, Sanville B. The use of ivacaftor in an adult with severe lung disease due to cystic fibrosis (DeltaF508/G551D). J Cyst Fibros 2013;12(5):530–531.

49. Taylor-Cousar J, Niknian M, Gilmartin G, et al. Effect of ivacaftor in patients with advanced cystic fibrosis and a G551D-CFTR mutation: Safety and efficacy in an expanded access program in the United States. J Cyst Fibros 2016;15(1):116–122.

50. Salvatore D, Terlizzi V, Francalanci M, et al. Ivacaftor improves lung disease in patients with advanced CF carrying CFTR mutations that confer residual function. Respir Med 2020;171:106073.

51. Keating D, Marigowda G, Burr L, et al. VX-445-Tezacaftor-Ivacaftor in Patients with Cystic Fibrosis and One or Two Phe508del Alleles. N Engl J Med 2018;379(17):1612–1620.

52. Middleton PG, Mall MA, Drevinek P, et al. Elexacaftor-Tezacaftor-Ivacaftor for Cystic Fibrosis with a Single Phe508del Allele. N Engl J Med 2019;381(19):1809–1819.

53. Heijerman HGM, McKone EF, Downey DG, et al. Efficacy and safety of the elexacaftor plus tezacaftor plus ivacaftor combination regimen in people with cystic fibrosis homozygous for the F508del mutation:a double-blind, randomised, phase 3 trial. Lancet 2019;394(10212):1940–1948.

54. Burgel PR, Durieu I, Chiron R, et al. Rapid Improvement after Starting Elexacaftor-Tezacaftor-Ivacaftor in Patients with Cystic Fibrosis and Advanced Pulmonary Disease. Am J Respir Crit Care Med 2021;204(1):64–73.

55. Volkova N, Moy K, Evans J, et al. Disease progression in patients with cystic fibrosis treated with ivacaftor: Data from national US and UK registries. J Cyst Fibros 2020;19(1):68–79.

56. Ramos KJ, Quon BS, Heltshe SL, et al. Heterogeneity in Survival in Adult Patients With Cystic Fibrosis With $FEV1 < 30\%$ of Predicted in the United States. Chest 2017;151(6):1320–1328.

57. Trimble AT, Donaldson SH. Ivacaftor withdrawal syndrome in cystic fibrosis patients with the G551D

mutation. J Cyst Fibros 2018;17(2):e13–16.

58. Hassoun PM. Pulmonary Arterial Hypertension. N Engl J Med 2021;385(25):2361–2376.
59. Kuntz CL, Hadjiliadis D, Ahya VN, et al. Risk factors for early primary graft dysfunction after lung transplantation: a registry study. Clin Transpl 2009;23(6):819–830.
60. Diamond JM, Lee JC, Kawut SM, et al. Clinical risk factors for primary graft dysfunction after lung transplantation. Am J Respir Crit Care Med 2013;187(5):527–534.
61. Baillie TJ, Granton JT. Lung Transplantation for Pulmonary Hypertension and Strategies to Bridge to Transplant. Semin Respir Crit Care Med 2017;38(5):701–710.
62. Campo A, Mathai SC, Le Pavec J, et al. Outcomes of hospitalisation for right heart failure in pulmonary arterial hypertension. Eur Respir J 2011;38(2):359–367.
63. Sandoval J, Gomez-Arroyo J, Gaspar J, et al. Interventional and surgical therapeutic strategies for pulmonary arterial hypertension: Beyond palliative treatments. J Cardiol 2015;66(4):304–314.
64. Goldstein JN, Refaai MA, Milling TJ Jr, et al. Fourfactor prothrombin complex concentrate versus plasmafor rapid vitamin K antagonist reversal in patients needing urgent surgical or invasive interventions: a phase 3b, open-label, non-inferiority, randomised trial. Lancet 2015;385(9982):2077–2087.
65. Refaai MA, Goldstein JN, Lee ML, et al. Increased risk of volume overload with plasma compared with four-factor prothrombin complex concentrate for urgent vitamin K antagonist reversal. Transfusion 2015;55(11):2722–2729.
66. Harano T, Rivosecchi RM, Morrell MR, et al. Dabigatran reversal with idarucizumab prior to lung transplantation. Clin Transpl 2021;35(1):e14142.
67. Crespo-Leiro MG, Lopez-Vilella R, Lopez Granados A, et al. Use of Idarucizumab to reversethe anticoagulant effect of dabigatran in cardiac transplant surgery. A multicentric experience in Spain. Clin Transpl 2019;33(12):e13748.

# 第 2 章　急性失代偿肺移植候选者的住院管理

Stephan A. Soder, Eduardo Fontena, Juan C. Salgado, Abbas Shahmohammadi,
Marcos N. Samano, Tiago N. Machuca　著

李聪　周伟　译

周建平　校

【关键词】
- 危重症　• 肺移植　• 体外膜肺氧合　• 康复

【要点】
- 基于紧急程度的肺分配制度增加了等待肺移植候选者的病情复杂性与危重性，最终影响其接受移植的可能性。
- 移植团队通常需处理晚期肺病候选者的急性病情恶化。
- 需通过多学科团队审慎选择患者，以避免无效治疗，并为可能通过肺移植（LTx）获得良好预后的患者提供支持。
- 体外生命支持（ECLS）系统可作为肺移植的有效过渡治疗，接受过渡治疗与未过渡治疗受体的长期条件生存率相当。
- 康复在筛选和准备过渡至移植的患者中发挥着关键作用。

## 2.1 引　言

近 15 年前，美国肺分配的优先级依据由候捐者在等待名单上累积的时间，改为根据疾病严重程度和移植后预期生存率，用肺源分配评分（LAS）表示。值得注意的是，1 年内死亡风险在评分计算中比移植后生存率所占地位更重要[1]。虽然这一变化与候捐者死亡率预期下降有关（最近报告为 14.6%），但可以预见移植团队将不得不照顾日益年长、病情复杂的受体和患者[2]。这种基于紧急程度的分配也导致移植中心常规考虑为病情更危重、通常已住院，且不少在 ICU 的患者进行移植。根据器官移植科学登记处的数据，

# 肺移植：胸外科临床问题

2009—2019 年，移植时已住院和入住 ICU 的肺移植（LTx）受体比例分别从 18.9% 增加至 26.8% 以及从 9.2% 增加至 16.5%[2,3]。

此外，随着基于紧急程度分配制度的实施，越来越多的间质性肺病（ILD）患者而非慢性阻塞性肺疾病（COPD）患者被列入等待名单并接受移植。2009—2019 年，因 COPD 接受移植的受体比例从 33% 下降至 22.9%，而因 ILD 接受移植的比例从 44.5% 上升至 63.5%[2,3]。ILD 组患者往往病情复杂、不稳定，慢性肺疾病轨迹难以预测。为日益增长的病情严重的复杂受体提供肺移植，要求移植团队必须熟悉慢性肺病急性失代偿的识别和管理[4]。此类患者通常需要住院，在 ICU 升级护理，最终需要就是否继续保留移植资格或从候补名单中除名进行艰难的讨论（图 2-1）。本章我们将回顾急性失代偿肺移植受体的管理，包括潜在的挽救策略、桥接、康复以及除名指征。

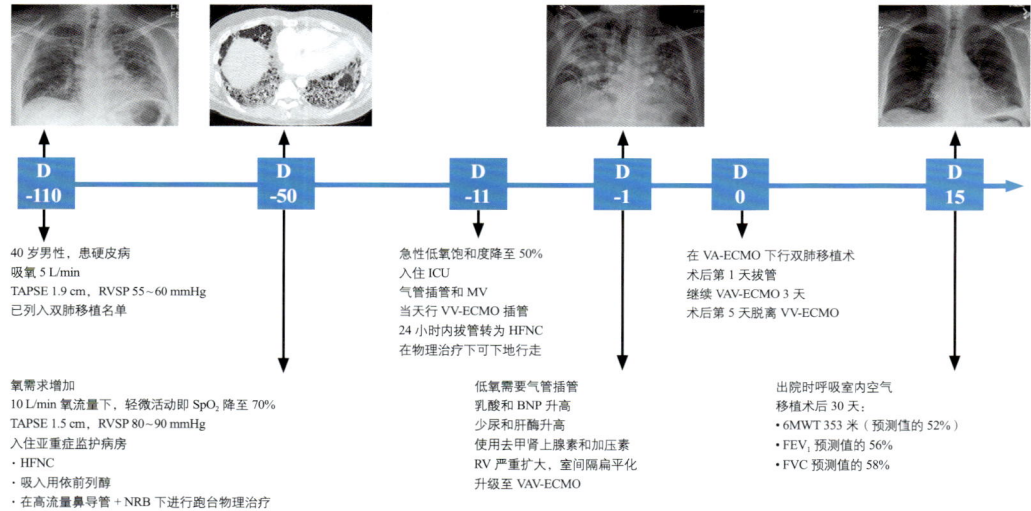

图 2-1 临床图示详细描述了一位终末期肺部疾病患者病情进行性恶化和急性恶化的演变过程

注：1：入院；2：入住步行病房；3：入住重症监护室（ICU）；4：升级 ECLS 策略；5：双肺移植；6：出院。6MWT，6 分钟步行测试；BNP，脑钠肽；DC，出院；ECMO，体外膜肺氧合；$FEV_1$，第一秒用力呼气容积；FVC，用力肺活量；HFNC，经鼻高流量氧疗；ICU，重症监护病房；MV，机械通气；NRB，非再呼吸氧面罩；POD，术后日；PRED，预测值；RV，右心室；RVSP，右心室收缩压；TAPSE，三尖瓣环收缩期位移；VA-ECMO，静脉-动脉 ECMO；VAV-ECMO，静脉-动脉-静脉 ECMO；VV-ECMO，静脉-静脉 ECMO

## 2.2 疾病严重程度对肺移植后预后的影响

如预期的那样，在 LAS 实施的早期，候捐者死亡率有所下降，但病情最危重的患者从移植中获得的生存获益最低。在分析 2005 年 5 月至 2009 年 5 月之间的 6082 例器官共享联合网络（the United Network for Organ Sharing，UNOS）数据库患者时发现，LAS 为 50~59 分的患者净生存获益为 3.44 年，LAS > 90 分的患者仅为 1.95 年[5]。同一研究团队分析了 2006—2007 年 UNOS 数据，发现随着 LAS 增加，移植后 1 年生存率显著下降，LAS < 50、50~74 和 > 75 患者的生存率分别为 83%、79% 和 64%[6]。危重症组的发病率也增加，包括需要肾脏替代治疗和并发感染。随着医疗进步、桥接策略改进以及术中管理措施的优化，危重症患者的预后已有显著改善。在 2005—2014 年间 3548 例 LAS 上四分位成年患者中，尽管平均 LAS 从 63 增加到 79，但移植后 1 年生存率从 2005—2008 年间的 77% 提高至 2011—2014 年间的 84%[7]。

2007 年，法国实施了"高度紧急肺移植"制度，优先将供肺分配给急性失代偿的患者。这一复杂人群的 1 年生存率仅为 67%，3 年生存率为 59%[8]。某中心收治的囊性纤维化（CF）患者比例较高（37 例中占 81%），其预后较佳，与非高紧急状态患者队列相当，机械通气时间：15.5 天 vs. 11 天，而肺移植后 1 年生存率：81% vs. 80%[9]。

在斯堪的纳维亚经验中，随着 2009 年实施的紧急分配，基于疾病严重程度对受体进行优先排序大大缩短了移植等待时间。在列为紧急状态的受体中，81% 在 4 周内接受移植，而常规状态组仅为 4.3%。紧急组 1 年生存率为 81.3%，常规组为 85.5%，无显著统计学差异。紧急组候捐者死亡主要与体外膜肺氧合（extracorporeal membrane oxygenation，ECMO）桥接相关[10]。

天普大学报告了 37 例特发性肺纤维化急性加重（acute exacerbation of idiopathic pulmonary fibrosis，AE-IPF）患者与 52 例稳定特发性肺纤维化（IPF）患者的治疗经验[11]。37 例 AE-IPF 患者中仅 28 例接受了移植（候捐名单死亡率 32%）。AE-IPF 患者的 1 年生存率为 71%，稳定期患者为 94%。

同样，佛罗里达大学报告了 27 例因 ILD 急性失代偿入院的移植候选者与 69 例病情稳定的 ILD 候选者的预后[12]。每组仅有 2 例候捐者死亡，移植后 1 年生存率相当，急性失代偿组为 96%，稳定组为 92.5%。作者推测急性加重组的良好生存可能与以下因素有关：①急性加重期列名患者在胸外科移植医疗团队管理的专科病房接受治疗；②供者肺源充足，急性加重患者中位移植等待时间仅 10 天；③术中更多使用静脉 - 动脉

ECMO 而非体外循环；④与天普队列相比，患者相对年轻（60 岁 vs. 67 岁）。

此外，紧急列名患者（定义为在同一次住院期间列名并移植）的预后情况令人满意。在克利夫兰医学中心 2006—2017 年移植的 201 例患者队列中[13]，紧急列名患者更年轻（54 岁 vs. 57 岁），ILD 患者更多（76% vs. 48%），上呼吸机（49% vs. 1%）或体外生命支持（extracorporeal life support，ECLS）（22% vs. 0.14%）的比例更高。尽管紧急组候捐者死亡率高达 32%，年龄较大、胆红素升高以及从外院转入为早期候捐者死亡的显著预测因素，但移植后总体并发症发生率相似，72 小时原发性移植物功能不全（PGD）发生率也相当（紧急组 17% vs. 选择性组 12%）。此外，移植后生存率相当（住院死亡率 13% vs. 11%），移植后 6 年内的移植物功能也相似。这项研究凸显了即使是转入时病情极其危重的患者，如果能够在有丰富经验的中心治疗，也有可能获得良好预后。

医院容量对住院受体预后的影响仍有争议。一项对 2007—2017 年 18 416 例成人肺移植患者的 UNOS 数据库分析发现，移植时已有 20% 的患者住院[14]。这些患者更年轻（55 岁 vs. 60 岁），COPD 患者更少（10% vs. 22%），LAS 评分更高（70 vs. 38）。这些患者的等待时间预期可能会更短（27 天 vs. 73 天）；但他们更常经历延长的机械通气（mechanical ventilation，MV）（56.7% vs. 30%），住院时间中位数更长（22 天 vs. 15 天）。与入住小体量中心相比，入住大体量中心（研究期间年均移植量 25 例）生存率更高，这种差异在 CF 患者中更为明显。这些结果提示，鉴定更适合管理高危重患者的移植中心，甚至在不同专业水平和风险承受能力的移植中心之间开放二次会诊的可能窗口，可能会带来潜在获益。

在考虑为高危重患者进行移植时，需要考虑资源利用问题。Arnaoutakis 等在 2011 年报告，LAS 最高四分位患者的住院费用显著较高，不仅是首次入院费用（Q4 27.6668 万美元 vs. Q1-3 的 18.8342 万美元），移植后 1 年内的费用也更高（Q4 29.2247 万美元 vs. Q1-3 的 18.8342 万美元）[15]。最近，梅奥医学中心的研究显示，随着 LAS 增加，住院和移植后费用稳步上升[16]。在多因素模型中，他们发现 LAS 每增加 10 分，首次入院费用增加 12%。

上述研究结果凸显了全球肺移植项目面临的挑战，同时也提示我们需要：①制定更有效的策略，为病情突然恶化的移植候选者提供更好的支持；②扩大现有的供体库；③改进围术期管理，以延长移植后生存期；④优化候选者的筛选，避免徒劳无益的列名或移植。

## 2.3 急性失代偿肺移植候选者的医疗管理

肺移植候选者的门诊随访频率取决于疾病严重程度。在我们中心，稳定患者通常每1~2个月来一次门诊，评估其健康状况并更新 LAS。LAS > 50 分的患者需每 2 周就诊 1 次。虽然没有明确的入院标准，但我们可以参考一些指标，如需氧量突然增加 50% 以上，需要 8~10 L/min 以上的氧气，无法继续使用家中的常规低流量供氧设备进行体力活动[12]。

### 2.3.1 间质性疾病

ILD 包括各种肺实质疾病，其临床病程通常是多变且不可预测的。少部分患者会出现 ILD 急性加重，住院病死率高达 90%[17,18]。这可能是由于迅速进展的成纤维增生过程，也可能由诸如感染等因素引发[17]。这些患者存在慢性低氧性呼吸衰竭急性加重，随着病情进展，晚期阶段还可出现高碳酸血症。由于缺乏有效疗法，ILD 加重期的治疗以支持疗法为主；虽然高剂量激素使用较为普遍，但疗效尚无定论[19]。最重要的治疗途径是加快对可移植患者的评估。

呼吸支持可逐步升级，从鼻管到面罩、经鼻高流量氧疗（high-flow nasal cannula，HFNC）、无创正压通气（noninvasive positive pressure ventilation，NPPV）、MV 和 ECLS[20]。与传统低流量吸氧相比，HFNC 可能提供以下生理学益处：改善氧合，减少解剖无效腔，降低呼吸代谢成本，产生鼻咽和气管正压，减轻呼吸功，预先调节吸入气体，改善分泌物清除，提高舒适度[21]。在急性呼吸衰竭患者的随机临床试验中，与传统低流量吸氧或 NPPV 相比，HFNC 与气管插管需求的减少和病死率的降低有关[22,23]。虽然支持 ILD 患者使用 HFNC 的数据很少，但对需要更高流量和(或)浓度氧气的患者而言，HFNC 可能是一种合适的替代疗法[20]。同样，在进行有创的 MV 前，可尝试使用 NPPV 稳定呼吸状态。鉴于 MV 相关的病死率较高，美国胸科学会建议不对这些患者进行气管插管，除了某些特殊人群，如肺移植候选者或出现明确可逆性恶化原因的患者[19]。

如使用 HFNC 和 NPPV 呼吸衰竭仍在进展，可考虑加用吸入性肺血管扩张剂（如一氧化氮吸入、前列环素吸入）。吸入性肺血管扩张剂可改善氧合，支持 ILD 患者常见的右心室（right ventricular，RV）功能障碍/肺动脉高压（pulmonary hypertension，PH），同时避免静脉（intravenous，IV）给药肺血管扩张剂常见的肺通气/血流灌注（ventilation/perfusion，V/Q）失调[24]。

### 2.3.2 慢性阻塞性肺疾病

自 LAS 实施以来，COPD 患者移植等待时间延长，因此可能出现急性失代偿。BODE 指数（体重指数、气流受限、呼吸困难和运动能力）是一个有用的预后工具，显示最高四分位患者可从移植中获益。2021 版《肺移植候选者筛选共识文件》继续依靠该评分作为转诊和列名时机的指导[25]。COPD 候选者入选移植通常 BODE 评分＞7 分，并伴有频繁急性加重史，第一秒用力呼气容积（$FEV_1$）≤ 20% 预测值，PH 和（或）高碳酸血症。

随着 COPD 进展，调整氧气补充对于维持等待移植患者可接受水平的体能锻炼和充足营养状态至关重要。此外，还需要教育患者使用缩唇呼吸和步调，以尽量避免运动诱发的肺过度充气。

晚期 COPD 的急性加重通常由感染、无法代偿呼吸性酸中毒、PH 和胃食管反流病引起。支气管扩张剂、类固醇、抗微生物药物（必要时包括抗病毒药）等药物治疗，以及支持治疗（包括补充氧气和无创/有创通气）是短暂支持的主要策略。HFNC 和 NPPV 已成为支持和避免 MV 的首选方法。尽管关于 HFNC 治疗 COPD 急性加重的预后数据有限，但一些小型前瞻性病例系列研究显示，呼吸频率明显减慢，$PaCO_2$ 下降[26,27]。此外，患者可能比无创通气（NIV）更容易耐受 HFNC[28]。尽管如此，鉴于现有数据有限，欧洲呼吸学会最近建议，对于 COPD 加重引起的高碳酸血症性呼吸衰竭，在使用 HFNC 之前，先试用 NIV[29]。

### 2.3.3 肺动脉高压

在 PH 患者中，肺动脉高压（PAH）和慢性血栓栓塞性肺高压（chronic thromboembolic pulmonary hypertension，CTEPH）患者因右心衰竭失代偿而就诊更为常见，伴随着高发病率和死亡率[30]。法国一家转诊中心最近的一份报告显示，PAH 失代偿后 3 个月和 1 年病死率分别为 31% 和 41%。当肺移植不可行时，病死率甚至更高，分别为 46% 和 56%[31]。随着 PH 治疗的进展，使得生活质量（quality of life，QoL）改善，疾病相关发病率和病死率降低，收入 ICU 的失代偿 PH 伴右心衰竭的患者往往是那些已经接受最大药物治疗且用尽所有治疗选择的患者[30]。由于这些患者治疗复杂，理想情况下应在具有 PAH、ECLS 和肺移植专业知识的高级肺衰竭中心进行管理。

失代偿的诱因多种多样，包括感染、妊娠和手术等应激情况、心律失常和用药依从性差等。除了处理诱因外，还应注意优化前负荷/液体平衡。静脉前列腺素如依前列素，磷酸二酯酶（phosphodiesterase，PDE）抑制剂，以及一氧化氮吸入或依前列素吸入等吸入性肺血管扩张剂均可用于降低右心室后负荷。对于无反应者，可考虑使用强心药如多巴酚丁胺和肌苷类如米力农，以增强右心室收缩，使心排出量大于 2 L/（min·m²），静脉血氧饱和度（venous oxygen saturation，$SvO_2$）> 65%。血管加压素是首选的升压药，因为它具有肺血管扩张作用。由于其对右心室/肺动脉循环耦联的有益影响和正性肌力作用，去甲肾上腺素也是较好的选择。

与 ILD 急性加重类似，低氧性呼吸衰竭采用补充氧气、HFNC 和 NPPV 治疗。然而，应尽量努力避免气管插管和 MV。气管插管和镇静可能在右心室衰竭晚期诱发血流动力学衰竭，因为它们会抑制心肌收缩力并引起血管扩张。通常需要采用清醒纤维支气管镜插管，谨慎镇静，并适当使用血流动力学支持和升压药。

如上述治疗未能改善临床状态，应考虑 ECLS。在考虑 ECLS 之前，需要回答两个问题：①患者是否存在 PAH 失代偿的可逆原因；②患者是否为潜在的肺/心肺移植候选者。

### 2.3.4 囊性纤维化

CF 仍然是北美和欧洲肺移植的常见适应证，在过去的 10 年中略有下降，这归因于 CF 跨膜传导调节因子（CFTR）调节剂的出现，这是一类新型药物，通过改善受损 CFTR 蛋白的产生、细胞内加工和（或）功能而发挥作用[32]。研究表明，它们可以改善 $FEV_1$ 和症状相关的 QoL，减少急性加重，主要见于轻中度 CF 肺病患者，也有新的数据显示其对晚期肺病患者的益处[33]。相当一部分患者并未携带任何一种已批准使用 CFTR 调节剂的突变。这一类别约占非西班牙裔白种人 CF 患者的 8%，西班牙裔患者的 25%，黑种人/非裔美国人患者的 30%[34]。

CF 列名患者出现急性加重的处理包括根据已知肺微生物群进行经验性抗生素治疗和强化气道清除。常见做法是至少选择一种抗生素覆盖从呼吸道分泌物培养出的每种细菌分离株，铜绿假单胞菌感染则选用两种抗生素。抗生素疗程根据初始反应而定，对于反应迅速者为 10 天，对于反应较慢和需要 ICU 级别护理的患者为 14 天或更长。对于此类患者，抗生素持续到症状和 $FEV_1$ 改善达平台期（通常疗程为 14~21 天）[35]。关于气道清除策略，建议继续进行门诊治疗，包括吸入剂（如高渗盐水），以及机械胸部物理治疗（如震动治疗或更新型的肺内震荡通气装置）[36]。对于肺实质严重损坏的 CF 患者，急性加重可并发大咯血。在这种情况下,紧急支气管镜检查可有助于识别和填塞出血肺段,但最终可能需要进行体循环动脉栓塞术。

## 2.4 移植前桥接

危重的肺移植候选者在等待合适供体器官期间死亡风险高。在特定患者中可能需要使用支持装置作为桥接治疗,以避免进一步恶化并维持移植候选资格。此外,越来越多的移植是针对急性或亚急性不可逆性肺损伤疾病,如 COVID-19 ARDS,可在移植入选的同时使用桥接治疗[37]。

几十年来,MV 一直被用作一种桥接手段。然而,由于需要镇静、身体功能退化、无法达到移植,以及移植后生存率较低[38,39],加之人们对 ECLS 经验日益丰富,使得如今 MV 这种桥接方式不再那么吸引人[40]。

### 2.4.1 体外生命支持作为移植前桥接的经验

使用 ECLS 移植桥接(bridge to transplantation,BTT)依赖于尽量避免或减少对 MV 的需求,减少镇静,便于患者下床活动,同时维持移植资格。ECLS 支持的患者危重病肌病(critical illness myopathy,CIM)的发病率差异很大,范围为 30%~75%[41,42]。减少镇静方案和早期活动与预后改善相关[43,44],此类患者的积极康复可缩短移植后 MV 时间、ICU 和住院时间[45]。在若干病例系列中,脱离 MV、活动和行走与更高的 BTT 成功率相关[46-48]。

在大多数已发表的研究中,成功桥接到肺移植的比例为 56%[49]~89%[47,50],某单中心 1 年时间内报告的成功率为 100%[51]。在一项大型队列研究中,简化急性生理学评分Ⅱ、ECLS 支持期间计划外气管插管肾脏替代治疗和脑血管意外被确定为 BTT 不成功的独立预测因素。相反,下床活动与 BTT 成功相关[48]。文献报道的桥接时间中位数为 2~17 天[51,52],静脉-静脉体外膜肺氧合(veno-venous extracorporeal membrane oxygenation,VV-ECMO)是最常用的配置。

BTT 患者移植 72 小时后 3 级 PGD 的发生率差异很大,可低至 5.6%[50]。通常,术后会维持 ECLS,此时应将 PGD 分类为"无法评分"。预计桥接患者在移植后的早期会有较长的住院时间[51]和较高的死亡率[50,52],这是由临床严重性和潜在的去适应作用造成的。然而,有研究证明那些实现移植的桥接患者条件生存率与非桥接移植患者相当[46-48,53,54],

尤其是在大型中心，1年、3年和5年的生存率分别为58%~100%[51,52]、63%~83%[47,48]，以及55%~65%[47,50]。此外，ECLS桥接患者的真实生存获益必须考虑到该队列没有移植的情况下的明确死亡率。

### 2.4.2 移植适应证与预后

评估可能影响肺移植候选者和进行ECLS的BTT患者预后的相关临床因素，对决策过程和管理至关重要。囊性纤维化患者可能会有更好的BTT预后[47,55,56]。一个大型CF患者移植系列报告称，移植后1年的条件生存率在桥接患者中为81%，与非桥接患者相比没有统计学差异[56]。有病例报告称，未被控制的肺部感染通过双侧肺切除并成功采用体外生命支持系统进行了移植前桥接治疗[57]。相反，患特发性PAH和右心室功能不全的患者与较差的生存率相关[47,58]。间质性肺病的患者在不同研究系列中的预后表现出很大的差异性[47,55,58]。

再移植的桥接是另一个不利的预后因素。多伦多研究小组的一个病例系列显示，首次移植的患者的中位存活时间明显优于再移植桥接患者（60个月 *vs.* 15个月，$P=0.041$），后者的5年总生存率为39%[47]。

### 2.4.3 体外生命支持系统的启动及配置选择

ECLS的应用不仅是为了更好地支持使用呼吸机的患者，而且还能避免对迅速恶化的患者使用插管。当今方法学的一个主要概念是边走边桥接（ambulatory bridging）。ECLS必须以尽可能保持患者清醒为目标，并且最好是使患者可以下床行走。2012年，汉诺威团队报告显示，与机械通气（MV）相比，体外膜肺氧合（ECMO）不仅改善了预后，而且在患者无需插管保持清醒状态下置管时效果更佳[59]。随后，若干项研究展示了与日益改善的预后相关的不断增长的经验[47,48,60,61]。

清醒插管的部位与活动能力密切相关，插管必须安装和固定好，以避免移位并在允许活动的同时维持血流。尽管传统上认为股动脉插管与有限的床外物理治疗相关[62]，但经良好训练的团队报告的能够行走的病例越来越多[62-66]。Pasrija及其同事报告了使用股静脉-动脉ECMO（veno-arterial ECMO，VA-ECMO）的经验，14%的患者可能可以行走。在行走期间或之后没有血流受限，没有重大出血或血管并发症[66]。一个大型系列研究评估了与ECMO支持患者床外物理治疗相关的因素，研究期间活动频率增加，51%的股部插管患者实现了行走[62]。

迄今为止，对于启动 ECLS 作为 BTT 的确切时机尚无共识。积极参与康复治疗的移植候选者，如果出现难以用标准药物治疗控制的急性失代偿，或尽管给予最大程度的无创通气支持，但运动耐力仍持续恶化至无法行走，则可考虑使用 ECLS 作为 BTT[47]。对于尽管给予持续气道正压通气，但动脉血二氧化碳分压（$PCO_2$）仍持续升高（> 70 mmHg）[50]，以及已插管、镇静且无法脱离 MV 但有康复可能的患者，可以考虑使用 ECLS。此外，出现心源性休克、右心衰竭或肺动脉收缩压过高，也提示需要给予右心室支持。

一旦患者被认为适合接受 ECLS BTT，ECLS 的配置应针对患者的潜在病理生理状态，恢复生命需求，在确保床旁管理的简便性和安全性的同时，实现最佳的活动能力。首先，应将呼吸功能不全分为以高碳酸血症为主的衰竭以及伴有或不伴有高碳酸血症的低氧血症性衰竭。其次，识别出右心室受压迫征兆以及即将发生的右心室衰竭非常重要。大多数出现急性呼吸恶化的患者也可能存在血流动力学不稳定的情况。然而，只要使用 VV-ECMO 纠正低氧血症和（或）酸中毒，血流动力学状态通常会显著改善。重要的是，某些患者可能需要根据临床进展情况，在桥接过程中改变 ECLS 的配置。图 2-2 提出了一个 ECLS BTT 的方案。

### 2.4.4 抗凝

接受 ECLS 支持的患者因血液与管路的接触而出现凝血功能受损。可能发生血栓和出血等严重事件。然而，随着 ECMO 技术的改进，生物相容性管路不太可能激活凝血和先天免疫反应，从而能够延长 ECMO 运行时间，减少血制品消耗，并减轻表面引发的炎症[67]。

使用肝素涂层管路，高流量 VV-ECMO 可以在不需要强制性抗凝的情况下安全维持，从而预防出血并发症，尽管理论上这可能会加快因纤维蛋白形成和凝血而继发的膜老化。在最近一项研究中，Kurihara 等比较了其机构 38 例接受抗凝（肝素或比伐卢定）患者与 36 例仅接受抗血栓预防治疗患者的经验。前一组胃肠道出血发生率更高，输血需求量更大，而两组均未发生管路血栓[68]。对于接受 VA-ECMO 支持的患者，由于动脉血栓栓塞风险高，相关发病率高，抗凝治疗仍然是标准做法。然而，最近一项包含 75 例患者的报告指出，不使用抗凝的 VA-ECMO 的可行性和益处[69]。

# 第2章  急性失代偿肺移植候选者的住院管理

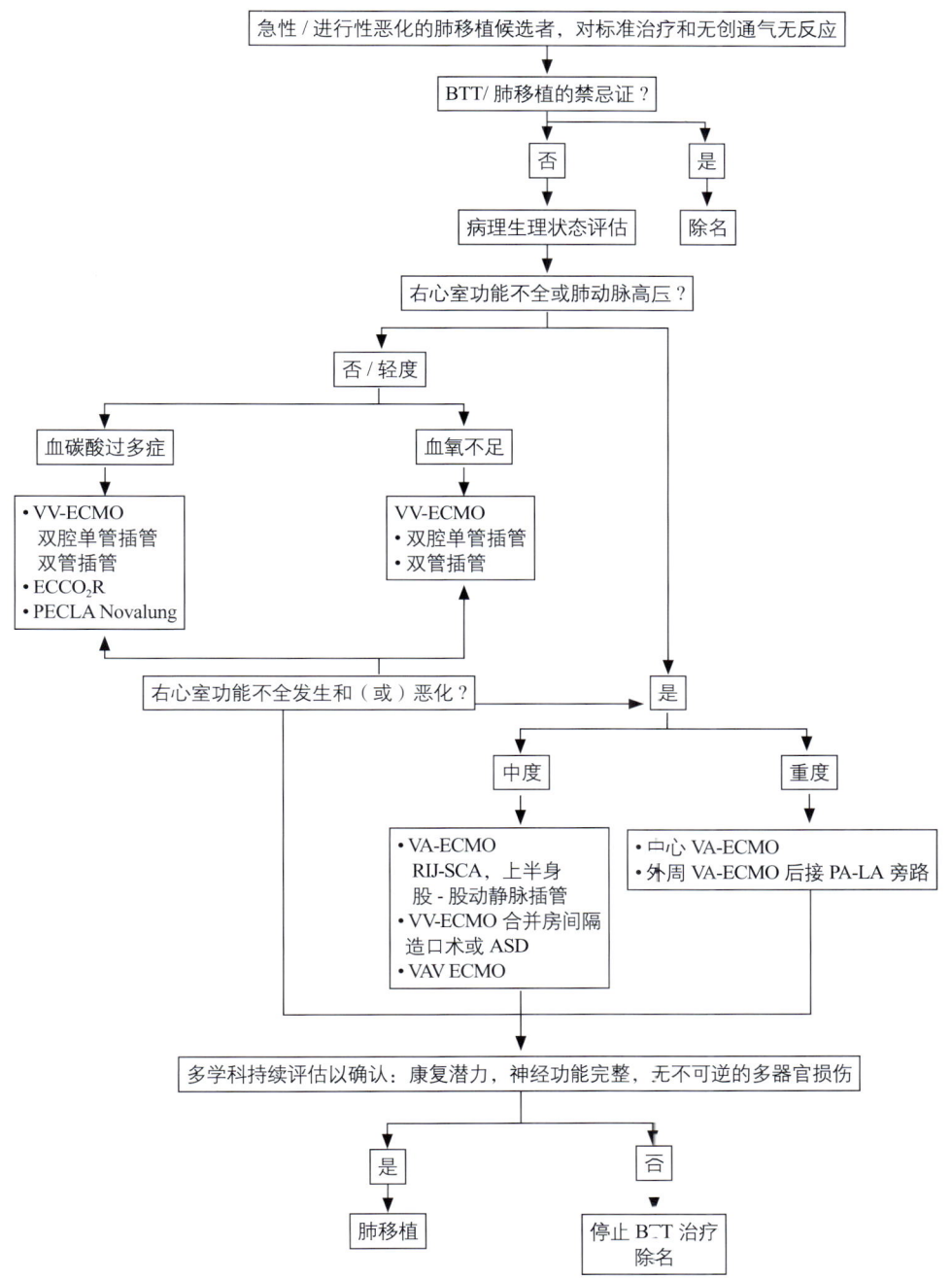

**图 2-2  失代偿肺移植候选者中移植桥接治疗的 ECLS 总结算法**

注：该图重点说明了在 BTT 潜在候选者中 ECLS 方式和插管的选择。该图提供了高度复杂的临床评估和决策过程的快捷方式，治疗方案的选择取决于资源可用性、当地专业知识以及相关多学科团队的培训。ASD，房间隔缺损；$ECCO_2R$，体外二氧化碳清除；ECLS BTT，作为移植桥接的体外生命支持；ECMO，体外膜肺氧合；PA-LA 旁路，肺动脉-左心房旁路；PECLA，无泵体外肺辅助装置；PH，肺动脉高压；RIJ-SCA，右颈内静脉-锁骨下动脉配置；RV，右心室；VA-ECMO，静脉-动脉 ECMO；VAV-ECMO，静脉-动脉-静脉 ECMO；VV-ECMO，静脉-静脉 ECMO

## 2.5 急性失代偿期间的康复

对于出现急性失代偿的移植候选者，积极康复至关重要，因为虚弱或机能退化是导致除名或转为舒适治疗的主要因素之一。尽管这些患者显然是早期康复以维持移植候选资格的目标人群，但历史上，一般认为 ECLS 支持的患者病情太不稳定，无法进行积极的物理治疗，通常采取镇静和肌肉松弛治疗。然而，随着体外循环技术的进步和多学科团队专业知识的不断提高，清醒 ECLS 联合早期活动的能力正在迅速发展[70]。

建议在整个等待期间进行移植前运动训练，以防止活动缺乏和身体机能退化。康复指南可根据疾病严重程度进行修改。如果疾病进展或功能恶化，应不断对物理治疗目标进行重新评估，并进行氧气滴定。训练强度应与运动时氧饱和度、心率、呼吸困难和疲劳症状相关联。肺移植康复指南建议在运动过程中维持至少 88% 的氧饱和度（$SO_2$）。由于 BTT 患者有 CIM 的风险，因此康复应侧重于保持近端肌肉和下肢力量。

保持患者自主呼吸的基本原理包括减少 V/Q 失调，保护呼吸肌和膈肌张力。此外，自主呼吸对静脉回流和心脏充盈有一定的改善[71]。了解自主呼吸患者中心肺 ECMO 的相互作用对于清醒 ECMO 的应用至关重要（表 2-1）。

关于清醒体外膜肺氧合期间的康复，为避免肺移植候选者插管和深度镇静，首选经外周 ECMO 插管。在意识镇静和经皮技术下进行插管是可行的，并逐渐成为标准。在最初 24~48 小时内，如果患者已插管，其目标是达到呼吸和血流动力学稳定，并减少所有神经肌肉阻滞药物。一旦患者状态稳定，应逐渐减少镇静，以确保平稳醒来和脱离机械通气地实现。可能需要进行芬太尼或右美托咪定输液来控制疼痛和谵妄，以促进这一过程。

使用 NPPV 或 HFNC 可促进拔管成功。对于那些身体状况太差而无法脱离机械通气或出现明显不同步的患者，早期行气管切开十分有益[72-74]。气管切开的优点包括减少气道阻力、减少镇静需求、促进气道清除等。此外，与经口插管相比，患者可以经口进食并更安全地活动。

镇静方案应根据患者需求制定，并进行早期活动。许多中心已采用基于团队的方法对 ECLS BTT 患者进行康复。其中包括与物理和作业治疗师、床旁护士、执业护士、呼吸治疗师、ECMO 专家、重症监护团队以及由外科医生、肺科医生和高级执业医师组成的肺移植团队之间的协作和联合查房。

## 第2章 急性失代偿肺移植候选者的住院管理

表 2-1 清醒 ECLS 支持患者的优势、挑战和管理

| 清醒、自主呼吸患者的优势 | 清醒 ECMO 的潜在挑战 | 应对挑战的策略 |
| --- | --- | --- |
| 呼吸肌和膈肌张力改善 | 由于呼吸功增加，导致需氧量增加和 $PaCO_2$ 升高；自发通气增加的肺泡内压力可能引发自发性肺损伤 | 调整镇静以防止疲劳并避免呼吸窘迫症状；从 ETT 改为气管切开；调整吹气流量 |
| 吸气负压增加，导致静脉回流和心排血量增加，有利于淋巴引流 | 间歇性 IVC 在引流管周围塌陷，引发管路震颤 | 低血容量如果导致管路震颤，需要矫正；调整镇静和 ECMO 流量 |
| 舒适度提高 | 分泌物清除能力下降 | 对于留置管的患者，首选气管切开而非拔管，以便进行分泌物清洁 |
| 让患者积极参与锻炼和物理治疗 | 插管脱落；设备故障 | 随时准备应急设备用于插管和严重事件的复苏；当患者进行物理治疗/活动时，应有足够的多学科人员协助 |
| ICU 精神病/谵妄减少 | 如出现其他并发症，可能难以停止清醒患者的生命支持 | 在整个护理过程中持续让家属参与 |

注：ECMO，体外膜肺氧合；ETT，气管插管；ICU，重症监护病房；IVC，下控静脉

# 2.6 除名触发因素

对于尽管给予最佳支持但病情持续恶化的桥接患者，不同机构在多学科决策方面有不同的方案。严格的患者选择和定期重新评估移植候选资格与成功实现 BTT 和移植后生存的可能性直接相关。对身体状况和多器官功能提出更严格的要求，可能导致桥接治疗中断更多及移植后生存率更高[48]。对于那些无法行走且肾功能障碍可逆的患者，维持其移植资格的机构 BTT 比例较高，但可能存在更高的围术期死亡率[47,50]。

随着我们不断努力为危重肺移植患者扩大移植机会，我们始终需要认识到"过度桥接"的问题。例如，急性失代偿的肺移植候选者中衰弱现象普遍存在，并与肺移植后早期死亡风险增加相关[75]。衰弱可定义为一种表型状态，包括缓慢、虚弱、体力活动低下、萎缩和乏力，可通过 Fried 衰弱表型（fried frailty phenotype，FFP）[76] 和简易体能状况量表（short physical performance battery，SPPB）[77] 等工具进行评估，如表 2-2 所示[76-79]。衰弱评分目前适用于危重症情况，据此将患者分为健康、易感、衰弱和临终[80]。与非衰弱患者相比，衰弱患者在 1 年内除名或死亡的风险增加（使用 SPPB 为 36% vs. 16%，使

用 FFP 为 27% vs. 13%)[81]。目前的挑战是确定如何将这些发现纳入日常临床实践，以评估肺移植候选者并优化器官分配。

表 2-2 目前用于临床评估患者衰弱程度的工具

| 评估工具 | 特征 |
| --- | --- |
| Fried 衰弱表型（Fried 等，2001）[76] | 体重减轻（超过 4.54 kg）；无力（握力）；乏力（自述）；步行速度（4.57 m）；体力活动（千卡/周） |
| 衰弱累积指数（Mitnitski 等，2015）[78] | 基于 70 个项目的临床病症和疾病清单；个体存在的衰弱项目与考虑的总衰弱项目数之比 |
| Frail Scale 衰弱评估量表（Van Kan 等，2008）[79] | 疲劳（你感到疲劳吗？）；耐力（你能爬一层楼梯吗？）；步行（你能走一个街区吗？）；疾病（超过 5 种）；体重减轻（超过 5%） |
| 简易体能状况量表（SPPB）（Singer JP 等，2018）[77] | 三项评估：步速、椅子站立、平衡 |

注：每种方法都使用特征来评分和分类衰弱程度

在出现其他器官衰竭的情况下，患者也可能被除名。然而，有报道在远定的"年轻"候选者感染 COVID-19 后进行了肺肾和心肺联合移植[82,83]。除此之外，肺肝和心肺移植大多局限于慢性病。泛耐药菌也是失代偿患者除名的潜在原因。

无论出现上述何种情况，在这些困难情景中，姑息治疗/团队都有可能改善生活质量，缓解症状负担，优化医疗资源利用[84]。此外，由于急性恶化患者（无论是否使用 ECLS）的临床状况每天都在变化，姑息团队的早期介入对支持患者和家属至关重要。

## 2.7 总 结

尽管终末期肺病患者病情高度复杂，且需要入院和高级别支持的急性恶化患者数量不断增加，但在有经验的中心，经过严格筛选的患者在接受肺移植后仍可获得满意的结果。多学科团队协作在持续移植资格评估、关注潜在疾病特点的最佳药物管理以及积极康复方面发挥着至关重要的作用。严格的筛选标准对于识别合适的 BTT 候选者至关重要。针对患者/疾病特点的 ECLS 策略可以为患者提供支持，并允许候选者在等待肺移植期间进行康复。

## 第2章 急性失代偿肺移植候选者的住院管理

【临床护理要点】

- 对急性失代偿性肺移植候选者的管理应关注潜在疾病的特点,同时在候选者处于等待名单期间根据需要提供必要的生命支持。
- 将危重患者纳入积极康复计划至关重要,并与移植后生存相关。
- 接受 ECLS 桥接治疗的患者在进行肺移植后,其生存率与未桥接患者相当。
- 长期 ECMO 支持是可行的,可以为危重患者提供支持,同时维持其移植资格并进行康复。

# 参考文献

1. Eberlein M, Garrity ER, Orens JB. Lung allocation in the united states. Clin Chest Med 2011; 32(2): 213–222.
2. Valapour M, Lehr CJ, Skeans MA, et al. OPTN/SRTR2019 annual data report: lung. Am J Transplant 2021;21(S2):441–520.
3. Organ procurement and transplantation network and scientific registry of transplant recipients 2010 data report. Am J Transplant 2012;12(SUPPL. 1): 1–156.
4. Shigemura N, Toyoda Y. Elderly patients with multiple comorbidities: insights from the bedside to the bench and programmatic directions for this new challenge in lung transplantation. Transpl Int 2020;33(4):347–355.
5. Russo MJ, Worku B, Iribarne A, et al. Does lung allocation score maximize survival benefit from lung transplantation? J Thorac Cardiovasc Surg 2011;141(5):1270–1277.
6. Russo MJ, Iribarne A, Hong KN, et al. High lung allocation score is associated with increased morbidity and mortality following transplantation. Chest 2010;137(3):651–657.
7. Crawford TC, Grimm JC, Magruder JT, et al. Lung transplant mortality is improving in recipients with a lung allocation score in the upper quartile. Ann Thorac Surg 2017;103(5):1607–1613.
8. Orsini B, Sage E, Olland A, et al. High-emergency waiting list for lung transplantation: early results of a nation-based study. Eur J Cardiothorac Surg. 2014;46(3):e41–47. discussion e47.
9. Roux A, Beaumont-Azuar L, Hamid AM, et al. High emergency lung transplantation: dramatic decrease of waiting list death rate without relevant higher posttransplant mortality. Transpl Int 2015;28(9): 1092–1101.
10. Auråen H, Schultz HHL, Hämmäinen P, et al. Urgent lung allocation system in the Scandiatransplant countries. J Hear Lung Transplant 2018;37(12):1403–1409.
11. Dotan Y, Vaidy A, Shapiro WB, et al. Effect of acute exacerbation of idiopathic pulmonary fibrosis on lung transplantation outcome. Chest 2018;154(4):818–826.
12. Chizinga M, Machuca TN, Shahmohammadi A, et al. Lung transplantation for acute exacerbation of interstitial lung disease. Thorax 2021.

13. Tang A, Thuita L, Siddiqui HU, et al. Urgently listed lung transplant patients have outcomes similar to those of electively listed patients. J Thorac Cardiovasc Surg 2021;161(1):306–317. e8.
14. Ranganath NK, Malas J, Chen S, et al. High lung transplant center volume is associated with increased survival in hospitalized patients. Ann Thorac Surg 2021;111(5):1652–1658.
15. Arnaoutakis GJ, Allen JG, Merlo CA, et al. Impact of the lung allocation score on resource utilization after lung transplantation in the United States. J Hear Lung Transplant 2011;30(1):14–21.
16. Keller CA, Gonwa TA, White LJ, et al. Utilization and cost analysis of lung transplantation and survival after 10 years of adapting the lung allocation score. Transplantation 2019;103(3):638–646.
17. Collard HR, Ryerson CJ, Corte TJ, et al. Acute exacerbation of idiopathic pulmonary fibrosis an international working group report. Am J Respir Crit Care Med 2016;194(3):265–275.
18. Leuschner G, Behr J. Acute exacerbation in interstitial lung disease. Front Med 2017;4(OCT).
19. Raghu G, Collard HR, Egan JJ, et al. An Official ATS/ERS/JRS/ALAT Statement: Idiopathic pulmonary fibrosis: Evidence-based guidelines for diagnosis and management. Am J Respir Crit Care Med 2011;183(6):788–824.
20. Faverio P, De Giacomi F, Sardella L, et al. Management of acute respiratory failure in interstitial lung diseases: Overview and clinical insights. BMC Pulm Med 2018;18(1):70.
21. Drake MG. High-flow nasal cannula oxygen in adults: An evidence-based assessment. Ann Am Thorac Soc 2018;15(2):145–155.
22. Frat J-P, Thille AW, Mercat A, et al. High-flow oxygen through nasal cannula in acute hypoxemic respiratory failure. N Engl J Med 2015;372(23):2185–2196.
23. Jones PG, Kamona S, Doran O, Sawtell F, Wilsher M. Randomized controlled trial of humidified high-flow nasal oxygen for acute respiratory distress in the emergency department: the HOT-ER study. Respir Care 2016;61(3):291–299.
24. Ventetuolo CE, Klinger JR. Management of acute right ventricular failure in the intensive care unit. Ann Am Thorac Soc 2014;11(5):811–822.
25. Leard LE, Holm AM, Valapour M, et al. Consensus document for the selection of lung transplant candidates: an update from the international society for heart and lung transplantation. J Hear Lung Transplant 2021;40(11):1349–1379.
26. Plotnikow GA, Accoce M, Fredes S, et al. High-flow oxygen therapy application in chronic obstructive pulmonary disease patients with acute hypercapnic respiratory failure: a multicenter study. Crit Care Explor 2021;3(2):e0337.
27. Pisani L, Betti S, Biglia C, et al. Effects of high-flow nasal cannula in patients with persistent hypercapnia after an acute COPD exacerbation: a prospective pilot study. BMC Pulm Med 2020; 20(1):12.
28. Pisani L, Astuto M, Prediletto I, Longhini F. High flow through nasal cannula in exacerbated COPD patients: a systematic review. Pulmonology 2019; 25(6):348–354.
29. Oczkowski S, Ergan B, Bos L, et al. ERS clinical practice guidelines: high-flow nasal cannula in acute respiratory failure. Eur Respir J 2021;2101574.
30. Hoeper MM, Granton J. Intensive care unit management of patients with severe pulmonary hypertension and right heart failure. Am J Respir Crit Care Med 2011;184(10):1114–1124.

31. Savale L, Vuillard C, Pichon J, et al. Five-year survival after an acute episode of decompensated pulmonary arterial hypertension in the modern management era of right heart failure. Eur Respir J 2021;58(3).
32. Davis PB. Therapy for cystic fibrosis — the end of the beginning? N Engl J Med 2011; 365(18):1734–1735.
33. Shteinberg M, Taylor-Cousar JL. Impact of cftr modulator use on outcomes in people with severe cystic fibrosis lung disease. Eur Respir Rev 2020;29(155).
34. McGarry ME, McColley SA. Cystic fibrosis patients of minority race and ethnicity less likely eligible for CFTR modulators based on CFTR genotype. Pediatr Pulmonol 2021;56(6):1496–1503.
35. Wagener JS, Williams MJ, Millar SJ, Morgan WJ, Pasta DJ, Konstan MW. Pulmonary exacerbations and acute declines in lung function in patients with cystic fibrosis. J Cyst Fibros 2018;17(4): 496–502.
36. Hassan A, Milross M, Lai W, Shetty D, Alison J, Huang S. Feasibility and safety of intrapulmonary percussive ventilation in spontaneously breathing, non-ventilated patients in critical care: a retrospective pilot study. J Intensive Care Soc 2021;22(2):111–119.
37. Bharat A, Machuca TN, Querrey M, et al. Early outcomes after lung transplantation for severe COVID-19: a series of the first consecutive cases from four countries. Lancet Respir Med 2021;9(5):487–497.
38. Elizur A, Sweet SC, Huddleston CB, et al. Pre-transplant mechanical ventilation increases short-term morbidity and mortality in pediatric patients with cystic fibrosis. J Hear Lung Transplant 2007;26(2):127–131.
39. Mason DP, Thuita L, Nowicki ER, Murthy SC, Pettersson GB, Blackstone EH. Should lung transplantation be performed for patients on mechanical respiratory support? The US experience. J Thorac Cardiovasc Surg 2010;139(3):765–773.
40. Hayanga JWA, Hayanga HK, Holmes SD, et al. Mechanical ventilation and extracorporeal membrane oxygenation as a bridge to lung transplantation: closing the gap. J Hear Lung Transplant 2019; 38(10):1104–1111.
41. Dellgren G, Riise GC, Swärd K, et al. Extracorporeal membrane oxygenation as a bridge to lung transplantation: a long-term study. Eur J Cardiothorac Surg 2015;47(1):95–100.
42. Crotti S, Iotti GA, Lissoni A, et al. Organ allocation waiting time during extracorporeal bridge to lung transplant affects outcomes. Chest 2013;144(3):1018–1025.
43. Brahmbhatt N, Murugan R, Milbrandt EB. Early mobilization improves functional outcomes in critically ill patients. Crit Care 2010;14(5):321.
44. Polastri M, Loforte A, Dell'Amore A, Nava S. Physiotherapy for patients on awake extracorporeal membrane oxygenation: a systematic review. Physiother Res Int 2016;21(4):203–209.
45. Rehder KJ, Turner DA, Hartwig MG, et al. Active rehabilitation during extracorporeal membrane oxygenation as a bridge to lung transplantation. Respir Care 2013;58(8):1291–1298.
46. Hoopes CW, Kukreja J, Golden J, Davenport DL, Diaz-Guzman E, Zwischenberger JB. Extracorporeal membrane oxygenation as a bridge to pulmonary transplantation. J Thorac Cardiovasc Surg 2013; 145(3):862–868.
47. Hoetzenecker K, Donahoe L, Yeung JC, et al. Extracorporeal life support as a bridge to lung transplantation–experience of a high-volume transplant center. J Thorac Cardiovasc Surg 2018; 155(3):1316–1328. e1.
48. Tipograf Y, Salna M, Minko E, et al. Outcomes of extracorporeal membrane oxygenation as a bridge to lung transplantation. Ann Thorac Surg 2019; 107(5):1456–1463.
49. Biscotti M, Gannon WD, Agerstrand C, et al. Awake extracorporeal membrane oxygenation as bridge to lung

transplantation: a 9-year experience. Ann Thorac Surg 2017;104(2):412–419.

50. Benazzo A, Schwarz S, Frommlet F, et al. Twentyyear experience with extracorporeal life support as bridge to lung transplantation. J Thorac Cardiovasc Surg 2019;157(6):2515–2525. e10.

51. Todd EM, Biswas Roy S, Hashimi AS, et al. Extracorporeal membrane oxygenation as a bridge to lung transplantation: A single-center experience in the present era. J Thorac Cardiovasc Surg 2017; 154(5):1798–1809.

52. Yeo HJ, Lee S, Yoon SH, et al. Extracorporeal life support as a bridge to lung transplantation in patients with acute respiratory failure. Transplant Proc 2017;49(6):1430–1435.

53. Toyoda Y, Bhama JK, Shigemura N, et al. Efficacy of extracorporeal membrane oxygenation as a bridge to lung transplantation. J Thorac Cardiovasc Surg 2013;145(4):1065–1071.

54. Langer F, Aliyev P, Schäfers HJ, et al. Improving outcomes in bridge-to-transplant: Extended extracorporeal membrane oxygenation support to obtain optimal donor lungs for marginal recipients. ASAIO J 2019;65(5):516–521.

55. Lafarge M, Mordant P, Thabut G, et al. Experience of extracorporeal membrane oxygenation as a bridge to lung transplantation in France. J Hear Lung Transplant 2013;32(9):905–913.

56. Yeung JC, Machuca TN, Chaparro C, et al. Lung transplantation for cystic fibrosis. J Hear Lung Transplant 2020;39(6):553–560.

57. Cypel M, Waddell T, Singer LG, et al. Bilateral pneumonectomy to treat uncontrolled sepsis in a patient awaiting lung transplantation. J Thorac Cardiovasc Surg 2017;153(4):e67–69.

58. Kukreja J, Tsou S, Chen J, et al. Risk factors and outcomes of extracorporeal membrane oxygenation as a bridge to lung transplantation. Semin Thorac Cardiovasc Surg 2020;32(4):772–785.

59. Fuehner T, Kuehn C, Hadem J, et al. Extracorporeal membrane oxygenation in awake patients as bridge to lung transplantation. Am J Respir Crit Care Med 2012;185(7):763–768.

60. Lang G, Kim D, Aigner C, et al. Awake extracorporeal membrane oxygenation bridging for pulmonary retransplantation provides comparable results to elective retransplantation. J Hear Lung Transplant 2014;33(12):1264–1272.

61. Schechter MA, Ganapathi AM, Englum BR, et al. Spontaneously breathing extracorporeal membrane oxygenation support provides the optimal bridge to lung transplantation. Transplantation 2016; 00(00):1.

62. Abrams D, Madahar P, Eckhardt CM, et al. Early mobilization during extracorporeal membrane oxygenation for cardiopulmonary failure in adults: factors associated with intensity of treatment. Ann Am Thorac Soc 2022;19(1):90–98.

63. Schmidt F, Jack T, Sasse M, et al. Back to the roots? dual cannulation strategy for ambulatory ECMO in adolescent lung transplant candidates: an alternative? Pediatr Transplant 2017;21(4):e12907.

64. Wells CL, Forrester J, Vogel J, et al. Safety and feasibility of early physical therapy for patients on extracorporeal membrane oxygenator: university of maryland medical center experience. Crit Care Med 2018;46(1):53–59.

65. Shudo Y, Kasinpila P, Lee AM, et al. Ambulating femoral venoarterial extracorporeal membrane oxygenation bridge to heart-lung transplant. J Thorac Cardiovasc Surg 2018;156(3):e135–137.

66. Pasrija C, Mackowick KM, Raithel M, et al. Ambulation with femoral arterial cannulation can be safely performed on venoarterial extracorporeal membrane oxygenation. Ann Thorac Surg 2019;107(5):1389–1394.

67. Thomas J, Kostousov V, Teruya J. Bleeding and thrombotic complications in the use of extracorporeal membrane oxygenation. Semin Thromb Hemost 2018;44(01):020–029.
68. Kurihara C, Walter JM, Karim A, et al. Feasibility of venovenous extracorporeal membrane oxygenation without systemic anticoagulation. Ann Thorac Surg 2020;110(4):1209–1215.
69. Wood KL, Ayers B, Gosev I, et al. venoarterial-extracorporeal membrane oxygenation without routine systemic anticoagulation decreases adverse events. Ann Thorac Surg 2020;109(5):1458–1466.
70. Abrams D, Javidfar J, Farrand E, et al. Early mobilization of patients receiving extracorporeal membrane oxygenation: a retrospective cohort study. Crit Care 2014;18(1):R38.
71. Langer T, Vecchi V, Belenkiy SM, et al. Extracorporeal gas exchange and spontaneous breathing for the treatment of acute respiratory distress syndrome: an alternative to mechanical ventilation? Crit Care Med 2014;42(3).
72. DiChiacchio L, Boulos FM, Brigante F, et al. Early tracheostomy after initiation of venovenous extracorporeal membrane oxygenation is associated with decreased duration of extracorporeal membrane oxygenation support. Perfusion 2020;35(6):509–514.
73. Swol J, Strauch JT, Schildhauer TA. Tracheostomy as a bridge to spontaneous breathing and awakeECMO in non-transplant surgical patients. Eur J Heart Fail 2017;19:120–123.
74. Salna M, Tipograf Y, Liou P, et al. Tracheostomy is safe during extracorporeal membrane oxygenation support. ASAIO J 2020;66(6):652–656.
75. Schaenman JM, Diamond JM, Greenland JR, et al. Frailty and aging-associated syndromes in lung transplant candidates and recipients. Am J Transplant 2021;21(6):2018–2024.
76. Fried LP, Tangen CM, Walston J, et al. Frailty in older adults: evidence for a phenotype. J Gerontol A Biol Sci Med Sci 2001;56(3):M146–157.
77. Singer JP, Diamond JM, Anderson MR, et al. Frailty phenotypes and mortality after lung transplantation: a prospective cohort study. Am J Transplant 2018; 18(8):1995–2004.
78. Mitnitski A, Rockwood K. Aging as a process of deficit accumulation: Its utility and origin. Interdiscip Top Gerontol 2014;40:85–98.
79. van Kan GA, Rolland YM, Morley JE, Vellas B. Frailty: toward a clinical definition. J Am Med Dir Assoc 2008;9(2):71–72.
80. De Biasio JC, Mittel AM, Mueller AL, Ferrante LE, Kim DH, Shaefi S. Frailty in critical care medicine: a review. Anesth Analg 2020;130(6):1462–1473.
81. Singer JP, Diamond JM, Gries CJ, et al. Frailty phenotypes, disability, and outcomes in adult candidates for lung transplantation. Am J Respir Crit Care Med 2015;192(11):1325–1334.
82. Guenthart BA, Krishnan A, Alassar A, et al. First lung and kidney multi-organ transplant following COVID-19 infection. J Heart Lung Transplant 2021;40(8): 856–859.
83. COVID patient's heart-lung transplant is world's first. Available at. https://news.vumc.org/2020/10/08/covid-patients-heart-lung-transplant-is-worlds-first/.
84. Wentlandt K, Weiss A, O'Connor E, Kaya E. Palliative and end of life care in solid organ transplantation. Am J Transplant 2017;17(12):3008–3019.

# 第3章　急性呼吸窘迫综合征的肺移植

Ankit Bharat, Konrad Hoetzenecker　著

李聪　周伟　译

周建平　校

【关键词】
- 急性呼吸窘迫综合征　• 肺移植　• 急性肺损伤　• 肺功能衰竭

【要点】
- 尽管药物治疗经过优化，但严重急性呼吸窘迫综合征（ARDS）患者的病死率仍然很高。
- 肺移植是经过严格筛选的 ARDS 患者的挽救性治疗。
- 尽管移植前病程复杂，但 ARDS 患者移植后生存率极佳。

## 3.1 引　言

据世界卫生组织（WHO）报告，呼吸系统疾病是全球五大死亡原因之一。例如，仅在美国，每年流感就导致 4000 万~6000 万新发感染，其中死亡人数高达 4 万~6 万，绝大多数病例死于肺损伤和急性呼吸窘迫综合征（acute respiratory distress syndrome，ARDS）。感染性和非感染性病因都可引起 ARDS。对 ARDS 发病率的全球人群估计仅为近似值，可能为 3.65/10 万 ~86.0/10 万[1,2]。美国的发病率最高，范围为 64.2/10 万~86.0/10 万，即每年约 20 万例[3]。据估计，重症监护病房（ICU）收治患者中占 10%~15%，机械通气（MV）患者高达 23% 符合 ARDS 的定义[4-7]。在一项近 3 万名 ICU 患者的国际研究中，10% 的 ICU 入院是由于 ARDS[8]。根据柏林定义，ARDS 根据动脉血氧分压（arterial partial pressure of oxygen，$PaO_2$）与吸入氧浓度（fraction of inspired oxygen，$FiO_2$）的比值分为轻度（300 mmHg）、中度（200 mmHg）和重度（100 mmHg）[9]。仅约 25% 的 ARDS 患者最初被归类为轻度，而 75% 为中度至重度。1/3 的轻度病例会进展为中度或重度。轻度、中度和重度 ARDS 的病死率分别为 27%、32% 和 45%，总病死率约为 43%[10,11]。

因此，ARDS带来的疾病负担巨大。

## 3.1.1 导致终末期肺病的急性呼吸窘迫综合征的病理生理学机制

ARDS是一种常见的终末期肺损伤，可由各种病因引起，病程高度可变。它始于肺泡毛细血管损伤，引发常伴有肺部愈合和肺功能改善的增殖状态，并最终导致纤维化期，标志着急性损伤的终止。主要的组织学改变包括肺泡水肿、内皮和上皮损伤以及含蛋白质的液体和血液渗入肺泡腔。ARDS患者易患院内并发症、多器官功能障碍和压力/容量创伤，加上其基础健康状况和并发症，可影响预后，结果从自发恢复到严重肺实质坏死、支气管扩张或纤维增生不等。随着ICU护理的进步，重度ARDS患者的病死率已经有所下降，但仍然很高[12]。重度ARDS病程早期的死亡与肺炎、脓毒症和多器官功能障碍等并发症有关。然而，在那些存活下来的患者中，纤维增生的发展可能导致院内并发症、无法脱离机械通气，最终导致大部分患者的治疗目标转为舒适护理[13]。

研究表明，大量纤维增生导致肺功能不全在ARDS患者中很常见[14-16]。ARDS发作后72小时内即可见广泛胶原沉积的证据[17,18]，且胶原产物如前胶原肽Ⅲ与致命转归相关[19]。研究表明，ARDS患者体内释放促纤维化化学物质如TGF-β1和胰岛素样生长因子-Ⅰ可能促进纤维增生反应[20]。即使采用小潮气量通气，临床上明显的纤维增生也很常见[21]。肺纤维化的特征是肺实质内胶原沉积异常和紊乱，尤其影响肺泡腔，类似于某些慢性终末期肺病。

我们最近对正常人肺与重度COVID-19 ARDS患者或因终末期特发性肺纤维化需要移植的患者肺的三维基质组织进行了比较。正常人肺显示出良好的复杂基质，而COVID-19 ARDS患者的肺则完全缺乏基质组织，在纤维化气道周围有斑片状的细胞岛。这种模式与终末期特发性肺纤维化患者的肺相似[22,23]。利用单细胞RNA测序（RNA-Seq）创建的转录图谱[24-27]已经鉴定出纤维化肺中独特的细胞群，可能与纤维化的发生有因果关系[28-31]。使用迁移学习方法[32]比较终末期肺纤维化[25]和COVID-19 ARDS患者肺组织的单细胞RNA-Seq数据，我们发现两者在许多细胞群中有显著的同源性。我们还发现，一群表达*TP63*、*KRT5*、*KRT17*、*LAMB3*、*LAMC2*、*VIM*、*CHD2*、*FN1*、*COL1A1*、*TNC*、*HMGA2*和几个衰老标志物（*CDKN1A*、*CDKN2A*、*CCND1*、*CCND2*、*MDM2*、*SERPINE1*）的细胞会在纤维化过程中积累，可能通过表达*TGFB1*、*ITGAV*和*ITGB6*促进疾病发生[26,27]。在正常肺中，*KRT17*的表达仅限于近端气道的基底细胞、club细胞和纤毛细胞，但在远端气道中不存在表达[24,26]。与正常肺相比，在COVID-19终末期和肺纤维化患者的远端气道中可以很容易观察到这些细胞。此外，直接比较肺纤维化和COVID-19患者KRT17+细胞的差异基因表达，未发现任一疾病特有的基因，进一步凸显了这两种疾病的相似性。此外，比较肺纤维化和COVID-19 ARDS患者巨噬细胞的差异基因表达，结果也显示出这两种疾病之间有相当大的相似性。我们的分析还发现，在COVID-19 ARDS患者中观察到一小群细胞，其特征是表达参与钙（*AK5*、*SIGLEC15*、*CKB*和*SLC9B2*）、铁（*SLC40A1*、*CD163*）和脂质（*MERTK*、*PLTP*、*ABCA1*）代谢以及运动和免疫信号（*MARCKS*、*TLR2*、*CCL20*）的基因，可能反映了ARDS患者的继发感染和持续炎症[22,23]。促纤维化巨噬细胞通过形成自我维持的回路刺激成纤维细胞，该回路由自分泌的生长因子促进[33,34]。我们的数据表明，肺纤维化患者和重度COVID-19患者的成纤维细胞在很大程度上相似。总的来说，这些数据表明，一些COVID-19 ARDS患者会发展为终末期肺病，与其他疾病（如肺纤维化）相似。

遗憾的是，目前尚无针对纤维增生的有效药物治疗。类固醇也未能显示出对ARDS相关纤维增生患者预后的改善[35]。其他药物如酪氨酸激酶抑制剂[36]、靶向细胞外基质蛋白的化合物[37]和针对TGF-β的靶向治疗[38]仍处于探索阶段，其在预防纤维增生中的作用尚不清楚。因此，对于筛选出的ARDS终末期肺纤维化患者，肺移植（LTx）可能是唯一可行的解决方案。

### 3.1.2 肺移植的临床考虑

关于ARDS患者使用肺移植的医学争论主要集中在"获益"和"候选资格"两个话题上。关注的问题包括移植物中诱发感染的复发可能性，原生肺的急性损伤带来的技术挑战，以及与呼吸机相关的肺炎病原体感染移植肺的潜在风险。更重要的是，原生肺可能会恢复，其长期预后可能优于移植。我们认为，以下两大标准可用于确定ARDS患者进行移植的需求。首先，在ARDS发作后经过充分时间和优化的药物治疗后，肺部损伤大到患者难以脱离机械通气和(或)体外膜肺氧合（ECMO）支持等机械生命支持。其次，出现了药物难以治疗的肺部或胸膜并发症。与这些标准相关的一些常见情况包括纤维增生性ARDS、肺坏死伴空洞或气囊，或严重支气管扩张。如何准确识别那些不会自发恢复、可以从肺移植中获益的患者尚不清楚。根据我们的经验，首选方法是在肺恢复被认为可能的情况下，继续为患者提供药物治疗，因为已有报道称患者在长期体外生命支持（ECLS）后可自发恢复[22,23]。当ARDS发作后经过足够时间且认为不太可能发生肺恢复时，应考虑进行肺移植。在病程中过早考虑肺移植可能会使护理路径偏离自发恢复，降低其可能性。虽然目前不可逆所需的时间尚不清楚，但我们建议至少应在 ARDS 发作后等待 4~6 周，再考虑进行肺移植。然而，当有严重的肺部并发症，如伴右心室衰竭的肺动脉高压、难治性院内感染肺炎或反复气胸出现，无法通过有或无 ECMO 的药物治疗时，可以例外。对于 COVID-19 相关的 ARDS，在规定时间后，我们发现以下指标有助于肺移植的医疗决策：①上述肺部后遗症的发展；②肺坏死伴空洞，尤其是与败血症相关时；③存在显著肺动脉高压；④肺顺应性小于 20 mL/cm $H_2O$；⑤弥漫性肺纤维化的证据。对于表现出肺恢复迹象的患者，如肺顺应性、胸片和气体交换的改善，应推迟移植。我们先前提出了一种针对重度 COVID-19 相关 ARDS 患者的移植考虑方法[22,39]。鉴于 COVID-19 与非 COVID-19 ARDS 的相似性，我们认为同样的原则可用于所有 ARDS 患者。

### 3.1.3 急性呼吸窘迫综合征的肺移植文献回顾和已报道预后

尽管慢性肺病术后预后已明确，但 ARDS 肺移植的获益仍在不断显现[40]。当认为不太可能发生肺恢复且考虑移植时，重度 ARDS 患者病情通常比较危重，并会发展出相当多的 ICU 相关并发症。重度 ARDS 的病程也经常有肺部并发症出现，如气胸、血胸、脓胸、肺坏死和院内感染性肺炎[41]。因此，人们担心这些患者肺移植的技术可行性，衰弱可能导致术后预后较差，以及移植后院内感染病原体的复发。除了少数病例报告外，迄今已有 3 个较大的 ARDS 肺移植病例系列发表（表 3-2）。第一个系列报告了韩国患者中的实践经验。2008—2013 年间，共评估 14 例患者，最终有 9 例接受移植[40]。由于左心室衰竭、右心功能不全或重度肺动脉高压，其中 3 例移植实际上是心肺联合移植。2021 年，Harano 及其同事进行了回顾性 UNOS 注册分析。这是迄今为止最大的病例队列，包括 2005—2018 年间列入肺移植的 65 例患者[42]。61%（$n=39$）进行了移植，其余患者因进一步恶化或原生肺最终恢复而被除名。最近，Frick 等报告了来自 3 个欧洲大体量肺移植中心（奥地利维也纳、比利时鲁汶、荷兰格罗宁根）的联合报告[43]。1998—2018 年间，13 例患者因 ARDS 接受移植。虽然所有发表的患者群体均包括重度 ARDS 患者，但 ARDS 的潜在病因在已发表队列之间存在很大差异。在韩国研究中，一半患者（$n=7$）是因吸入加湿器消毒剂而导致肺衰竭，其次最常见的原因是肺炎（$n=5$）。在欧洲队列中，病毒感染（$n=7$）和细菌感染（$n=5$）是 ARDS 的主要原因[43]。UNOS 数据库研究无法提供 ARDS 原因的详细数据。

表 3-1　ARDS 的肺移植的研究报道

| 作者 | Chang 等<br>（韩国单中心） | Harano 等<br>（UNOS 数据库） | Frick 等<br>（欧洲多中心） |
| --- | --- | --- | --- |
| 研究时段 | 2008 年 10 月至<br>2013 年 10 月 | 2005 年 5 月至<br>2018 年 12 月 | 1998 年 8 月至<br>2020 年 5 月 |
| 移植患者人数/所列人数（N） | 9/14 | 39/63 | 13/-[a] |
| ARDS 病因（N） | 吸入消毒剂（4 例）/肺炎（4 例）/溺水（1 例） | n/a | 病毒感染（7 例）/细菌感染（5 例）/术后感染（1 例） |
| 移植受体中位年龄 | 39 | 35 | 29 |
| MV 中位时间（天）[b] | 11 | n/a | 33 |
| 中位住院时间（天） | 56 | 33 | 54 |
| 住院死亡率 | 11.1% | 10.3% | 7.7% |
| 1 年生存率 | 78% | 82.1% | 71.6% |
| 3 年生存率 | 78% | 69.2% | n/a |
| 5 年生存率 | n/a | n/a | 54.2% |

注：n/a，无数据；[a] 未报道；[b] MV，机械通气

普遍认为，ARDS 的肺移植是复杂的，术中和术后管理具有挑战性。因此，很难达到与其他适应证（ILD、CF、COPD）类似的预后。事实上，上述 3 项队列研究的数据证实了这一假设。3 项系列均报告了肺移植后机械通气时间延长，机械通气时间（length of mechanical ventilation，LMV）中位数为 11~33 天[40,43]，住院时间延长，中位数为 33~56 天（见表 3-1）[40,42,43]。然而，这些预后与其他复杂患者组相当，尤其是那些需要 ECLS 桥接到肺移植的急性或慢性肺病患者[44-48]。与当代基准相比，ARDS 肺移植后的长期生存率也较低。韩国研究组报告的 1 年和 3 年生存率均为 78%。9 例患者中有 1 例（11.1%）在术后即刻死亡[40]。Harano 等的 UNOS 系列报告了 1 年和 3 年生存率分别为 82.1% 和 69.2%。作者还提供了倾向性评分匹配分析，将 ARDS 患者与 79 例限制性肺病对照组进行比较。2∶1 匹配包括肺源分配评分、性别、年龄和移植类型，确保对照组具有同等复杂性。倾向性匹配队列显示出与 ARDS 队列相似的长期预后，1 年生存率为 85.9%，3 年生存率为 65.4%。无论是 ARDS 或非 ARDS 诊断，对桥接与非桥接患者进行进一步比较结果也没有显示出显著差异[42]。在 Frick 及其同事报告的欧洲队列中，13 例患

者中有 1 例在术后早期死亡，院内死亡率为 7.7%，1 年生存率为 71.6%，5 年生存率为 54.2%。由于这些研究纳入的患者可追溯至 1993 年，因此应考虑时代效应对结局的影响，特别是欧洲组报告 2016 年后 ARDS 移植患者的结局有所改善[43]。尽管如此，ECMO 桥接到移植的患者 1 年生存率可达 76%~88%，3 年生存率为 61%~83%，5 年生存率为 55%~68%[44-50]。事实上，我们最近一项 COVID-19 ARDS 国际患者队列研究显示，即使对于接受 ECMO 支持的患者，肺移植可能是重度 COVID-19 相关 ARDS 患者的可行挽救性治疗选择。总的来说，目前的证据得出结论，经过精心筛选的 ARDS 患者可获得与其他病情同样严重的患者相当的肺移植结局。

### 3.1.4 肺移植术前检查

在 ARDS 的急性期，必须放弃一些常规用于确定肺移植候选资格的检查。例如，由于大多数考虑移植的 ARDS 患者较为年轻，有未发现的恶性肿瘤或显著心血管并发症的可能性较低。以下是我们认为很重要的检查：

- 胸腹部计算机断层扫描（computed tomography，CT）；
- 病毒学检查（Epstein-Barr 病毒、巨细胞病毒、甲型/乙型肝炎、人类免疫缺陷病毒）；
- 对于高敏患者，进行群体反应性抗体（panel reactive antibody，PRA）检测和不可接受的 HLA 抗原检测；
- 外周血管超声检查，评估静脉血栓；
- 对于非清醒桥接，进行脑部 CT 扫描以排除大出血/缺血（尽管我们承认这可能是某些中心的相对禁忌证）；
- 超声心动图；
- 对于 50 岁以上患者，进行 CT 冠状动脉造影或左心导管检查；
- 肝脏超声/纤维化扫描；
- 不做乳腺 X 线检查、冠状动脉造影、结肠镜检查、胃镜检查。

### 3.1.5 清醒或镇静状态下桥接急性呼吸窘迫综合征患者

在肺移植中，使桥接患者保持清醒已成为越来越常使用的做法。在某些中心，患者清醒甚至是移植的先决条件。我们认为主要有 2 个原因：①若干研究表明，与镇静桥接的患者相比，清醒桥接患者的预后显著更好[45,51,52]；②肺移植的决定十分重要，因此需要患者本人同意。

我们认为这 2 个论点仅适用于需要 ECLS 桥接的慢性肺病患者，可能不适用于 ARDS。唤醒 ARDS 患者通常是不可能的，因为与需要 ECLS 桥接的纤维化患者不同，ARDS 患者病情通常严重[43]。他们的肺顺应性极差，潮气量不到 100 mL。这些独特的挑战通常会导致严重应激和脱氧发作。

我们的观点是，考虑到疾病的严重程度和移植候选者缺乏替代治疗，在许多欧洲国家可以豁免本人同意。这需要医疗代理人或成年代表的同意。然而，如果这种代表（由法院指定）的实施耗时过长，则须遵循镇静患者的推定意愿，并在假设患者希望接受挽救其生命的治疗的情况下，由亲属同意移植是可以接受的。在考虑对 ARDS 患者进行肺移植时，"正确的时机"至关重要。一旦确认肺损伤不可逆，我们不建议为了获取本人同意试图唤醒镇静患者。在危重患者中，ECLS 时间越长，并发症发生率越高，阻碍移植的成功[53]。在讨论 ARDS 患者的最佳列名时机时，必须考虑这个"机会之窗"。

### 3.1.6 病情恶化时除名的考虑

由于已发表的证据仅限于少数病例报告和 3 个小型病例队列，因此对于将恶化患者除名的时机和情况尚无明确建议。理想情况下，ARDS 移植候选者应处于稳定状态，仅有单器官功能衰竭。然而，其他器官的功能障碍也经常出现。我们中心通常不认为在既往肾功能正常的患者中出现暂时性肾衰竭是肺移植的禁忌证。因此，在等待期间需要肾脏替代治疗的患者不应被除名。然而，胆汁淤积性肝功能障碍可能会造成重大挑战。继发性硬化性胆管炎（secondary sclerosing cholangitis，SCC）是需要长期 ECLS 治疗 ARDS 患者的可怕并发症[54,55]。由于 SCC 患者的治疗选择有限，死亡率极高，因此我们认为胆汁淤积参数升高是 ARDS 患者肺移植的禁忌证。ARDS 肺移植的另外 2 个主要禁忌证是 ECLS 期间出现不可控制的弥漫性出血或感染性休克。然而，如果感染性休克的原因明显是肺部，且患者病情无法稳定，可考虑双侧全肺切除联合中心 Novalung/VA-ECMO 桥接概念[56]。

## 3.2 总　结

尽管与其他适应证相比，ARDS 移植数量仍然较低，但肺移植已成为未恢复患者亚群的既定治疗方法。然而，必须给予足够的 ECLS 时间来确定原生肺的再生潜力。患者选择至关重要，移植应保留给那些没有恢复前景的患者。这通常将肺移植的选择限制在

# 第3章 急性呼吸窘迫综合征的肺移植

ARDS 发作前相对健康的患者。在经过严格筛选的 ARDS 患者队列中，肺移植后显示出良好的长期预后。

> 【临床护理要点】
> - 重度急性呼吸窘迫综合征（ARDS）患者的病死率仍然很高。
> - 相当一部分重度 ARDS 患者出现不可逆的肺损伤，无法脱离机械生命支持。
> - 对于某些因重度 ARDS 导致不可逆肺损伤的患者，肺移植可能是一种挽救生命的治疗方法。

### 声明

本文作者 Ankit Bharat 获得美国国立卫生研究院科研经费支持（基金号：NIH HL145478、HL147290 和 HL147575）。

## 参考文献

1. Pham T, Rubenfeld GD. Fifty Years of Research in ARDS. The Epidemiology of Acute Respiratory Distress Syndrome. A 50th Birthday Review. Am J Respir Crit Care Med 2017 195(7):860–870.
2. Rubenfeld GD, Caldwell E, Peabody E, et al. Incidence and outcomes of acute lung injury. N Engl J Med 2005;353(16):1685–1693.
3. Diamond M, Peniston Feliciano HL, Sanghavi D, et al. Acute Respiratory Distress Syndrome. StatPearls, Treasure Island: FL); 2021.
4. Frutos-Vivar F, Nin N, Esteban A. Epidemiology of acute lung injury and acute respiratory distress syndrome. Curr Opin Crit Care 2004;10(1):1–6.
5. Estenssoro E, Dubin A, Laffaire E, et al. Incidence, clinical course, and outcome in 217 patients with acute respiratory distress syndrome. Crit Care Med 2002;30(11):2450–2456.
6. Esteban A, Anzueto A, Frutos F, et al. Mechanical Ventilation International Study, G. , Characteristics and outcomes in adult patients receiving mechanical ventilation: a 28-day international study. JAMA 2002;287(3):345–355.
7. Zaccardelli DS, Pattishall EN. Clinical diagnostic criteria of the adult respiratory distress syndrome in the intensive care unit. Crit Care Med 1996; 24(2):247–251.
8. Bellani G, Laffey JG, Pham T, et al. Epidemiology, Patterns of Care, and Mortality for Patients With Acute Respiratory Distress Syndrome in Intensive Care Units in 50 Countries. JAMA 2016;315(8):788–800.
9. Force ADT, Ranieri VM, Rubenfeld GD, et al. Acute respiratory distress syndrome: the Berlin Definition.

JAMA 2012;307(23):2526–2533.

10. Sedhai YR, Yuan M, Ketcham SW, et al. Validating Measures of Disease Severity in Acute Respiratory Distress Syndrome. Ann Am Thorac Soc 2021; 18(7):1211–1218.
11. Zambon M, Vincent JL. Mortality rates for patients with acute lung injury/ARDS have decreased over time. Chest 2008;133(5):1120–1127.
12. Burnham EL, Janssen WJ, Riches DW, et al. The fibroproliferative response in acute respiratory distress syndrome: mechanisms and clinical significance. Eur Respir J 2014;43(1):276–285.
13. Ketcham SW, Sedhai YR, Miller HC, et al. Causes and characteristics of death in patients with acute hypoxemic respiratory failure and acute respiratory distress syndrome: a retrospective cohort study. Crit Care 2020;24(1):391.
14. Bulpa PA, Dive AM, Mertens L, et al. Combined bronchoalveolar lavage and transbronchial lung biopsy: safety and yield in ventilated patients. Eur Respir J 2003;21(3):489–494.
15. Patel SR, Karmpaliotis D, Ayas NT, et al. The role of open-lung biopsy in ARDS. Chest 2004;125(1):197–202.
16. Papazian L, Doddoli C, Chetaille B, et al. A contributive result of open-lung biopsy improves survival in acute respiratory distress syndrome patients. Crit Care Med 2007;35(3):755–762.
17. Farjanel J, Hartmann DJ, Guidet B, et al. Four markers of collagen metabolism as possible indicators of disease in the adult respiratory distress syndrome. Am Rev Respir Dis 1993;147(5):1091–1099.
18. Meduri GU, Tolley EA, Chinn A, et al. Procollagen types I and III aminoterminal propeptide levels during acute respiratory distress syndrome and in response to methylprednisolone treatment. Am J Respir Crit Care Med 1998;158(5 Pt 1):1432–1441.
19. Clark JG, Milberg JA, Steinberg KP, et al. Type III procollagen peptide in the adult respiratory distress syndrome. Association of increased peptide levels in bronchoalveolar lavage fluid with increased risk for death. Ann Intern Med 1995;122(1):17–23.
20. Krein PM, Sabatini PJ, Tinmouth W, et al. Localization of insulin-like growth factor-I in lung tissues of patients with fibroproliferative acute respiratory distress syndrome. Am J Respir Crit Care Med 2003;167(1):83–90.
21. Marshall RP, Bellingan G, Webb S, et al. Fibroproliferation occurs early in the acute respiratory distress syndrome and impacts on outcome. Am J Respir Crit Care Med 2000;162(5):1783–1788.
22. Bharat A, Machuca TN, Querrey M, et al. Early outcomes after lung transplantation for severe COVID-19: a series of the first consecutive cases from four countries. Lancet Respir Med 2021;9(5):487–497.
23. Bharat A, Querrey M, Markov NS, et al. Lung transplantation for patients with severe COVID-19. Sci Transl Med 2020;12(574).
24. Reyfman PA, Walter JM, Joshi N, et al. Single-Cell Transcriptomic Analysis of Human Lung Provides Insights into the Pathobiology of Pulmonary Fibrosis. Am J Respir Crit Care Med 2019;199(12):1517–1536.
25. Valenzi E, Bulik M, Tabib T, et al. Single-cell analysisreveals fibroblast heterogeneity and myofibroblasts in systemic sclerosis-associated interstitial lung disease. Ann Rheum Dis 2019;78(10):1379–1387.
26. Habermann AC, Gutierrez AJ, Bui LT, et al. Singlecell RNA sequencing reveals profibrotic roles of distinct epithelial and mesenchymal lineages in pulmonary fibrosis. Sci Adv 2020;6(28) :eaba1972.

27. Adams TS, Schupp JC, Poli S, et al. Single-cell RNAseq reveals ectopic and aberrant lung-resident cell populations in idiopathic pulmonary fibrosis. Sci Adv 2020;6(28):eaba1983.
28. Strunz M, Simon LM, Ansari M, et al. Alveolar regeneration through a Krt81 transitional stem cell state that persists in human lung fibrosis. Nat Commun 2020;11(1):3559.
29. Kobayashi Y, Tata A, Konkimalla A, et al. Persistence of a regeneration-associated, transitional alveolar epithelial cell state in pulmonary fibrosis. Nat Cell Biol 2020;22(8):934–946.
30. Jiang P, Gil de Rubio R, Hrycaj SM, et al. Ineffectual Type 2-to-Type 1 Alveolar Epithelial Cell Differentiation in Idiopathic Pulmonary Fibrosis: Persistence of the KRT8(hi) Transitional State. Am J Respir Crit Care Med 2020;201(11):1443–1447.
31. Wu H, Yu Y, Huang H, et al. Progressive Pulmonary Fibrosis Is Caused by Elevated Mechanical Tension on Alveolar Stem Cells. Cell 2020;180(1): 107–121. e17.
32. Lotfollahi M, Naghipourfar M, Luecken MD, et al. Query to reference single-cell integration with transfer learning. bioRxiv 2020;2020.
33. Joshi N, Watanabe S, Verma R, et al. A spatially restricted fibrotic niche in pulmonary fibrosis is sustained by M-CSF/M-CSFR signalling in monocytederived alveolar macrophages. Eur Respir J 2020;55(1).
34. Zhou X, Franklin RA, Adler M, et al. Circuit Design Features of a Stable Two-Cell System. Cell 2018; 172(4):744–757. e17.
35. Steinberg KP, Hudson LD, Goodman RB, et al. Blood Institute Acute Respiratory Distress Syndrome Clinical Trials, N. , Efficacy and safety of corticosteroids for persistent acute respiratory distress syndrome. N Engl J Med 2006;354(16):1671–1684.
36. Beyer C, Distler JH. Tyrosine kinase signaling in fibrotic disorders: Translation of basic research to human disease. Biochim Biophys Acta 2013; 1832(7):897–904.
37. Yamaguchi Y, Takihara T, Chambers RA, et al. A peptide derived from endostatin ameliorates organ fibrosis. Sci Transl Med 2012;4(136):136ra71.
38. Wrighton KH, Lin X, Feng XH. Phospho-control of TGF-beta superfamily signaling. Cell Res 2009;19(1):8–20.
39. Machuca TN, Cypel M, Bharat A. Comment on Let's Build Bridges to Recovery in COVID-19 ARDS, not Burn Them! Ann Surg 2020;274(6):e870–871.
40. Chang Y, Lee SO, Shim TS, et al. Lung Transplantation as a Therapeutic Option in Acute Respiratory Distress Syndrome. Transplantation 2018;102(5): 829–837.
41. Botta M, Tsonas AM, Pillay J, et al. Ventilation management and clinical outcomes in invasively ventilated patients with COVID-19 (PRoVENT-COVID): a national, multicentre, observational cohort study. Lancet Respir Med 2020;9(2):139–148.
42. Harano T, Ryan JP, Chan EG, et al. Lung transplantation for the treatment of irreversible acute respiratory distress syndrome. Clin Transplant 2021;35(2):e14182.
43. Frick AE, Gan CT, Vos R, et al. Lung transplantation for acute respiratory distress syndrome: A multicenter experience. Am J Transplant 2021;22(1): 144–153.
44. Abdelnour-Berchtold E, Federici S, Wurlod DA, et al. Outcome after extracorporeal membrane oxygenation-bridged lung retransplants: a singlecentre experience. Interact Cardiovasc Thorac Surg 2019;28(6):922–928.

45. Benazzo A, Schwarz S, Frommlet F, et al. Twenty-year experience with extracorporeal life support as bridge to lung transplantation. J Thorac Cardiovasc Surg 2019;157(6):2515–2525 e10.

46. Hoetzenecker K, Donahoe L, Yeung JC, et al. Extracorporeal life support as a bridge to lung transplantation-experience of a high-volume transplant center. J Thorac Cardiovasc Surg 2018; 155(3):1316–1328 e1.

47. Ius F, Natanov R, Salman J, et al. Extracorporeal membrane oxygenation as a bridge to lung transplantation may not impact overall mortality risk after transplantation: results from a 7-year single-centre experience. Eur J Cardiothorac Surg 2018;54(2):334–340.

48. Langer F, Aliyev P, Schafers HJ, et al. Improving Outcomes in Bridge-to-Transplant: Extended Extracorporeal Membrane Oxygenation Support to Obtain Optimal Donor Lungs for Marginal Recipients. ASAIO J 2019;65(5):516–521.

49. Hayanga JWA, Hayanga HK, Holmes SD, et al. Mechanical ventilation and extracorporeal membrane oxygenation as a bridge to lung transplantation: Closing the gap. J Heart Lung Transplant 2019; 38(10):1104–1111.

50. Tipograf Y, Salna M, Minko E, et al. Outcomes of Extracorporeal Membrane Oxygenation as a Bridge to Lung Transplantation. Ann Thorac Surg 2019; 107(5):1456–1463.

51. Biscotti M, Gannon WD, Agerstrand C, et al. Awake Extracorporeal Membrane Oxygenation as Bridge to Lung Transplantation: A 9-Year Experience. Ann Thorac Surg 2017;104(2):412–419.

52. Fuehner T, Kuehn C, Hadem J, et al. Extracorporeal membrane oxygenation in awake patients as bridge to lung transplantation. Am J Respir Crit Care Med 2012;185(7):763–768.

53. Oh DK, Hong SB, Shim TS, et al. Effects of the duration of bridge to lung transplantation with extracorporeal membrane oxygenation. PLoS One 2021; 16(7):e0253520.

54. Patel KV, Zaman S, Chang F, et al. Rare case of severe cholangiopathy following critical illness. BMJ Case Rep 2014;2014.

55. Tunney R, Scott J, Rudralingam V, et al. Secondary sclerosing cholangitis following extracorporeal membrane oxygenation for acute respiratory distress in polytrauma. Clin Case Rep 2018;6(9): 1849–1853.

56. Cypel M, Waddell T, Singer LG, et al. Bilateral pneumonectomy to treat uncontrolled sepsis in a patient awaiting lung transplantation. J Thorac Cardiovasc Surg 2017;153(4):e67–69.

# 第 4 章 潜在肺捐献者的管理

Ashwini Arjuna, Anna Teresa Mazzeo, Tommaso Tonetti, Rajat Walia, Luciana Mascia 著

周永巧 谢锐文 译

周建平 校

【关键词】

- 肺供体管理
- 神经学死亡判定后的捐献
- 循环死亡判定后的捐献
- 器官捐献
- 肺保护性通气
- COVID 捐献者筛查
- 对死亡供体进行 SARS-CoV-2 评估
- 捐献者重症监护管理

【要点】

- 潜在的供肺管理涉及优化患者和器官相关因素,以增加移植物存活成功率。
- 通过优化边缘器官捐献者可以扩大肺移植捐献者库,以确保移植成功。
- 肺供体管理应包括基于保护方案的策略,以改善肺及肺外生理功能。
- COVID-19 疫情为捐献者库的选择、筛选和管理策略增加了新的管理维度。

## 4.1 引　言

肺移植（LTx）可以作为延长终末期呼吸衰竭患者生命的治疗方法。然而,尽管捐献者管理不断改进,供体器官短缺仍然是一个主要的问题。器官功能的优化和保护是重症监护医学的支柱。这一理念也适用于潜在器官捐献者的护理。当不可逆脑损伤患者发展为脑死亡时,临床重点可以从脑保护转移到潜在器官捐献者的护理上。改善器官功能的机会窗口从入住重症监护病房（ICU）的那一刻开始,涵盖 ICU 护理直至脑死亡诊断的所有阶段。在实质器官中,肺是最重要的,也是很难维持的,因此,只有 15%~20% 多器官捐献者能够恢复[1]。Miñambres 及其同事提出,虽然年龄或吸烟史等因素无法改变,但床边管理策略中应考虑其他可改变的因素[2,3]。大部分移植肺来自神经学死亡判定（neurologic determination of death, DNDD, 以前称为脑死亡）后的供体。与传统的 DNDD 供体相比,使用循环死亡判定（circulatory determination of death, DCDD）供体

器官实现的长期生存率更高[4]。实施集束化护理是 ICU 供体管理的主要内容。DNDD 供体会因神经源性肺水肿而出现特殊的病理生理变化,并且保护性机械通气(MV)是控制这种情况的基础。其他管理策略旨在通过与器官获取组织和移植团队合作进行细致而积极的护理来保护器官功能,包括利尿、治疗性支气管镜检查、胸部物理治疗、预防误吸、肺保护性通气和定期肺复张操作,以潜在地改善氧合并提高总体恢复(也称为获取)率。为扩大捐献者库正在探索的一个新方向是利用新冠病毒阳性捐献者来扩大捐献者队列。在本章中,我们将对肺捐献者管理策略进行讨论,以保留捐献候选资格并在恢复前优化生理参数。

## 4.2 通气管理和血气交换

过去 20 年来,关于潜在 DNDD 捐献者通气管理的建议发生了巨大变化,重点是避免呼吸机引起肺损伤以保护肺功能,并尽量减少多器官功能障碍。DNDD 供体的病理生理学涉及复杂的系统性紊乱,主要由颅内高压和释放大量内源性儿茶酚胺引起,导致自主神经血管张力丧失以及低血压。因此,脑死亡的特征是心肌损伤和多器官缺血导致的心血管衰竭以及神经源性肺水肿(neurogenic pulmonary edema,NPE)。NPE 的特点是儿茶酚胺大量释放、肺毛细血管通透性增加和细胞因子释放增加。事实上,NPE 在放射学和临床特征方面与急性呼吸窘迫综合征(ARDS)相似,如出现动脉低氧血症和双侧胸部 X 线透视浸润[5]。

经实验和临床数据验证的双重打击模型解释了毁灭性脑损伤后发生的肺衰竭的发展,并演变成脑死亡[5-7]。第一次打击是由脑损伤引发交感神经风暴和促炎级联反应的结果。一旦启动,呼吸系统就很容易受到通气机械应力引起的进一步炎症损伤[8]。呼吸功能的恶化会进一步损害中枢神经系统,形成恶性循环[7]。脑损伤启动的炎症反应可能会使肺部因连续的伤害性刺激而进一步受损。由于第一次打击与损伤的严重程度有关,因此临床干预措施有限且不太可能成功。另一方面,适当的通气设置可能会影响二次打击,从而损害远端器官功能。

事实上,已经确定创伤性脑损伤为 ARDS 的诱发因素[9]。最近,Rincon 及其同事[10]的报告称,这种并发症会导致脑损伤后院内死亡的风险较高。在一项针对重度脑损伤患者的前瞻性观察研究中,损伤性机械通气是导致 ARDS 发生的因素,与较长时间的呼吸机依赖和较长的 ICU 住院时间有关[11]。

## 第4章 潜在肺捐献者的管理

在重度脑损伤演变为脑死亡的情况下，潜在器官捐献者的重症监护管理需从"脑保护"策略转向"器官保护"策略，以优化器官捐献。肺部负责维持全身系统内稳态——最佳氧合和最佳酸碱平衡（pH），而心脏则负责外周器官的最佳灌注。传统上，潜在器官捐献者的临床管理旨在保证最佳氧合和灌注，而不是主要保护心胸器官。从这个角度来看，心胸器官在器官捐献中发挥着双重作用，因为它们既需要保护周围器官，又是潜在的供体器官（图 4-1）。因此，在捐献过程中，器官功能进行连续重新评估对结合不同器官的临床优先级别至关重要，同时要记住适宜性参数可能会随着时间的推移而改变。

**心胸器官的双重作用**

| 保护供体器官的周围器官 | 保护心肺以供捐赠 |
|---|---|
| • 最佳灌注<br> - 中性液体平衡<br> - 适度的儿茶酚胺水平<br> - 低水平的 PEEP | • 心脏保护<br> - 最佳的液体平衡<br> - 低儿茶酚胺水平<br> - 低水平的 PEEP |
| • 最佳氧合和 pH<br> - 没有具体的策略 | • 肺部保护：<br> - 低 $FiO_2$<br> - 适度的 PEEP<br> - 低潮气量<br> - 液体负平衡 |

**图 4-1 心胸器官在器官捐献中发挥双重作用**
注：肺保证最佳的氧合和酸碱平衡，心脏保证周围器官的最佳灌注，但两者均是潜在的供体器官

在一项针对潜在器官捐献者的多中心、随机、对照试验中，与使用传统呼吸机方案相比，使用肺保护策略可以使肺恢复率翻倍（54% vs. 27%；$P < 0.005$）[12]。采用的方案是潮气量为 6~8 mL/kg 预计体重（predicted body weight，PBW）、呼气末正压（positive end-expiratory pressure，PEEP）8~10 cm $H_2O$、闭合回路吸痰、持续气道正压等于之前的 PEEP 进行呼吸暂停测试，以及与呼吸机断开连接后的肺复张操作。根据这一证据，Rech 及其同事[13]得出结论，器官捐献者管理中的最佳证据支持采用保护性机械通气，而激素替代等其他策略的证据则很薄弱。Slutsky 和 Ranieri[8]最近得出了类似的结论，他们建议对有心跳的器官捐献者使用肺部保护性策略。

因此，最新的供体管理共识声明[14]，建议采用保护性通气策略，即应用 6~8 mL/kg PBW 之间的潮气量，降低驱动压，并将 PEEP 优化至 8~10 cm $H_2O$，使气道峰值压力低于 35 mmHg[2,4,14,15]。肺复张操作应在气管抽吸或吸痰后断开呼吸机回路，并始终提供

回路湿化[16]。如果患者需要高 PEEP，则应仅进行气管抽吸以清除分泌物，避免肺复张[6]。气管插管套囊应充气至足够高的压力以防止误吸，床头高度应为 30°[17]。应使用最低限度的吸入氧浓度（$FiO_2$），将动脉血氧分压（$PaO_2$）浓度维持在 80~100 mmHg，不仅可以保证氧气输送，还可以避免受者肺因高氧引起的损伤。应纠正酸中毒确保正常二氧化碳水平（$PaCO_2$ 为 35~45 mmHg）。谨慎使用利尿剂，以进一步减少通气灌注不匹配和弥散异常，从而增加 $PaCO_2/FiO_2$ 比值[18]。这种强化肺供体方案与肺恢复率的增加相关，而不会对肺受体的早期生存率或原发性移植物功能不全（PGD）产生负面影响。

总之，强有力的证据表明：①脑损伤发展为脑死亡是 ARDS 的诱发因素；②有害的机械通气策略会增加潜在器官捐献者肺损伤的风险，导致呼吸机诱导的肺损伤；③保护性通气策略可以显著增加供体肺的数量，而不会影响其他器官的功能。器官获取组织的现有指南不再建议使用高潮气量和低水平 PEEP，同时有强有力的证据支持对潜在器官捐献者采用保护性机械通气[19]。

## 4.3 液体管理

器官恢复链中的一个关键点是早期识别患有毁灭性脑损伤的患者。事实上，及时诊断和转诊潜在的器官捐献者是恢复的关键。自主神经功能障碍、外周血管张力丧失、炎症介质释放以及液体平衡改变会导致前负荷、收缩性和后负荷受损。识别血流动力学不稳定的致病因素对于液体管理尤为重要[20]。

当颅内压升高威胁到大脑灌注时，就会发生进行性脑干缺血，导致心血管功能迅速变化，称为自主神经风暴。预计全身性炎症反应对肺部水平有多种影响。急性脑损伤后强烈的心肺相互作用在脑死亡时达到顶峰。当脑灌注停止时，会发生严重周围血管舒张，并有相对血容量减少出现。尿崩症常常由亢利尿素缺失引起，导致利尿不适当、高钠血症和低血容量恶化。在这些变化开始发生时，须密切监测、早期发现和及时治疗。低渗性多尿、高钠血症、血清渗透压高于 295 mmol/kg $H_2O$ 和尿液渗透压低于 200 mmol/kg $H_2O$ 是尿崩症的诊断标准，结合临床怀疑，需要立即补液以及补充缺失的激素。

因此，在护理潜在的器官捐献者时，血容量正常是首要治疗目的，而及时纠正低血容量是治疗的目标。最近关于供体心肺获取的共识声明[14]表明，对于前负荷降低的供体，等渗晶体溶液是液体补充和维持的首选。对于纠正低血容量后仍存在高钠血症的患者，应使用含葡萄糖溶液或低渗溶液，如 0.45% 氯化钠。

DNDD 时的潜在捐献者可能与 ARDS 患者的生理功能非常相似[21]。传统的血流动力学指标，如平均动脉压（mean arterial pressure，MAP）、中心静脉压（central venous pressure，CVP）和尿量，很容易在床边测量。近年来，超声心动图已被引入重症监护，以评估床边的血流动力学状态，在心肌顿抑、NPE 以及心脏或肺挫伤可能妨碍胸部器官捐献时尤其有用[14]。

经肺热稀释法衍生的实时脉搏波结果，例如被动抬腿试验引起的心输出量增加（>10%），或呼气末闭塞测试引起的心输出量增加（>5%），以及呼吸测量连续脉压变化和每搏输出量变化是最近引入的床边液体反应性动态指数，可以指导临床医生优化液体管理，以保证氧气输送，同时避免肺水肿增加。在一项小型单中心研究中，48% 的捐献者检测到通过脉压变化评估的液体反应性，并且前负荷反应性捐献者的移植器官数量更高[22]。最近，在脑死亡捐献者中进行的第一项大型多中心随机（MOnIToR）试验验证了一个假设，即针对心脏指数、平均动脉压和脉压变化的"协议引导液体治疗"算法会增加器官移植的数量。然而，并没有发现显著差异，这强调需要进行更大规模的研究来评估基于液体反应性的供体管理的有效性[23]。

通过严格调节体液状态来预防肺水肿，同时保持周围器官充分的全身灌注是潜在肺供体管理中的另一个关键点。限制性输液策略与自由输液策略是这些利益冲突的典型例子，并且对 ARDS 患者和潜在器官捐献者的护理都提出了挑战。尽管如此，Minãmbres 及其同事[24]表明，严格的液体平衡可以预防 NPE 并增加适合移植的肺的数量，同时还能维持肾移植物的存活。同一研究小组还在一项更大规模的研究中表明，使用强化肺捐献者治疗策略不会对心脏、肝脏、肾脏和胰腺的获取率产生负面影响[3]。满足捐献者管理目标[25]的概念适用于所有器官，也包括肺部；主要目标是 MAP 60~80 mmHg、CVP 6~10 mmHg、$PaO_2$ 80~100 mmHg（最低 $FiO_2$）、温度 36~37.5℃、尿量每小时 0.5~2 mL/kg，以及血清 $Na^+$ 浓度 135~150 mmol/L。如果需要血管加压药，应当使用最小剂量。关于血管加压药的选择尚未达成共识，但去甲肾上腺素或去氧肾上腺素可能是治疗分布性休克的首选，血管加压素用于难治性休克，并且多巴胺、多巴酚丁胺或肾上腺素用于治疗原发性心泵功能障碍[14,19]。最近的研究发现，满足捐献者管理目标是每个捐献者移植超过 4 个器官的独立预测因素[25]，并且当扩大供体标准（年龄较大且有并发症）时移植 3 个或更多器官的概率高达 90%[26]。

## 4.4 死亡原因及其影响

供体肺的接受率为15%~20%（在所有实质器官中最低）[1]。需要对DNDD进行临床评估，包括全身和神经系统以及是否存在昏迷、是否存在脑干反射的记录以及呼吸暂停测试（根据指南进行）[19]。若临床检查无法确诊可能需要辅助检测［如脑电图、计算机断层扫描（CT）血管造影和MRI/血管造影］。外伤和脑血管意外（cerebrovascular accident，CVA）仍然是脑死亡最常见的原因[14]。脑死亡的原因与胸部器官的特定并发症有关，如NPE、心肺挫伤或创伤捐献者的心肌损伤。CVA捐献者应考虑多种全身性疾病，包括左心室肥厚、动脉血管性疾病和高血压。药物相关死亡可能对心肌收缩力有一定影响。来自DCDD供体的器官的使用越来越多，特别是在引入体外灌注技术之后。最常关注的是热缺血性损伤以及与此类捐赠相关的伦理困境。热缺血时间定义为从心脏骤停到器官原位灌注的时间，应低于150分钟[27]。必须满足心肺无循环标准。考虑到肺部对热缺血时间的相对耐受性，从撤除生命支持到死亡的时间可以延长至90分钟，在某些方案中甚至可以延长至120~180分钟[28]。最近的美国器官共享联合网络研究[4]并未显示DNDD和DCDD受者之间在围术期死亡率、气道裂开、透析需求、术后住院时间或总生存率方面存在显著差异。

## 4.5 支气管镜检查

支气管镜检查是一种治疗和诊断工具，应在所有潜在的肺捐献者中进行，包括X线片和$PaO_2$正常的捐献者。在供体肺招募开始时进行早期支气管镜检查可以帮助记录支气管内解剖结构，并评估吸入的胃内容物或血液、感染、炎症和脓性分泌物。支气管肺泡灌洗样本可以帮助指导下呼吸道感染的抗微生物治疗[29]。根据我们的经验，如果在第一次检查时发现大量分泌物，重新评估支气管树对帮助清除分泌物及降低病原体负荷非常重要。重复检查的频率取决于最初支气管镜检查的结果、检查的质量以及随后胸部成像的变化和对新感染的担忧。如果怀疑有肺不张，初始支气管镜检查可以指导是否需要重复抽吸、物理治疗、调整抗生素治疗方案及肺复张策略。

建议在DNDD捐献者进行供肺移植之前对支气管树至少进行一次检查[19]。存在气道红斑或分泌物不应妨碍器官取出。在DCDD捐献者中，撤除支持前的气道检查是基于中心特定的方案。越来越多的器官获取组织开始要求在器官分配前进行支气管镜检查，以最大限度地实现器官安置。

## 4.6 胸部放射成像

清晰的胸部 X 线片通常被列为接受供体肺的先决条件；然而，仅异常的胸部 X 线片不应排除肺恢复的适宜性[4]。胸部 X 线片可以帮助估计总肺容量[30] 并识别血管充血、水肿、浸润和挫伤，同时还提示是否需要专用成像（如 CT），或进行进一步感染检查，如痰液、气管抽吸物取样、支气管镜检查和灌洗。在供体器官恢复计划到位之前，每日常规进行便携式胸部 X 线检查。当前，在美国和欧洲都实行至少使用一台胸部 CT 来对供体肺进行评估，以识别胸部 X 线片上遗漏的结节或浸润，筛查结构性病变，肺部疾病和解剖异常，并估计肺容量[31]。

## 4.7 微生物培养结果与抗生素

供肺同种异体移植感染率高达 50%[32]，并且插管持续时间的增加与支气管树定植率较高相关[29]。然而，供体肺定植率与移植后肺炎发生率及移植物预后无关[33]。多重耐药菌株感染和侵袭性真菌及分枝杆菌感染仍然是肺移植的相对禁忌证，而活动性结核分枝杆菌感染仍然是绝对禁忌证。在经验性广谱抗生素使用的时代，大多数患有活动性细菌感染的供体肺都可以通过积极的抗生素治疗来挽救[34]。应组织感染病专家会诊以处理非典型感染。在重度假丝酵母菌感染的供体肺中，抗真菌预防可以降低侵袭性假丝酵母菌病的发生率。然而，最近的研究并未显示预防性使用抗真菌药物与移植后同种异体移植感染率或定植率降低之间存在关联。相反，感染继发的低氧血症程度可能是供体肺可挽救性的更准确指标。此外，通常不认为供体菌血症或败血症是器官捐献的绝对禁忌证，除非有影像学和微生物学数据强烈支持感染性结节存在。

## 4.8 输血对供肺管理的影响

即使在低危受者中，大量输血（定义为短时间内输注 > 10 单位的血液制品）也与肺移植后 30 天和 90 天[35] 的死亡率相关。具体而言，供体输血已被确定为原发性移植物功能不全的潜在危险因素。尽管尚不清楚其机制，但在原发性移植物功能不全和输血相关急性肺损伤（transfusion-related acute lung injury，TRALI）[36] 患者中已检测出生物标志物。例如，晚期糖基化终末产物可溶性受体（sRAGE），为急性肺损伤与 TRALI

之间的相关性提供了依据，从而反映了与输血相关的死亡风险。年轻创伤患者的早期稳定需要大量输血，其是供体库的主要贡献者。由于创伤和受损的血液制品会增加原发性移植物功能不全发生的风险，因此，中心特定的风险承受能力和积极管理原发性移植物功能不全的经验应该为选择接受大量输血的供体肺的决定提供依据。

## 4.9 2019 冠状病毒病（COVID-19）筛查指南

国际心肺移植学会（ISHLT）[37]建议避免使用以下供体的器官进行移植：①严重急性呼吸综合征冠状病毒2（severe acute respiratory syndrome coronavirus 2，SARS-CoV-2）聚合酶链反应（polymerase chain reaction，PCR）检测阳性的供体；②当前患有2019 冠状病毒病（coronavirus disease 2019，COVID-19）临床症状的供体[38]；③胸部影像学显示 COVID-19 肺炎但无症状的供体。但对于过去 14 天内已知接触过 COVID-19 确诊或疑似病例且无 COVID 19 临床表现的供体，仍可考虑使用。目前关于抗原检测用于肺供体评估的数据有限[38]。由于移植后免疫抑制剂可能会引发受体严重感染，因此所有潜在供体都必须在器官获取前接受严重急性呼吸综合征冠状病毒2（severe acute respiratory syndrome coronavirus 2，SARS-CoV-2）感染风险评估。具体包括：①详细询问病史以分层评估供体 SARS-CoV-2 暴露风险；②对潜在肺供体进行胸部影像学检查和微生物学采样。逆转录 PCR（RT-PCR）仍是活动性感染检测的金标准[39]。供体的 COVID-19 疫苗接种状态不影响上述建议[38]。对于 DCDD 供体，需至少采集一份呼吸道样本。欧洲指南与 ISHLT 建议一致。

### 4.9.1 死亡供体 COVID-19 评估与检测

美国疾病控制与预防中心（Centers for Disease Control and Prevention，CDC）报告了 3 例供体上呼吸道样本 SARS-CoV-2 阴性但肺受体仍发生感染的案例，事后追溯发现供体下呼吸道样本检测呈阳性[38,40-42]。为最大限度降低供体源性 SARS-CoV-2 感染风险，同时提高供体利用率，器官获取与移植网络（Organ Procurement and Transplantation Network，OPTN）建议：对所有死亡供体进行核酸检测（nucleic acid test，NAT），样本应取自上下呼吸道（包括鼻咽拭子、鼻咽冲洗液、鼻咽抽吸物、鼻腔冲洗液、鼻腔抽吸物、中鼻甲拭子、口咽拭子、气管抽吸物、支气管抽吸液/冲洗液、支气管肺泡灌洗液或肺活检组织），检测时间需在器官获取前 72 小时内（以接近获取时间最佳）。

OPTN 政策进一步规定了在供体肺恢复进行移植时对下呼吸道样本进行前瞻性检测。呼吸道样本 NAT 阴性可降低潜在感染传播风险，但以下情况的安全性尚未明确：①仅依赖 SARS-CoV-2 抗体检测；②非呼吸道样本 NAT 检测；③仅通过影像学检查诊断。此外，目前 COVID-19 既往感染与活动性感染的区别、供体 SARS-CoV-2 疫苗接种状态对传播风险的影响仍不明确。

### 4.9.2 COVID-19 康复期供体的定义与风险评估

COVID-19 康复期供体定义为有 COVID-19 确诊史的免疫活性供体，自发病之日起 21 天以上，症状缓解。OPTN 指出[42]，若此类供体在评估时 SARS-CoV-2 NAT 呈阴性，则传播感染的风险极低。但关于移植物质量与长期预后的数据仍有限，是否选用此类供体需综合评估受者在等待名单中的死亡风险。此外，以下两类供体也被认为传播风险较低：①轻度 COVID-19 病史供体（无需氧疗或住院治疗），发病后 10~21 天且症状已缓解；② COVID 19 康复期供体，发病后 21~90 天内 SARS-CoV-2 NAT 检测阳性[43]。

### 4.9.3 COVID-19 活动期供体评估

COVID-19 活动期供体的定义需满足以下条件[42,44]：①免疫功能正常；②有 COVID-19 确诊病史；③呼吸道样本 SARS-CoV-2 NAT 阳性；④发病时间不足 21 天。传播风险评估与欧洲实践风险特征：①此类供体向受体及移植团队传播病毒的风险尚不明确；②肺移植受体的感染风险显著高于其他实体器官受体[44]。欧洲指南仅考虑将此类供体器官用于符合以下全部条件的受者：①当前 SARS-CoV-2 阳性或既往感染史；②临床状况危重；③等待期间死亡风险高于潜在感染传播风险。附加要求：①建议检测受体抗体效价（即使移植后检测）；②需签署充分知情同意书。例外案例与伦理考量：2021 年 6 月，意大利某移植中心在伦理委员会特批下[45]，为两例 SARS-CoV-2 阴性且无抗体的受体（64 岁与 15 岁）实施了心脏移植，供体 SARS-CoV-2 检测阳性。决策依据：①受体等待期间死亡风险极高；②术后随访显示两例受体均未发生 SARS-CoV-2 感染。

### 4.9.4 活体供体评估与检测

建议活体捐赠者采用感染控制措施，在器官恢复前 14 天进行自我隔离，使用接近器官恢复时间的 NAT 检测呼吸道样本的 SARS-CoV-2（但在 72 小时内），以减少对受赠者的传播风险。然而，目前尚缺乏长期的结果数据。

## 4.10 总　结

移植是院内外多学科团队共同努力的结果，多器官移植的目标需要协作团队的共同努力才能实现。供体管理的最终目标实际上是保留捐献机会，并最大限度地增加和优化用于移植的供体器官的数量和质量。

## 4.11 未来发展方向

尽管全球器官捐献者数量有所增加，但器官利用率仍然不够理想，面临多重挑战。最佳的重症监护管理是器官捐献计划成功的基础。管理边缘供体将有助于增加可用于移植的器官数量，同时保持受者安全、可接受的同种异体移植结果和受者生存率。成功的器官恢复需要有效的团队方法、积极的复苏策略、标准化的捐献者管理方案、清晰的沟通、家庭支持、社区意识以及持续的教育和培训[46]。展望未来，常规胸部 CT 和下呼吸道检查 RT-PCR SARS-CoV-2 检测仍是护理标准。离体肺灌注的使用将扩大供体库，有助于弥补肺移植的供需缺口。我们对 COVID-19 大流行影响肺移植的认知将持续深化。

【临床护理要点】

- 每位重症监护室中的患者都是潜在的供体，采用多学科闭环沟通方法，可以挽救肺和其他器官。
- 脑死亡后捐献和循环死亡后捐献的术后生存率相当，应鼓励中心采纳短期和长期两种捐献方式，以满足肺移植中的供需缺口。
- 早期保护性通气策略、根据需要进行的持续肺复张操作以及良好的液体平衡仍然是管理潜在肺捐献的治疗基石。
- 胸部成像和支气管镜检查结果将进一步有助于供体的医疗管理，包括利尿的需要、扩展抗生素的使用以及治疗性分泌物抽吸。
- 随着大流行为供体库增加了一个新的维度，通过详细病史采集、下呼吸道样本检测、影像学检查和临床判断充分筛查供体的 COVID 感染，有助于获取更多肺源。

## 致谢

感谢迪皮卡·拉齐亚博士对撰写本章的帮助。

## 声明

作者没有任何需要声明的事项。

# 参考文献

1. Wey A, Valapour M, Skeans MA, et al. Heart and lung organ offer acceptance practices of transplant programs are associated with waitlist mortality and organ yield. Am J Transplant 2018;18(8):2061–2067.
2. Minãmbres E, Pérez-Villares JM, Chico-Fernández M, et al. Lung donor treatment protocol in brain dead-donors: a multicenter study. J Heart Lung Transplant 2015;34(6):773–780.
3. Minãmbres E, Pérez-Villares JM, Terceros-Almanza L, et al. An intensive lung donor treatment protocol does not have negative influence on other grafts: a multicentre study. Eur J Cardiothorac Surg 2016;49(6):1719–724.
4. Van Raemdonck D, Neyrinck A, Verleden GM, et al. Lung donor selection and management. Proc Am Thorac Soc 2009;6(1):28–38.
5. Busl KM, Bleck TP. Neurogenic pulmonary edema. Crit Care Med 2015;43(8):1710–1715.
6. Mascia L, Mastromauro I, Viberti S, et al. Management to optimize organ procurement in brain dead donors. Minerva Anestesiol 2009;75(3):125–133.
7. Pelosi P, Rocco PR. The lung and the brain: a dangerous cross-talk. Crit Care 2011;15(3):168.
8. Slutsky AS, Ranieri VM. Ventilator-induced lung injury. N Engl J Med 2013;369(22):2126–2136.
9. Gajic O, Dabbagh O, Park PK, et al. Early identification of patients at risk of acute lung injury: evaluation of lung injury prediction score in a multicenter cohort study. Am J Respir Crit Care Med 2011;183(4):462–470.
10. Rincon F, Ghosh S, Dey S, et al. Impact of acute lung injury and acute respiratory distress syndrome after traumatic brain injury in the United States. Neurosurgery 2012;71(4):795–803.
11. Mascia L, Zavala E, Bosma K, et al. High tidal volume is associated with the development of acute lung injury after severe brain injury: an international observational study. Crit Care Med 2007;35(8): 1815–1820.
12. Mascia L, Pasero D, Slutsky AS, et al. Effect of a lung protective strategy for organ donors on eligibility and availability of lungs for transplantation: a randomized controlled trial. JAMA 2010;304(23): 2620–2627.
13. Rech TH, Moraes RB, Crispim D, et al. Management of the brain-dead organ donor: a systematic review and meta-analysis. Transplantation 2013;95(7):966–974.
14. Copeland H, Hayanga JWA, Neyrinck A, et al. Donor heart and lung procurement: a consensus statement. J Heart Lung Transplant 2020;39(6):501–517.
15. Botha P, Rostron AJ, Fisher AJ, et al. Current strategies in donor selection and management. Semin Thorac Cardiovasc Surg 2008;20(2):143–151.

16. Philpot SJ, Pilcher DV, Graham SM, et al. Lung recruitment manoeuvres should be considered when assessing suitability for lung donation. Crit Care Resusc 2012;14(3):244–245.
17. Lorente L, Blot S, Rello J. New issues and controversies in the prevention of ventilator-associated pneumonia. Am J Respir Crit Care Med 2010; 182(7):870–876.
18. Powner DJ, Hewitt MJ, Levine RL. Interventions during donor care before lung transplantation. Prog Transplant 2005;15(2):141–148.
19. Kotloff RM, Blosser S, Fulda GJ, et al. Management of the potential organ donor in the ICU: Society of Critical Care Medicine/American College of Chest Physicians/Association of Organ Procurement Organizations Consensus Statement. Crit Care Med 2015;43(6):1291–1325.
20. Meyfroidt G, Gunst J, Martin-Loeches I, et al. Management of the brain-dead donor in the ICU: general and specific therapy to improve transplantable organ quality. Intensive Care Med 2019;45(3):343–353.
21. Keddissi JI, Youness HA, Jones KR, et al. Fluid management in acute respiratory distress syndrome: a narrative review. Can J Respir Ther 2019;55:1–8.
22. Murugan R, Venkataraman R, Wahed AS, et al. Preload responsiveness is associated with increased interleukin-6 and lower organ yield from brain-dead donors. Crit Care Med 2009;37(8):2387–2393.
23. Al-Khafaji A, Elder M, Lebovitz DJ, et al. Protocolized fluid therapy in brain-dead donors: the multicenter randomized MOnIToR trial. Intensive Care Med 2015;41(3):418–426.
24. Miñambres E, Rodrigo E, Ballesteros MA, et al. Impact of restrictive fluid balance focused to increase lung procurement on renal function after kidney transplantation. Nephrol Dial Transplant 2010; 25(7):2352–2356.
25. Malinoski DJ, Patel MS, Daly MC, et al. The impact of meeting donor management goals on the number of organs transplanted per donor: results from the United Network for Organ Sharing Region 5 prospective donor management goals study. Crit Care Med 2012;40(10):2773–2780.
26. Patel MS, Zatarain J, De La Cruz S, et al. The impact of meeting donor management goals on the number of organs transplanted per expanded criteria donor: a prospective study from the UNOS Region 5 Donor Management Goals Workgroup. JAMA Surg 2014;149(9):969–975.
27. Domínguez-Gil B, Duranteau J, Mateos A, et al. Uncontrolled donation after circulatory death: European practices and recommendations for the development and optimization of an effective programme. Transpl Int 2016;29(8):842–859.
28. Levvey B, Keshavjee S, Cypel M, et al. Influence of lung donor agonal and warm ischemic times on early mortality: analyses from the ISHLT DCD Lung Transplant Registry. J Heart Lung Transplant 2019; 38(1):26–34.
29. Avlonitis VS, Krause A, Luzzi L, et al. Bacterial colonization of the donor lower airways is a predictor of poor outcome in lung transplantation. Eur J Cardiothorac Surg 2003;24(4):601–607.
30. Schlesinger AE, White DK, Mallory GB, et al. Estimation of total lung capacity from chest radiography and chest CT in children: comparison with body plethysmography. AJR Am J Roentgenol 1995; 165(1):151–154.
31. Gauthier JM, Bierhals AJ, Liu J, et al. Chest computed tomography imaging improves potential lung donor assessment. The J Thorac Cardiovasc Surg 2019;157(4):1711–1718. e1.
32. Ruiz I, Gavaldà J, Monforte V, et al. Donor-to-host transmission of bacterial and fungal infections in lung transplantation. Am J Transplant 2006;6(1): 178–182.

33. Weill D, Dey GC, Hicks RA, et al. A positive donor gram stain does not predict outcome following lung transplantation. J Heart Lung Transplant 2002; 21(5):555–558.

34. Bonde PN, Patel ND, Borja MC, et al. Impact of donor lung organisms on post-lung transplant pneumonia. J Heart Lung Transplant 2006;25(1):99–105.

35. Borders CF, Suzuki Y, Lasky J, et al. Massive donor transfusion potentially increases recipient mortality after lung transplantation. J Thorac Cardiovasc Surg 2017;153(5):1197–1203. e2.

36. Shah RJ, Bellamy SL, Localio AR, et al. A panel of lung injury biomarkers enhances the definition of primary graft dysfunction (PGD) after lung transplantation. J Heart Lung Transplant 2012;31(9):942–949.

37. International Society of Heart and Lung Transplantation. Guidance from the International Society of Heart and Lung Transplantation regarding the SARS CoV-2 pandemic. 2021. Available at:https://ishlt.org/ishlt/media/documents/SARS-CoV-2Guidance-for-Cardiothoracic-Transplant-and-VAD center. pdf. Accessed June 18, 2021.

38. International Society of Heart and Lung Transplantation. Deceased donor and recipient selection for cardiothoracic transplantation during the COVID-19 pandemic. April 12, 2021. Available at: https://ishlt.org/ishlt/media/documents/COVID-19_Guidance Document_Deceased-donor-and-recipient-selectionfor-cardiothoracic-transplantation. pdf. Accessed June 18, 2021.

39. Halpern SE, Olaso DG, Krischak MK, et al. Lung transplantation during the COVID-19 pandemic: safely navigating the new "normal. Am J Transplant 2020;20(11):3094–3105.

40. Kaul DR, Valesano AL, Petrie JG, et al. Donor to recipient transmission of SARS-CoV-2 by lung transplantation despite negative donor upper respiratory tract testing. Am J Transplant 2021;21(8):2885–2889.

41. Kumar D, Humar A, Keshavjee S, et al. A call to routinely test lower respiratory tract samples for SARS-CoV-2 in lung donors. Am J Transplant 2021;21:2623–2624.

42. Organ Procurement and Transplantation Network. Summary of current evidence and information–donor SARS-CoV-2 testing & organ recovery from donors with a history of COVID-19. Version release date: April 26, 2021. Available at: https://optn. transplant. hrsa. gov/media/4424/sars-cov-2-summary-of-evidence. pdf. Accessed June 30, 2021. Accessed June 30, 2021.

43. American Society of Transplantation. COVID-19 information. Available at: https://www. myast.org/covid-19-information. Accessed August 12, 2021.

44. Michaels MG, La Hoz RM, Danziger-Isakov L, et al. Coronavirus disease 2019: Implications of emerging infections for transplantation. Am J Transplant 2020; 20(7):1768–1772.

45. World's 1st transplants from COVID-positive donors performed in Italy. Available at: https://www. ansa. it/english/news/2021/06/10/worlds-1st-transplantsfrom-covid-positive-donors_9079492d-1f77-468db61a-9af28a8bfaf8. html. Accessed 8/23/2021. ANSAit. June 10, 2021.

46. Wojda TR, Stawicki SP, Yandle KP, et al. Keys to successful organ procurement: an experience-based review of clinical practices at a high-performing health-care organization. Int J Crit Illn Inj Sci 2017; 7(2):91–100.

# 第 5 章 肺移植心脏死亡后的捐献

Dirk Van Raemdonck, Laurens J. Ceulemans, Arne Neyrinck, Bronwyn Levvey, Gregory I. Snell 著

陈晓渝 译

梁瑞茵 校

【关键词】
- 脑死亡后捐献
- 循环死亡后捐献
- 临终医疗护理
- 肺移植
- 常温局部灌注
- 原发性移植物功能不全
- 撤除生命维持治疗

【要点】
- 受控循环死亡后供体的肺移植短期及长期预后与脑死亡后供体相当。
- 经筛选的非受控循环死亡后供体的肺移植具有可行性,但需更多移植中心积累经验。
- 对于撤除生命维持治疗的受控供体,离体肺灌注(EVLP)可用于移植前肺质量评估(非强制);但对非受控供体及功能性热缺血时间较长的受控供体,离体肺灌注为必需的。
- 快速获取技术(无接触期后)是受控循环死亡供体肺获取的最简方法,可与腹部器官常温局部灌注联合使用。
- 胸腹常温局部灌注技术将获取过程转化为死亡后心脏跳动状态下的操作,从而无需在移植前通过机器灌注进行离体肺评估。

## 5.1 引　言

肺移植(LTx)可改善特定终末期肺部疾病患者的数量和生活质量,随着其应用不断增加,已经成为一种标准疗法[1]。遗憾的是,由于缺乏合适的器官,因此并非所有肺移植的受体都能从中受益。优化肺供体来源应成为肺移植的重中之重。除了通过更好的供体登记、检测、报告和管理来改进当前做法外,还应探索使用不符合供肺标准的替代供体[2]。从历史上看,最大的供体来源是神经学上确定脑死亡后进行的捐献(donation after brain death，DBD）。即使在扩大供肺标准之后，这些供体的平均肺产量仍然很低，为 20%~40%。最近，世界各地的许多移植项目都在探索使用来自额外的供体库，即在确定心脏死亡后进行捐献（donation after circulatory death，DCD）。英国、荷兰、比利时、西班牙、瑞士、澳大利亚、加拿大和美国现已出现 DCD LTx 成功的报告[3]。

## 5.2 DCD 的捐献类别

为了表示缺血程度以及移植器官的原发性功能丧失或功能障碍的风险，马斯特里赫特分类[4]描述了 4 类 DCD：Ⅰ类代表到达医院前死亡，Ⅱ类代表在医院复苏但不成功，Ⅲ类代表预期的心脏骤停，Ⅳ类是意外的心脏骤停。Ⅰ类和Ⅱ类被分组为"不可控型"DCD（"uncontrolled" DCDs，uDCD），而Ⅲ类和Ⅳ类代表"可控型"DCD（"controlled" DCDs，cDCD）。根据不断积累的经验，制定了修改后的分类和附加子类别，并在表 5-1 中进行了描述。

表 5-1 DCD 修正版马斯特里赫特分类

| 类别 | 描述 | 详细信息 |
|---|---|---|
| Ⅰ类，不可控 | 发现病人时已经死亡：Ⅰ A. 院外；Ⅰ B. 院内 | 不可预期的突发性 CA，未经任何复苏 |
| Ⅱ类，不可控 | 心跳停止在眼前发生：Ⅱ A. 院外；Ⅱ B. 院内 | 不可预期的突发性 CA，复苏不成功 |
| Ⅲ类，可控 | 撤除生命支持治疗 | 计划撤除生命支持治疗[a]，预期的 CA |
| Ⅳ类，不可控 | 心跳停止时判定脑死亡 | 诊断脑死亡后但在计划的器官恢复之前发生突然的 CA |
| Ⅴ类，可控 | 死刑或安乐死后心脏骤停：Ⅴ A. 院外；Ⅴ B. 院内 | 注射死刑后突然出现预期的 CA[b] |

注：CA，心跳停止；DCD，心脏死亡后捐献；[a] 这一类别主要是指撤除生命支持治疗的决定；[b] 一些国家立法允许安乐死或药物支持时的医疗援助及随后的器官捐献（称为第五类）；数据来自参考文献[4-6]

## 5.3 DCD 供体的评估

标准和扩展的 DBD 肺选择标准同样适用于 cDCD[7]。关于 uDCD 肺捐赠的临床标准很少，经验都基于西班牙[8-10]和加拿大[11]的小型病例系列研究以及来自意大利[12,13]的单病种分析。意外的心跳停止（circulatory arrest，CA）没有可用的供体信息和病史，并且无法通过标准成像、支气管镜检查和氧合测试工具提前评估供体肺质量。

DBD 捐献会发生全身炎症和神经源性肺水肿，从而导致供体肺损伤，而潜在的 DCD 供体则不存在这种情况。尽管如此，DBD 和 DCD 都面临着与插管和通气相关的肺部误吸和感染等损伤的风险，与入住重症监护病房（ICU）的所有患者类似。

## 5.4 可耐受的热缺血

从 DCD 中取出的器官很容易受到热缺血的影响，从而对移植后的结果产生潜在的重要影响。主要注意的是临终期之前和（不可预见的）心跳停止之后的心搏期时间，持续在肺动脉冷冲洗中保存。与 DCD 移植的其他实质器官相比，肺有利于维持缺血状态，因为肺泡在没有灌注的情况下仍充满氧气[14]。因此，与肾脏[15]和肝脏[16]等腹部器官相比，cDCD 肺取出可以用更轻松的方式进行。

临终阶段通常被认为是肺损伤最重要的触发因素，因为心跳停止会通过剪切应力的变化而不是缺氧诱导内皮反应[17]。国际心肺移植学会（ISHLT）定义了 cDCD 中撤除生命支持治疗（withdrawal from life-sustaining therapy，WLST）的不同时间和间隔点（表 5-2）[18]。

表 5-2 ISHLT 定义的 cDCD 撤除生命支持治疗后的时间点、间隔和阶段

| 时间点 | 描述 |
| --- | --- |
| T0 | 撤除生命支持治疗或安乐死 |
| T1 | 氧饱和度 < 80% |
| T2 | 收缩压 < 50 mmHg |
| T3 | 心输出量 / 心搏停止 |
| T4 | 恢复肺充气 / 通气 |
| T5 | 开始肺冲洗 |

注：cDCD，循环亡死后控制性捐献；ISHLT，国际心肺移植学会；T0～T5，总热缺血时间；T2～T5，功能性热缺血阶段；T0～T3，临终阶段；T3～T5，心脏停搏期；数据来自 Cypel M, Levvey B, Van Raemdonck D, et al. International Society for Heart and Lung Transplantation donation after circulatory death registry report. J Heart Lung Transplant 2015;34:1278-82

大多数移植中心可以接受 WLST 后长达 60～120 分钟的等待时间。然而，更重要的是定义功能性热缺血时间（warm ischemia time，WIT；比如 T2～T5）的低血压期时长。对 507 例 cDCD LTx 多中心多变量 ISHLT DCD 登记分析进行统计，未发现临终持续时

间或功能性 WIT 与 1 年内受者死亡率之间的关联[19]。同样，对单中心的 180 例 cDCD LTx 记录的患者临终期持续时间进行了评估，在短期和长期受者生存率、原发性移植物功能不全（PGD）、ICU 住院时间、机械通气（MV）天数或总住院时间方面没有发现显著差异[20]。得出的结论是，临终期超过 60 分钟的移植肺可安全使用。此外，多伦多小组还报告了从 WLST 到 CA（即 T0~T3）超过 120 分钟的良好研究结果[21]。他们描述了在 WLST 后 12 小时使用静态肺充气技术获得肺部，然后在手术室（operating room, OR）近 2 小时后使用冷冲洗方式进行肺取出[22]。捐献者直到 WLST 后 10 小时 54 分钟后，心跳停止 25 分钟后，血压才降至 50 mmHg 以下。因此 ISHLT DCD 登记中的功能性 WIT 应在先前病例报告的时间范围内[19]。来自墨尔本的研究人员最近报告了对其 DCD 肺供体库的统计，得出的结论是延长肺捐献时间途径（90 分钟至 24 小时）可以大幅扩大他们的肺供体库[23]。

## 5.5 WLST（包括 cDCD 中的安慰治疗）

停止药物治疗的决策可能因群体和地区而异。特别是对未完全恢复的危重患者，没有更多的治疗选择。当所有能改善患者身体状况的尝试都失败时，可以选择在近亲知情同意后进行 WLST。当后续治疗无法保证患者的生活质量时，可以做出停止治疗的决定[24]。如果处理得当，WLST 是人类共同的经历，尤其是在器官捐献的情况下，尽管对所有相关人员来说都很困难，但这种经历可以让人感到充实[25]。显然，移植医生与等候名单上的受者存在利益冲突，因此其在 WLST 的决定及实践中不承担任何作用或责任[26]。

中止手术的百分比可能取决于选择潜在供体的标准以及临终关怀期间给予的安慰治疗。在 WLST 后 120 分钟的时间窗口内未发生 CA 的捐献者数量估计约为 40%。因此，很多 LTx 团队都不愿意长途跋涉，因为徒劳的捐献会带来经济风险。目前已开发出一些算法，尝试预测病情恶化的可能性，但由于其并不准确而缺乏实用性[27,28]。根据我们在比利时使用 cDCD 的经验，只有不到 1% 的手术被中止（2021 年比利时移植协会未发表的数据）。

尽管证据尚不明确，但 WLST 期间对捐献者给予的安慰治疗可能会间接影响临终期的持续时间。人们担心接受 WLST 后给捐献者带来潜在的身体和心理痛苦。因此，在临终关怀和撤除阶段，应考虑对临终患者进行滴定安慰疗法（根据当地法律和临床实践的限制）。同时还可以采取器官保护措施。目前，没有有用的指南辅助停止治疗的方法，仅提供一般原则。镇静剂和镇痛剂的用量与死亡时间并无关联，但关于这方面的记录很少[28-30]。

总体而言，目前尚未达成共识，而且安慰疗法的问题引发了一场关于这种做法是否会间接导致同意捐献者寿命缩短的伦理争论[31]。可以说，在 WLST 认识到每天进行相同的治疗后，可以对潜在捐献者进行滴定安慰疗法。因为其他身患绝症的 ICU 患者每天都在接受同样的治疗，却没有进一步的治疗选择。缩短痛苦并不意味着缩短生命。制定关于 cDCD 临终关怀的国际指南将大有裨益。

## 5.6 DCD 肺恢复手术

与 DBD 相比，除了心脏已经停止跳动外，DCD 肺保存和恢复的手术技术没有显著差异。最近发表了关于供者心肺获取的 ISHLT 共识声明，对 DBD 和 DCD 的技术进行了描述[32]。建议在 WLST 时使用鼻胃管进行胃减压，以避免拔管后出现气道误吸。根据特定国家的法律，CA 后必须有一定的停滞期（3 分钟、5 分钟或 20 分钟），以符合死亡供体规则并排除自动复苏的可能性。胸骨正中切开术后，心前包膜和两侧胸膜被广泛打开。肺部会发生塌陷，可使用冷盐水进行局部降温。通过横切右心耳或下腔静脉，将充血的右心排出。需使用大口径引流管以引流静脉血并为肝脏减压。然后将气管插管插入肺动脉（pulmonary artery，PA），并在 PA 周围用荷包绳或结扎固定。也可以通过切开右心室流出道插入插管，并通过肺动脉瓣插入 PA 插管，以防心脏没有储存瓣膜。然后将插管拔出，并连接至肺静脉冲洗管。可以通过三通管将大量前列腺溶液直接注射到 PA 中。随后开始用 60 mL/kg 冷低钾右旋糖酐溶液顺行冲洗，横断左心耳使左心排气，同时重新为双肺通气，以确保保存溶液均匀分布。此时的支气管镜检查可确保所有肺叶完全扩张，然后可以在冲洗结束时在放气的同时仔细对肺部进行检查和触诊。心脏切除后可以通过 4 个肺静脉进行逆行冲洗，同时使肺部重新通气。或者首先，切除心肺块在后操作台上分离，然后进行逆行肺冲洗。

通常，在 DCD 取材过程中，肺移植的批准和接受要晚于 DBD 供体，因为后者在 CA 之前就已经可以对肺进行粗略评估和接受。如有疑问，可以通过离体肺灌注（ex-vivo lung perfusion，EVLP）进一步评估肺供体质量，详见下文。

cDCD 和 uDCD 肺恢复的实践在很大程度上因机构而异，并且始终需要符合现有的伦理和法律框架。

### 5.6.1 可控型供体

cDCD 的肺部标准通常可以在计划的手术前提前几个小时进行检查。不同国家和机构在 WLST 的位置（ICU 与 OR）、死前给予肝素、拔除气管插管、安慰治疗的实施、监测心脏活动、"无接触"期的时长、死亡宣告的时间以及死亡证明的法律要求上各不相同[33]。

在许多国家，WLST 是在有死亡认证的 ICU 中进行。然而在比利时，WLST 是在手术室或在重症监护医师或麻醉师的监督下进行的（图 5-1）。只要有要求，捐献者的亲属就可以进入手术室。捐献者死亡由 3 名未参与移植过程的独立医生证明。这种做法由于避免了额外的运输和供体铺巾时间，因此减少了心脏收缩期的总长度。

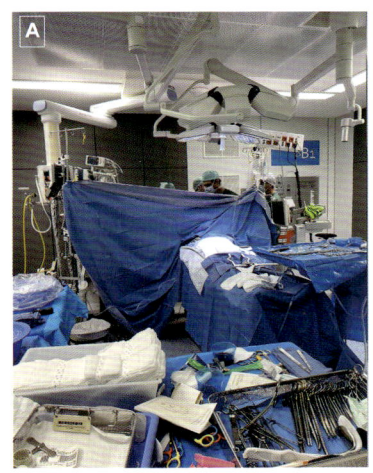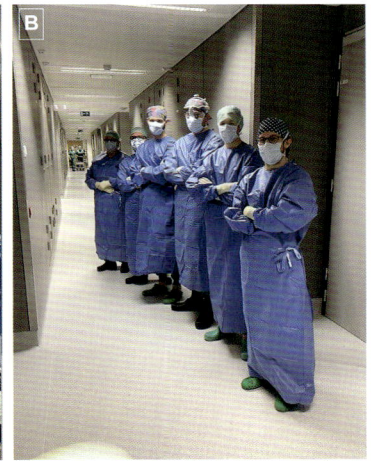

图 5-1　在比利时鲁汶从 cDCD 中取出多器官的手术室场景，捐献者已经完全准备好并披上了手术服

注：麻醉师确保滴定安慰疗法，（A）洗刷干净的取材团队正在手术室外等待 WLST 后心跳停止；（B）规定 5 分钟内不得接触捐献者，直到 3 名医生分别证实死亡后才可以开始手术

在 ISHLT DCD 登记处对欧洲、北美和澳大利亚的 22 个参与机构的 DCD 过程，1090 例 DCD 肺移植进行最大规模研究，发现其相关实践存在很大差异，包括肝素（53%）、皮质类固醇（58%）、纤溶药物（0.2%）、拔管（91%）、存在鼻胃管（62%）以及使用 EVLP（15%）移植后取出[34]。迄今为止，尚没有大型研究比较不同 cDCD 方案对 LTx 后的结果。

### 5.6.2 不可控型供体

与 cDCD 相比，uDCD 中因为没有手术室以及随时可用的工作人员，心脏复苏失败后的心跳停止与通过冷冲洗灌注保存之间的心脏停搏期将会更长。

不同的从死亡宣告后到肺恢复期间保护死者体内肺部免受热缺血性损伤的措施包括：隆德小组[35]和马德里小组[8]通过胸腔引流管插入冷溶液进行局部肺冷却，米兰小组[36]进行死后肺泡复张操作，以及多伦多小组[11]使用持续气道正压通气。在全球范围内 uDCD LTx 的经验仍然有限，评估不同技术对结果的影响有待进一步的研究。

## 5.7 死后肺移植前的质量评估

### 5.7.1 使用 EVLP 进行异位肺评估和保存

对于标准 cDCD LTx 患者使用移植前 EVLP 的确切作用仍不清楚。在 ISHLT DCD 登记的最大报告中，仅 15% 的病例使用了 EVLP，主要在 1 个机构进行[34]。在临终期短的总 WIT 病例中，证明供体肺在恢复时表现正常不一定需要使用 EVLP 进行 LTx 肺功能评估。Machuca 及其同事比较了 2007—2013 年间 55 例 cDCD 接受 LTx 后的结果，发现其中有 EVLP ($n=28$) 和无 EVLP ($n=27$) 之间生存率没有显著差异。然而，cDCD 联合 EVLP 病例的住院时间较短（中位数 18 天 vs. 23 天，$P=0.047$），机械通气的住院时间有缩短的趋势（2 天 vs. 3 天，$P=0.059$）[37]。对多伦多最近更新的 372 例 EVLP 病例多年来标准 cDCD[82%（40/49）]和高风险 cDCD[63%（69/109）]的肺利用率进行了比较[38]。结果显示在器官评估时没有明显问题的 DCD 肺移植中使用 EVLP 并不是常规做法，主要由外科医生自行决定。相比之下，对于扩展标准 DCD（包括 WLST 后 1 小时内未停止的供体）和不可控型 DCD 供体，EVLP 可能是移植安全又有用的要求。Bozoso 及其同事发布了一种选定 EVLP 使用的算法，认为它可以安全地增加 DCD 肺的使用[39]。尽管 EVLP 增加 DCD 肺供体使用似乎是合理的，但成本和资源利用率的相应增加可能会使 EVLP 令许多移植中心望而却步。

与 cDCD 相比，在移植前必须使用 EVLP 对 uDCD 肺进行评估，因为在恢复前无法获得有关肺移植功能和性能的信息。此外，在长时间的供体复苏和长时间的心脏停搏期间可能会发生严重的肺损伤。马德里小组描述了一种通过单次肺血冲洗对气体交换进行原位评估的技术[8]。同时，该小组还报告了在移植前使用肺装置对肺移植物进行原位评估和修复[9,40]。

### 5.7.2 常温区域灌注期间的原位肺评估和保存

事实证明，以简单冷藏作为DBD金标准的快速恢复对于保存DCD捐献者的腹部器官来说并不是最佳选择[15,16]。使用原位常温局部灌注（normothermic regional perfusion，NRP）和体外膜肺氧合（ECMO）技术进行DCD器官的恢复和保存正在整个欧洲慢慢得到采用[41]。因此，目前WLST后cDCD器官检索的做法可能在未来几年发生很大变化。

如果NRP仅限于腹部器官（abdominal NRP，A-NRF），肺部可以保留在温暖的胸膜腔中直至恢复。在此期间保护肺部的两种方法如下。首先，在持续腹部NRP期间，可以通过精心护理胸部止血来快速冲洗和切除肺部[42]。Santander[43]和Madrid[44]小组在一个病例系列中报告，采用这种技术进行LTx后取得了良好结果。或在等待腹部NRP完成时，可以通过插入胸膜腔的胸腔引流管对肺部进行局部冷却。其次，根据米兰小组[45,46]的报告，在腹部NRP期间通过原位保护性通气可以将肺保存在死者体内。

就胸腹NRP（thoracoabdominal NRP，TA-NRP）而言，其目的是重启停止跳动的心脏以进行DCD心脏移植[47]。一旦心脏恢复足够的心输出量，就可以断开ECMO，患者会变成有心跳的供体。这时，器官可以从WLST后最初的热缺血性损伤中复苏，并且可以按照类似于DBD的标准方式重新评估其功能，肺将以顺行冷冲洗灌注的标准方式进行保存。但迄今为止，关于TANRP捐献者肺移植的报道一直是传闻[48,49]。

NRP的使用引发了一系列关注和伦理问题，包括可能违反死亡供体规则原则、通过循环和呼吸功能永久或不可逆停止定义循环死亡，以及故意阻塞脑循环导致脑死亡[50,51]。非常重要的是，完成器官原位NRP的方法必须排除脑灌注的恢复，以免无法有效确定死亡。器官捐献死亡的统一概念要求脑循环永远停止，从而导致脑功能永久停止[52]。因此，在NRP期间监测脑灌注或功能的缺失是此类方案的重要组成部分。在A-NRP和TA-NRP期间用于将大脑与循环隔离的技术已有描述[53]。

## 5.8 DCD LTx 的结局

### 5.8.1 可控型供体

在过去的 10 年中，许多研究小组报告了他们的单中心 cDCD 经验。在大多数研究中，结果都与 DBD 的 LTx 进行了比较。Ceulemans 及其同事在之前的一篇综述中列出了截至 2019 年发表的最大规模研究的摘要[3]。总体而言，研究结果令人满意，大多数研究证实，cDCD LTx 后的结果在 PGD、总生存率和慢性肺同种异体移植物功能障碍（chronic lung allograft dysfunction，CLAD）生存期方面与 DBD 相当。

最大的研究于 2019 年由 ISHLT 胸部移植登记处发布，分析了来自欧洲、北美和澳大利亚的 22 个多中心提交的 DCD 数据[34]。研究队列包括 11 516 例 LTx，其中 1090 例（9.5%）是具有完整数据的 DCD-LTx，马斯特里赫特 Ⅲ 类 DCD 占 DCD 队列的 94.1%。在参与的中心中，每年进行 DCD-LTx 的比例从 2003 年的 0.6% 增加至 2016 年的 13.5%，从 WLST 到心跳停止的中位间隔时间为 15 分钟 [四分位距（interquartile range，IQR），11～22 分钟]，到冷冲洗的时间间隔为 32 分钟（IQR，26～41 分钟）（图 5-2）。与 DBD 相比，DCD 的供体年龄更高，分别为 46 岁（IQR，34～55 岁）和 40 岁（IQR，24～52 岁），双侧 LTx 进行的频率更高（88.3% vs. 76.6%），且受者更多有慢性阻塞性肺疾病或肺气肿作为移植指征。两者的 5 年生存率相当（63% vs. 61%；$P=0.72$）（图 5-3）。在多变量分析中，受者和供者的年龄、适应证诊断、手术类型（单次 LTx 与双侧/双 LTx）和移植年份（2003—2009 年 vs. 2010—2016 年）与生存率独立相关（所有 $P<0.001$）；但供体类型（DCD 与 DBD）则不然，风险比（hazard ratio，HR）为 1.04（0.90～1.19；$P=0.61$）。在 2019 年 ISHLT 登记处对 10 年死亡率风险因素的分析中，接受 DCD 捐献者与 10 年结果改善显著相关（$HR=0.65$；$P<0.01$）[1]。

迄今为止，已有 2 篇已发表数据的系统综述和荟萃分析报道。Krutsinger 及其同事于 2015 年发表的第一项研究中，对 11 项观察性队列研究进行了分析，其中 6 项符合荟萃分析的纳入标准[54]。在心脏死亡器官捐献（cDCD, $n=271$）与脑死亡器官捐献（DBD, $n=2369$）两组间，1 年死亡率无显著差异，相对风险（RR）为 0.88 [95% 置信区间（CI）：0.59～1.31；$P=0.52$；异质性（$I^2$）$=0$]。在对 5 项报告 PGD 的研究 [$RR=1.09$；95%$CI$: 0.68～1.73；$P=0.7$；$I^2=0$] 和 4 项报告急性排斥反应的研究（$RR=0.72$；95%$CI$: 0.49～1.05；$P=0.09$；$I^2=0$）进行的汇总分析中，cDCD 和 DBD 之间没有差异。Palleschi 及同事于 2020

# 第5章 肺移植心脏死亡后的捐献

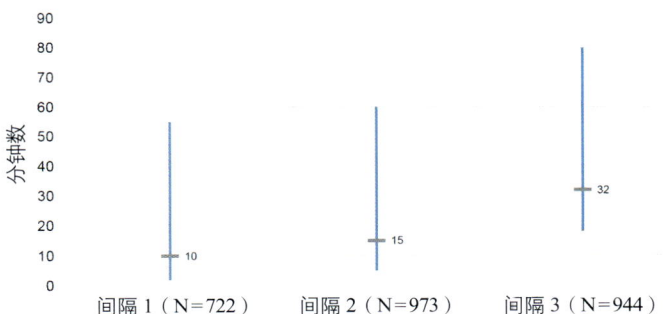

图 5-2 2003 年 1 月 1 日至 2017 年 6 月 30 日 DCD 肺移植中 DCD 过程的时间间隔分布

注：间隔 1= 从 WLST 到临终期开始的时间（由收缩压 < 50 mmHg 确定）；间隔 2= 从 WLST 到心输出量/心搏停止的时间；间隔 3= 从 WLST 到肺开始冷冲洗灌注的时间。水平线 = 中位数；竖条 = 第 5 到第 95 个百分位。来自 Van Raemdonck D, Keshavjee S, Levvey B, et al. Donation after circulatory death in lung transplantation - five-year follow-up from ISHLT Registry. J Heart Lung Transplant 2019;38:1235-45；经许可引用

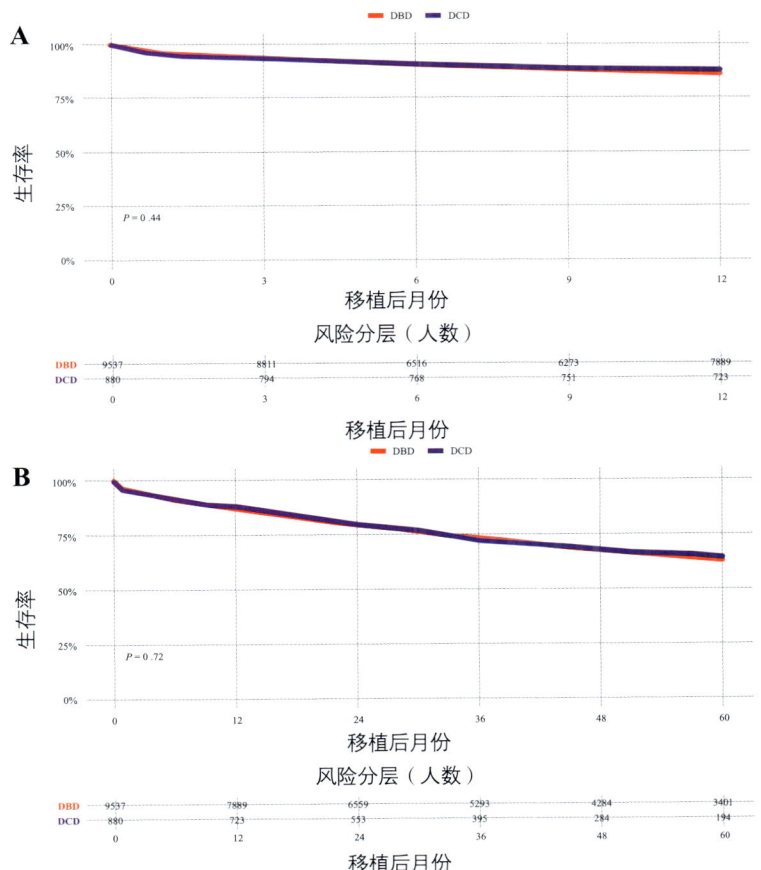

图 5-3 DCD 组与 DBD 组的移植后 1 年生存率（A）和 5 年生存率（B）

注：计算 2003 年 1 月至 2016 年 6 月期间进行的肺移植存活率，并且 DCD 组仅纳入马斯特里赫特Ⅲ类。来自 Van Raemdonck D, Keshavjee S, Levvey B, et al. Donation after circulatory death in lung transplantation - five-year follow-up from ISHLT Registry. J Heart Lung Transplant 2019;38:1235-45；经许可引用

年发表的第二项研究中,对 9 项观察性队列研究进行了分析,涉及 403 例 cDCD 和 2570 例 DBD 患者[55]。DBD 与 cDCD 的 1 年生存率($n=8$)和 5 年生存率($n=5$)的比值比分别为:1.00(95%$CI$:0.70~1.44;$P=0.973$;$I^2=19.2\%$)和 0.57(95%$CI$:0.43~0.76;$P<0.001$;$I^2=0$);2~3 级 PGD($n=7$)的 RR 为 1.03(95%$CI$:0.74~1.44;$P=0.867$;$I^2=0$);1 年无 CLAD 生存率($n=6$)的 RR 为 0.57(95%$CI$:0.19~1.72;$P=0.321$;$I^2=34.1\%$)。有趣的是,cDCD-LTx($n=6$)后观察到更多气道并发症($RR=2.07$;95%$CI$:1.09~3.94;$P=0.026$;$I^2=0$)。

总之,在观察性队列研究中,cDCD LTx 后的生存率与 DBD LTx 后的生存率相当。在气道并发症方面还需要进一步研究。cDCD 可能是扩大供体库安全有效的方法。

### 5.8.2 不可控型供体

uDCD-LTx 后的研究数据结果要少得多。在马德里小组的早期经验中,观察到的 PGD-3 发生率比预期更高(38%)和生存率更低(3 个月生存率为 78%,1 年生存率为 68%,5 年生存率为 51%)[8]。在其最新的 2002—2012 年间的论文结果中,对 DBD($n=292$)与 uDCD($n=38$)的结果进行了比较[9],除了性别不匹配(DBD 中男性受者女性供者为 17.8%,uDCD 中为 0%,$P<0.002$)、总缺血时间(DBD 中取出第一个肺和第二个肺分别为 309 分钟和 425 分钟,uDCD 中为 657 分钟和 822 分钟,$P<0.001$)和离体评估(分别为 1.4% 和 21.1%,$P<0.001$)外,两组结果相当。早期和晚期结局没有差异[ICU 住院时间分别为 9 天和 10.5 天、住院时间分别为 33.5 天和 35 天、PGD-3 分别为 24% 和 34.2%,CLAD($HR=1.19$;95%$CI$:0.61~2.32)],但 uDCD 移植患者的总体生存率较低($HR=1.67$;95%$CI$:1.06~2.64)。作者得出结论,uDCD-LTx 的生存率较低。

桑坦德小组[10]于 2019 年发表了他们使用 9 例 uDCD 中的 8 例 LTx 经验,平均无血流时间为(9.8±8.6)分钟。从心跳停止到局部冷却的时间为(96.8±16.8)分钟,保存时间为(159±31)分钟,在 LTx 前进行 EVLP 肺功能的评估患者仅 2 例,总缺血时间为(678±132)分钟,2 例(25%)PGD 3 级,1 个月、1 年和 5 年生存率分别为 100%、87.5% 和 87.5%。

多伦多小组[11]于 2020 年报告了北美第一个 5 uDCD LTx 研究。在 44 例潜在捐献者中,30 例(68%)获得了家属同意,16 例进行了现场评估,14 例在等待肺移植中进行了 EVLP 评估,EVLP 利用率为 35.7%。采用简单的原位肺充气法以防止热缺血损伤,平均时间为 2.8 小时。发现移植后 24、48 或 72 小时未观察到 PGD-3,中位 ICU 住院时间为 5 天（2~78 天），中位住院时间为 17 天（8~100 天）。30 天死亡率为 0。5 例患者中的 4 例达到平均存活时间为 651 天（121~1254 天），肺功能保存完好。这项研究概念验证并证明了通过简单的干预进行 uDCD 肺捐献的潜力。

总之，从 uDCD 中进行器官回收的工作具有挑战性。简单的供体干预和原位肺充气可有效地在心脏停搏期间保护肺部。与 cDCD 和 DBD 相比，uDCD-LTx 后的生存率似乎较低。然而，随着原位保存技术的改进和移植前肺移植物的异位评估，以及未来几年更多经验的积累，其生存率有望提高。

## 5.9 DCD LTx 的障碍

心脏死亡后的器官捐献在许多地区具有巨大潜力[56,57]。然而，人们已经认识到影响 DCD 机构的一些障碍，包括缺乏国家伦理、专业和法律框架来解决公众和专业人士对 DCD 途径各个方面的担忧。最近，一份国际合作声明的发布，旨在扩大 cDCD 器官在全球的使用[52]。该声明涉及 3 个基本方面：①描述了 WLST 公平性的确切预后过程，该决定应在器官捐献之前，并独立于任何器官捐赠考虑，且移植专业人员不得参与；②脑循环永久停止是判定心脏死亡的标准。观察 5 分钟后如果大脑没有循环，则可以宣布死亡，证实大脑循环的停止是永久的；③强调了灌注修复对于提高 cDCD 器官移植成功率的价值，无论各国实施的 cDCD 方案是进行原位或异位灌注。

此外，在现有 DCD 立法的国家中，cDCD 的器官产量比 DBD 低得多。有几个因素可以解释这种差异：直到现在人们还认为 DCD 的心脏无法成功移植，担心有额外的热缺血性损伤相关的器官质量下降，此外，还存在一种不确定性，即心脏死亡器官捐献（cDCD）可能在撤除生命支持治疗（WLST）后的预期时间内未出现心脏停搏。供体评分系统能够可靠地预测心搏停止的进展情况，或者根据肺质量、缺血时间等指标来预测早期移植物功能，这对于增加成功康复和移植的信心具有非凡的意义[58]。

大型审计工作表明，仍有大量未开发的 DCD 肺库，可能会进一步大幅增加肺移植数量。在一项回顾性图表审查中，弗吉尼亚大学的校长和同事分析了一家乡村转诊医院发生肺 DCD 的可能性，对 2014 年 8 月至 2015 年 6 月期间的所有院内死亡病例进行了分析。在总共 857 例死亡患者中，有 85 例符合 DCD 肺捐献条件[59]。不同地区和国家之间的肺产量也存在很大差异。尽管美国肺移植的总体利用率相对较高［2018 年：每百万人口（per million population，PMP）中有 7.8 名肺捐献者，澳大利亚为 8.9 名，英国为 2.8 名，荷兰为 5.2 名，西班牙为 8.0 名，比利时为 10.1 名］。然而，美国 DCD 肺的捐献率很低（2018 年：PMP 为 0.4，而澳大利亚为 2.3，英国为 0.6，荷兰为 1.8，西班牙为 1.4，比利时为 2.6）[60]。根据 2005—2019 年美国器官共享联合网络的数据，最近的一项研究调查了不使用 DCD 肺的预测因素[61]。在 30 916 个 DCD 肺中，只有 3.7%（1158 个）用于移植，72.8% 主要由于器官功能不良而被丢弃。在 8.4% 的案例中未要求获得同意，其中心脏死亡后捐献（DCD）是主要原因，占比达 73.4%。作者的结论是，丢弃率与捐献前因素（包括同意器官获取组织的行为）有关，这是潜在可改变的，以及捐献者因素（包括低氧血症）。增加患者同意和标准化 DCD 供体管理的干预措施（包括在低氧血症情况下选择性使用 EVLP），可能会增加 DCD 肺的使用。

DCD 肺供体的管理问题同样重要。EVLP 作为评估和肺复苏工具以及供体肺质量的生物标志物在临床领域都具有未来前景[62]。

uDCD 的阻碍在于物流后勤和伦理法律性质，以及人们对 uDCD 捐献者的移植结果缺乏信心。该步骤设计需要减少 uDCD 过程中固有的长时间热缺血影响，并处理其带来的伦理问题：终止高级救生心肺复苏与仅为了器官保存而延长支持、家庭捐献讨论的最佳时机、死亡判定标准或使用 NRP 进行器官原位保存的问题。

## 5.10 总　结

由于潜在 DBD 的肺移植持续短缺，人们对来自 DCD 的肺再次产生了兴趣。全球范围内使用可控型 DCD 肺移植的经验最多，而使用不可控型 DCD 肺移植的经验目前仅限于小型系列研究。在大型 ISHLT DCD 注册中心和两项系统性回顾和荟萃分析中，并未发现 DBD 与 cDCD-LTx 的结果有明显差异。

相较于其他 DCD 器官，供体肺不太容易受到冷热缺血过程的影响，而冷热缺血会威胁到其他 DCD 器官的存活。在 cDCD 中使用 NRP 进行原位肺保存，或在 uDCD 中使用肺泡募集，以及使用 EVLP 进行原位复苏和评估的新技术已经可用来在移植前选择质量良好的供体肺。

目前，仍有大量未开发的 DCD 肺库，它们可能会进一步大幅增加 LTx 的数量。人们已经认识到，一些潜在的可改变的障碍影响了来自 DCD 的器官的使用，包括缺乏国家伦理、专业和法律框架来解决公众和专业人员的担忧。如果想提高未充分利用的肺捐献者供体库的潜力，许多国家需要进一步努力解决 DCD 途径的这些方面的问题。

【临床护理要点】

- 来自 DCD 的供体肺应根据与目前用于 DBD 相同的标准和扩展标准进行选择。
- 来自 cDCD 的肺应始终由器官移植获取组织提供，并最大限度地由现场团队进行评估。
- 与从 cDCD 中获取腹部器官相比，不必要急于取肺。良好的抽吸装置和剪刀，是外科医生在安全引入肺动脉插管并在肺麻痹开始时为左心排气所需的唯一工具。取出后可以在后操作台上对肺部进行彻底检查。
- 如有疑问，可以通过 EVLP 进一步评估肺质量，以增加受体的信心。
- DCD 肺的交叉钳夹时间预计会稍长一些，因为无论是否使用 EVLP，最终接受移植都发生在取材过程的较晚阶段。

## 声明

D.Van Raemdonck 获得了 Broere 慈善基金会的支持。L.J.Ceulemans 获得了美敦力（Medtronic）资助的鲁汶大学指定主席以及鲁汶大学医院（KOOR）授予的博士后研究奖学金的支持。A.Neyrinck 获得了 KU Leuven 大学 C2 研究经费的支持。D.Van Raemdonck 和 G.Snell 设计了本章并撰写了初稿。该领域的专家 L.J.Ceulemans、A.Neyrinck 和 B.Levvey 对原始手稿进行了审阅。所有作者都批准了最终版本的发布。

# 参考文献

1. Chambers DC, Zuckermann A, Cherikh WS, et al. The International Thoracic Organ Transplant Registry of the International Society for Heart and Lung Transplantation: 37th adult lung transplantation report 2020; focus on deceased donor characteristics. J Heart Lung Transplant 2020;39:1016–1027.
2. Van Raemdonck D, Ceulemans LJ, Neyrinck A. Donor selection and management. In: Christie JD, editor. Chapter 11. Lung Transplant. 2nd edition. In: Janes S, editor. Encyclopedia of respiratory medicine. 2nd edition. Academic Press; 2021.
3. Ceulemans LJ, Inci I, Van Raemdonck D. Lung donation after circulatory death. Curr Opin Organ Transpl 2019;24:288–296.
4. Kootstra G, Daemen JH, Oomen AP. Categories of non-heart-beating donors. Transpl Proc 1995;27: 2893–2894.
5. Evrard, Belgian Working Group on DCD National Protocol. Belgian modified classification of Maastricht for

donors after circulatory death. Transpl Proc 2014;46:3138–3142.

6. Thuong M, Ruiz A, Evrard P, et al. New classification of donation after circulatory death donors definitions and terminology. Transpl Int 2016;29:749–759.
7. Orens J, Boehler A, de Perrot M, et al. A review of lung transplant donor acceptability criteria. J Heart Lung Transpl 2003;22:1183–1200.
8. Gomez-de-Antonio D, Campo-Canaveral JL, Crowley S, et al. Clinical lung transplantation from uncontrolled nonheart-beating donors revisited. J Heart Lung Transpl 2012;31:349–353.
9. Valdivia D, Gomez de Antonio D, Hoyoz L, et al. Expanding the horizons: uncontrolled donors after circulatory death for lung transplantation – first comparison with brain death donors. Clin Transplant 2019;33:e13561.
10. Suberviola B, Mons R, Ballesteros MA, et al. Excellent long-term outcome with lungs obtained from uncontrolled donation after circulatory death. Am J Transplant 2019;19:1195–1201.
11. Healey A, Watanabe Y, Milis C, et al. Initial lung transplantation experience with uncontrolled donation after cardiac death in North America. Am J Transplant 2020;20:1574–1581.
12. Musso V, Mendogni P, Scaravilli V, et al. Extended-criteria uncontrolled DCD donor for a fragile recipient:a case report about a challenging yet successful lung transplantation. Int J Surg Case Rep 2020;77S(Suppl):S67–71.
13. Palleschi A, Rosso L, Ruggeri GM, et al. Overcoming the limits of reconditioning: seventeen hours of ex-vivo lung perfusion (EVLP) with successful transplantation from uncontrolled circulatory death donor. Transplantation 2021;105(12):2620–2624.
14. Egan TM, Lambert CJ Jr, Reddick R, et al. A strategy to increase the donor pool: use of cadaver lungs for transplantation. Ann Thorac Surg 1991;52:1113–1120.
15. Heylen L, Jochmans I, Samuel U, et al. The duration of asystolic ischemia determines the risk of graft failure after circulatory-dead donor kidney transplantation: a Eurotransplant cohort study. Am J Transplant 2018;18:881–889.
16. Coffey JC, Wanis KN, Monbaliu D, et al. The influence of functional warm ischemia time on DCD liver transplant recipients' outcomes. Clin Transplant 2017;31.
17. Song C, Al-Mehdi AB, Fisher AB. An immediate endothelial cell signaling response to lung ischemia. Am J Physiol Lung Cell Mol Physiol 2001;281: L993–1000.
18. Cypel M, Levvey B, Van Raemdonck D, et al. International Society for Heart and Lung Transplantation donation after circulatory death registry report. J Heart Lung Transpl 2015;34:1278–1282.
19. Levvey B, Keshavjee S, Cypel M, et al. Influence of lung donor agonal and warm ischemic times on early mortality: analyses from the ISHLT DCD Lung Transplant Registry. J Heart Lung Transpl 2019;38:26–34.
20. Qaqish R, Watanabe Y, Hoetzenecker K, et al. Impact of donor time to cardiac arrest in lung donation after circulatory death. J Thorac Cardiovasc Surg 2021;161:1546–1555.
21. Reeb J, Keshavjee S, Cypel M. Successful lung transplantation from a donation after cardiocirculatory death donor taking more than 120 min to cardiac arrest after withdrawal of life support therapies. J Heart Lung Transpl 2016;35:258–259.
22. Donahoe LL, Kato T, Healey A, et al. Successful lung transplantation from lungs procured 12 hours after

withdrawal of life-sustaining therapy: changing the paradigm of controlled DCD donors? J Heart Lung Transpl 2021;40:1021.

23. Okahara S, Levvey B, McDonald M, et al. An audit of lung donor pool: optimal current donation strategies and the potential of novel time-extended donation after circulatory death donation. Heart Lung Circ 2021.

24. Kon AA, Shepard EK, Sederstrom NO, et al. Defining futile and potentially inappropriate interventions: a policy statement from the society of critical care medicine ethics committee. Crit Care Med 2016; 44:1769–1774.

25. Reynolds S, Cooper AB, McKneally M. Withdrawing life-sustaining treatment: ethical considerations. Thorac Surg Clin 2005;15:469–480.

26. Manara A. Bespoke end-of-life decision making in ICU: has the tailor got the right measurements? Crit Care Med 2015;43:909–910.

27. Munshi L, Dhanani S, Shemie SD, et al. Predicting time to death after withdrawal of life-sustaining treatment in potential donors after cardiac death. Crit Care Med 2012;40:1014–1028.

28. Wind J, Snoeijs MGJ, Brugman CA, et al. Prediction of time of death after withdrawal of life-sustaining treatment in potential donors after cardiac death. Crit Care Med 2012;40:766–769.

29. Chan JD, Treece PD, Engelbergh RA, et al. Narcotic and benzodiazepine use after withdrawal of life support: association with time to death. Chest 2004;126: 286–293.

30. Epker JL, Bakker J, Kompanje EJ. The use of opioids and sedatives and time until death after withdrawing mechanical ventilation and vasoactive drugs in a dutch intensive care unit. Anesth Analg 2011;112:628–634.

31. Ledoux D, Delbouille MH, Deroover A, et al. Does comfort therapy during controlled donation after circulatory death shorten the life of potential donors? Clin Transpl 2014;28:47–51.

32. Copeland H, Hayanga JWA, Neyrinck A, et al. Donor heart and lung procurement: a consensus statement. J Heart Lung Transpl 2020;39:501–517.

33. Gardiner D, Wind T, Cole B, et al. European vignettes in donation after circulatory death. Prog Transpl 2017;27:286–290.

34. Van Raemdonck D, Keshavjee S, Levvey B, et al. Donation after circulatory death in lung transplantation-five-year follow-up from ISHLT registry. J Heart Lung Transpl 2019;38:1235–1245.

35. Steen S, Sjöberg T, Pierre L, et al. Transplantation of lungs from a nonheart-beating donor. Lancet 2001; 357:825–829.

36. Valenza F, Citerio G, Palleschi A, et al. Successful transplantation of lungs from an uncontrolled donor after circulatory death preserved in situ by alveolar recruitment maneuvers and assessed by ex vivo lung perfusion. Am J Transplant 2016;16:1312–1318.

37. Machuca TN, Mercier O, Collaud S, et al. Lung transplantation with donation after circulatory determination of death donors and the impact of ex vivo lung perfusion. Am J Transplant 2015;15:993–1002.

38. Cypel M, Yeung JC, Donahoe L, et al. Normothermic ex vivo lung perfusion: does the indication impact organ utilization and patient outcomes after transplantation? J Thorac Cardiovasc Surg 2020;159: 346–355.

39. Bozso SJ, Nagendran J. Life after death: breathing life into lung transplantation from donation after circulatory death donors. Am J Transplant 2017;17: 2507–2508.

40. Moradiellos J, Naranjo JM, Cordoba M, et al. Clinical lung transplantation after ex vivo evaluation of

uncontrolled non heart-beating donor lungs: initial experience. J Heart Lung Transpl 2011;30:S38.

41. O'Neill S, Srinivasa S, Callaghan CJ, et al. Novel organ perfusion and preservation strategies in transplantation where are we going in the UK? Transplantation 2020;104:1813–1824.
42. Oniscu GC, Siddique A, Dark J. Dual temperature multi-organ recovery from a Maastricht category III donor after circulatory death. Am J Transplant 2014;14:2181.
43. Miñambres E, Ruiz P, Ballesteros MA, et al. Combined lung and liver procurement in controlled donation after circulatory death using normothermic abdominal perfusion. Initial experience in two Spanish centers. Am J Transplant 2020;20:231–240.
44. Tanaka S, Luis Campo-Cañaveral de la Cruz J, Crowley Carrasco S, et al. Effect on the donor lungs of using abdominal normothermic regional perfusion in controlled donation after circulatory death. Eur J Cardiothorac Surg 2021;60:590–597.
45. Palleschi A, Tosi D, Rosso L, et al. Successful preservation and transplant of warm ischemic lungs from donors after circulatory death by prolonged in situ ventilation during normothermic regional perfusion of abdominal organs. Interact Cardiovasc Surg 2019;29:699–705.
46. Zanierato M, Dondossola P, Palleschi A, et al. Donation after circulatory death: possible strategies for insitu organ preservation. Minerva Anesthesiol 2020; 86:984–991.
47. Tsui SSL, Oniscu GC. Extending normothermic regional perfusion to the thorax in donors after circulatory death. Curr Opin Organ Transpl 2017;22: 245–250.
48. Vandendriessche K, Tchana-Sato V, Ledoux D, et al. Transplantation of donor hearts after circulatory death using normothermic regional perfusion and cold storage preservation. Eur J Cardiothorac Surg 2021; 60(4):813–819.
49. Urban M, Castleberry AW, Markin NW, et al. Successful lung transplantation with graft recovered after thoracoabdominal normothermic perfusion from donor after circulatory death. Am J Transplant 2021. https://doi.org/10.1111/ajt.16806.
50. American College of Physicians. Ethics, determination of death, and organ transplantation in normothermic regional perfusion (NRP) with controlled donation after circulatory determination of death (cDCD): American College of Physicians statement of concern. Available at: https://www.acponline.org/acp_policy/policies/ethics_determination_of_death_and_organ_transplantation_in_nrp_2021.pdf. Accessed July 21, 2021.
51. McGee A, Gardiner D, Murphy P. Determination of death in donation after circulatory death: an ethical propriety. Curr Opin Organ Transpl 2018;23:114–119.
52. Dominguez-Gil B, Ascher N, Capron AM, et al. Expanding controlled donation after the circulatory determination of death: statement from an international collaborative. Intensive Care Med 2021;47: 265–281.
53. Manara A, Shemie SD, Large S, et al. Maintaining the permanence principle for death during in situ normothermic regional perfusion for donation after circulatory death organ recovery: a United Kingdom and Canadian proposal. Am J Transplant 2020;20: 2017–2025.
54. Krutsinger D, Reed RM, Blevins A, et al. Lung transplantation from donation after cardiocirculatory death: a systematic review and meta-analysis. J Heart Lung Transpl 2015;34:675–684.
55. Palleschi A, Rosso L, Musso V, et al. Lung transplantation from donation after controlled cardiocirculatory

death. Systematic review and meta-analysis. Transpl Rev (Orlando) 2020;34:100513.
56. Smith M, Dominguez-Gil B, Greer DM, et al. Organ donation after circulatory death: current status and future potential. Intensive Care Med 2019;45: 310–321.
57. Rakhra SS, Opdam HI, Gladkis L, et al. Untapped potential in Australian hospitals for organ donation after circulatory death. Med J Aust 2017;207: 294–301.
58. Okahara S, Levvey B, McDonald M, et al. Improving the predictability of time to death in controlled donation after circulatory death lung donors. Transpl Int 2021;34:906–915.
59. Chancellor WZ, Charles EJ, Mehaffey JH, et al. Expanding the donor lung pool: how many donations after circulatory death organs are we missing? J Surg Res 2018;223:58–63.
60. European Directorate for the Quality of Medicines & Health Care. Newsletter Transplant. International figures on donation and transplantation 2018, vol. 24, 2019. Available at: https://www. edqm. eu/en/news/just-released-newsletter-transplant-2019. Accessed July 21, 2021.
61. Choi AY, Jawitz OK, Raman V, et al. Predictors of nonuse of donation after circulatory death lung allografts. J Thorac Cardiovasc Surg 2021;161:458–466.
62. Snell GI, Levvey BJ, Levin K, et al. Donation after brain death versus donation after circulatory death: lung donor management issues. Semin Respir Crit Care Med 2018;39:138–147.

# 第6章 建立集中化供体器官获取和分配中心

Amit Bery, Aadil Ali, Marcelo Cypel, Daniel Kreisel  著

孙昊  译

周建平  校

【关键词】
- 肺移植  • 器官捐献  • 专门的供体护理机构  • 体外肺灌注

【要点】
- 与传统模型相比，SDCF 模式提供了高效、经济的供体管理和器官获取，从而提高了捐献器官产量，缩短了捐献器官缺血时间。
- SDCF 模式缩短了获取供体器官的进程、增加了日间移植手术量，提高了器官获取过程的安全性，减轻了外科医生的倦怠。
- 离体肺灌注（EVLP）可提高扩大标准供肺的使用率，目前正在研究该技术能否通过抗炎、抗细胞死亡及抗病毒等干预措施在移植前更好地预处理供肺。
- 集中的 EVLP 机构具有增加移植量和在特定地理区域的小型移植中心扩大标准供体器官的利用率的潜力。

## 6.1 引　言

肺移植（LTx）是治疗终末期肺部疾病的唯一治疗选择。在过去的 10 年里，肺移植手术的数量增加了 50%，肺供体的数量增加了 60%[1]。尽管供体管理和器官分配系统都有所改善，但器官移植等待者的死亡率仍然很高[1]。这些挑战使人们更加关注提高器官移植的效率和减少器官供体管理的成本。这种日益增加的关注导致了两种独立的供体管理和捐献器官获取模式的建立：传统的模式和标准化供体护理中心（specialized donor care facility，SDCF）模式[2-4]。

传统上，脑死亡供体是由宣布脑死亡诊断的医院在该区域器官获取组织（organ

# 第6章 建立集中化供体器官获取和分配中心

procurement organization，OPO）的帮助下来管理的[3-5]。在这个模式中，往往给予脑死亡供体较低的优先级，导致评估、管理和术间协调等方面的延迟[3,4,6]。供体器官获取的日程安排需要与移植中心的外科医生团队协调，而这些团队可能会来自多个医院，因此会导致供体器官获取延误[3]。供体器官获取时，移植外科医生必须日夜兼程从器官移植受者所在的医院赶往器官移植供体所在的医院进行器官获取手术。移植外科医生对供体所在医院的设施不甚熟悉，同时供体医院的工作人员也可能缺乏获取供体器官的经验[3,5,7]，这些问题都会导致供体器官获取不理想[3,4]。

中美洲移植中心（MTS，St. Louis，MO），在其移植中心的支持下，于2001年在美国成立了第一个SDCF[4,8]。该中心对最初将32 km范围内的25名血流动力学稳定的供体转移到MTS移植中心总部的手术室（OR）进行了经验的总结和评估，该评估显示与传统模式相比，在器官获取量和移植手术量相当的情况下，SDCF模式成本显著降低[8]。2008年，该中心建立了一个独立的2床位的重症监护病房（ICU），并配备了自己的手术室、组织获取室、心导管套件、实验室和计算机断层扫描仪（CT）。由于脑死亡供体数量的显著增加，2018年建成了一个功能齐备的6个床位的ICU。

在SDCF模式中，一个大规模的中心能够提供高效、及时和高性价比的供体器官管理和供体器官获取。在获得授权后，捐献者会尽早（平均7小时）被转移至标准化供体护理中心（SDCF），并在该中心接受中位时间为36小时的ICU监护。在2000多例脑死亡供体的转移过程中，只有2例心脏骤停发生，证实转运过程是安全的。截至2021年，美国和西班牙、加拿大的12家OPO中心使用了某种形式的SDCF来提供供体护理[9,10]。自2001年以来，有多项研究强调了SDCF模式的好处[4,5,11-14]。

## 6.2 器官获取模式的比较

### 6.2.1 医学专业知识要求

在传统模式中，供体由宣布脑死亡诊断的急症护理医院管理。这些医院的工作人员同时还要照顾各种各样的危重患者，而且他们通常缺乏相应的脑死亡供体的管理经验。这种模式在获取捐献器官时还需要医院手术室工作人员和麻醉医师的配合，但他们可能缺乏供体器官获取方面的经验。

在SDCF模式中，供体协调员在一名接受过危重病护理培训的内科医疗主任的监督下提供重症监护室级别的护理[3,4]。这些供体协调员一般是有 2 年以上 ICU 的护理经验的护士，专门提供供体护理[4]。以在供体管理方面经验丰富的团队为基础，SDCF 可以在器官获取前使用程序化的护理来优化供体，从而避免供体在危重患者多的大型 ICU 中经历护理延迟和变化的情况[4,6]。供体协调员在 SDCF 进行支气管镜检查、肺超声检查、中心/动脉置管和肝脏活检。此外，在供体器官获取手术期间，不需要麻醉医师的参与，而继续由供体协调员负责供体的管理[3]。

### 6.2.2 评估、管理和获取器官

在传统模式中，供体评估需要利用医院资源，进行供体评估的检查检验的顺序和时间需要与其他危重患者协调。

SDCF 模式中，机构可进行心导管检查、支气管镜检查、超声心动图检查、放射学研究（X 线、CT）、血库评估和其他实验室研究[3]。此外，SDCF 会单独雇佣专家顾问（病理学家、放射学家、心脏病学家等）完成对供体的诊断评估。一般来说，单独雇佣的专家顾问可以到现场完成紧急评估，但在某些情况下，也可以通过网络远程评估。因此，SDCF 可以通过将所有"评估要素"集中在现场，从而简化对供体的评估，避免在急症护理医院产生的有限的医疗资源竞争[3,9]。

脑死亡后，供体的生理变化可引起黏液堵塞、肺不张、神经源性肺水肿、负压吸引气道损伤和呼吸机诱导的肺损伤[15-20]。事实上，很大一部分脑死亡的供体会发展为急性肺损伤，阻碍肺利用[5,17,19,21]。一些研究表明，对供体进行程序化的管理可以提高肺的利用率[5,11,14,19,21-23]。SDCF 模式特别适用于制定和实施流程化的供体管理[5,11,14,24-26]。供体协调员使用护理流程来优化供体，而不像急症护理医院传统模式的差异性护理。先前的研究显示，与传统模式相比，SDCF 模式中的平均器官获取量更高，扩大标准供体和药物过量供体的使用也有所增加[4,27]。此外，SDCF ORs 专门用于供体器官的获取，并配备了经验丰富的供体协调员，简化了排期工作，提高了器官获取的效率[3-5]。事实上，已有研究证明随着冷缺血时间减少，供体在 SDCF 处的获取更有效[3]。

### 6.2.3 成本

在获得器官捐献授权后，区域 OPO 将负责供体管理和器官获取的费用。在传统模式中，供体管理在 ICU 时由重症监护医生负责，在手术室器官获取期间由麻醉医师负责。器官获取组织支付供体评估、管理和器官获取的医院费用[4,9]。OPO 随后向移植中心支

付器官获取费用（organ acquisition charge，OAC），其中包含移植后的平均每年供体护理费用[4,9]。

SDCF 模式需要大量的启动成本，用于建立一个能够提供器官护理和进行器官获取的机构。这一成本可通过提高供体护理的效率来抵消。在 SDCF 模式中，所有对供体的评估和管理都可以由供体协调员来完成，减少了对现场医生的需求度，并降低了成本[4,8,9]。此外，在供体器官获取期间进行供体管理，麻醉医师的工作可以由供体协调员来完成，成本进一步得到降低[4,8,9]。事实上，先前对 SDCF 模式的评估显示，与使用传统模式的器官获取组织相比，在 5 年的时间内，器官获取的成本降低了 50% 以上[4]。在此评估中，使用传统模式的器官获取组织显示出器官获取费用增加，而 SDCF 能够在 5 年内维持稳定的器官获取费用[4]。此外，经济模型表明，在美国普遍采用 SDCF 模式可以增加器官移植量，同时显著降低成本[9]。这一发现对胸部器官移植有重大影响，另外，评估调查显示采用 SDCF 模式进行 156 例移植可减少近 2500 万美元的成本[9]。

## 6.3 对外科医生倦怠的影响

高压的手术、长期和不可预测的工作时间、重要的岗位职责以及频繁奔波的工作要求都会导致移植外科医生的情绪疲惫、工作倦怠[28-31]。SDCF 模式解决了一些导致移植外科医生职业倦怠的主要原因[32]。

在传统模式中，多个获取器官小组协调安排手术室时间，并前往供体所在的医院获取器官。前往急症护理医院获取捐献器官会受到不定时、前往偏远地区和各种天气条件的影响。自 1954 年首次肾移植以来，这种器官获取方式一直使器官获取团队面临着重大风险[7,33-35]，已有超过 30 例与出行相关的死亡[3,7,34,35]。在 SDCF 模式中，可以降低与供体器官获取出行相关的风险。在十年间，某中心将其器官获取组织（OPO）捐献服务区域内非本地捐献者的转运需求减少了 93%。此外，尽管大多数器官获取仍是由受体中心的器官获取团队进行，但目前一些中心已经开始利用当地的外科团队进行器官获取。

在 SDCF 模式中，安排供体器官获取操作更有效，让器官获取和随后的移植在白天进行[4,32]。事实上，无论是器官获取手术还是器官移植手术，夜间手术都会增加术后并发症和受体死亡率的风险[36-41]。先前评估夜间手术对肺移植结果的影响的研究显示，气道裂开的风险增加，90 天死亡率增加[41]。另一项分析显示，与夜间手术相关的 5 年闭塞性毛细支气管炎术后并发症风险增加且总生存率降低[42]。通过限制夜间手术，SDCF 模式不仅有

### 肺移植：胸外科临床问题

助于改善治疗结果，而且还可以提高移植外科医生的生活质量并减少职业倦怠[32]。

## 6.4 体外肺灌注复苏设施

目前，正在使用的另一种模式是集中的体外肺评估和修复中心。扩大标准供体肺在常温离体肺灌注（EVLP）平台出现前是不能应用在肺移植手术中的，常温体外肺灌注平台的出现彻底改变了临床肺移植领域，允许增加扩大标准供体肺的使用[43]。该系统能扩大供体库、增加肺移植例数，因此使用 EVLP 已逐渐成为世界上几个大洲的临床实践的一部分[44-53]。临床 EVLP 可以通过建立单中心项目进行，也可以与专门的 EVLP 机构合作。根据地理标准（在大面积区域内只有少量移植中心）、医疗保健系统模式（在加拿大和美国，EVLP 是一种可报销的程序）以及建立肺移植研究项目的中心，通常单中心 EVLP 项目更受青睐。单中心 EVLP 项目的开发需要技术专长、巨额初始资金和基础设施，因此，主要局限于大规模的移植中心。

鉴于目前大多数中心每年进行的肺移植手术仍不到 40 例，且共享一个小的地理区域，为了克服以上困难，通过专门的器官获取机构集中化 EVLP 正在积极地探索[54]。这一概念的模式首先是供体肺被回收并运送到附近的 EVLP 专用机构。肺一旦到达 EVLP 中心便开始由器官灌注专家灌注。如果认为器官适合移植，会将提供给周围中心。接受移植的团队可以通过高质量的视频和网络平台很好地获取肺部评估信息。移植团队可根据要求向 EVLP 专家进行咨询。一旦器官受体医院接受该肺，它们则会被运输到器官受体医院并准备移植（图 6-1）。一项概念验证临床试验（标识符：NCT03641677）目前正在美国进行，该项目在佛罗里达州杰克逊维尔市和马里兰州巴尔的摩市建立了专门的机构，用来评估该方法的可行性。迄今为止，这些机构已经进行了 280 多例肺评估，其中近 200 例患者接受了移植（数据来源于与 United Therapeutics Corporation 的个人通信）。在适当的地理区域内建立这些集中式机构，主要为了对该模式进行验证，以及发现并克服相关的监管问题。证明"远程 EVLP"可行性的案例报告已经发表。

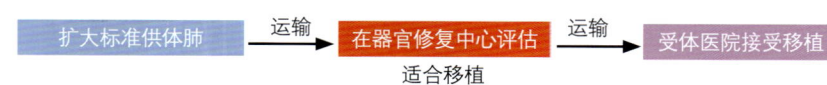

图 6-1　在器官修复中心进行 EVLP 检查的流程图

## 第6章 建立集中化供体器官获取和分配中心

在该报告中,扩大标准供体肺在芝加哥的一个三级医疗中心获得,随后被运送至多伦多进行 EVLP 评估[55]。经评估后,认为该肺适合进行移植,并将其运回芝加哥进行移植。虽然总缺血时间超过 15 小时,但未观察到原发性移植物功能不全(PGD)。这与最近的回顾性数据一致,即在长时间缺血时,注射 EVLP 可以保存超过 12 小时[56]。

建立这些机构有几个优势。首先,通过持续接触这些机构提供的高风险肺,不仅大型移植中心可以移植扩大标准供体肺,同时还促使较小的移植中心移植扩大标准供体肺。如前所述,专门的 EVLP 机构将专业知识集中化,将程序流程化,可能会增加这些地理区域内的移植量和捐献器官的利用率。其次,可以在这些 EVLP 设施中进行临床试验,研究在移植前对准备供体肺更好地干预措施,如抗炎、抗细胞死亡和抗病毒治疗。

对专用机构的成本结构和组织工作仍在探索和改进之中。对在个别中心或集中化机构执行 EVLP 的成本进行了个案比较,提出了不同的成本模型。然而,后者与购买 EVLP 设备和人员培训的初始资金成本无关。此外,在这些设施中进行 EVLP 治疗后,提高了肺利用率,增加了灌注/移植的比例,从而优化了财务模型。

## 6.5 讨 论

尽管 SDCF 模式与传统模式相比有许多优势,但更广泛的实施仍有障碍,其中包括巨大的启动成本、利用资源培训供体协调员,以及维持成本效益的最小捐献量(估计为 100 例捐献者/年)[9,10]。克服这些障碍的一些方法包括当地医疗中心的密切联系,外包检测以降低启动成本,以及逐步与移植中心建立长久融洽的合作关系[10]。2001 年,只有当地稳定的脑死亡供体被转移到 MTS SDCF,移植中心也仅仅只摘取到腹部器官[8]。供体协调员接受了 2 年的培训[10]。随着时间的推移,MTS SDCF 表现出了令人满意的结果,并与其服务的移植中心建立了信任,使其逐步扩展到目前存在的综合供体护理机构。

MTS 很幸运,它拥有一个城市所有的移植中心。针对移植中心相距较远,机构地点地皮价格高等客观情况的限制,一些其他的 OPO 已经对 SDCF 模式进行了调整,以适应特定的地理条件和医疗状况。一些 OPO 已经建立了独立的机构,如 MTS,而另一些则使用当地移植中心或外科中心内的设施。此外,许多带有 SDCF 的 OPO 在最初 24 小时内宣布脑死亡的医院管理供体,以完成 SDCF 可能无法进行的某些评估,如左右心导管检查。最近的一项评估表明,从成本效益的角度来看,38 个 OPO 有足够的供体量来支持 SDCF[9]。到目前为止,57 个 OPO 中有 12 个已经以某种形式采用了 SDCF 模式[9,10]。

然而，除 MTS 以外的 SDCF 的数据目前仍然有限。

OPO 由医疗保险和医疗补助服务中心（Centers for Medicare and Medicaid Services，CMS）和器官获取和移植网络（Organ Procurement and Transplantation Network，OPTN）监管。例如，CMS 和 OPTN 禁止 SDCF 管理活体供体，因此目前在 SDCF 模式中不可能在心源性死亡后进行捐献。虽然这些组织对 OPO 及其运营的 SDCP 进行监管，但目前尚无专门针对 SDCF 建立或管理的共识指南。

为了减少 OAC 还有一些替代模式，包括减少获取器官的路程的模式、器官获取团队的标准化和简化供体评估过程[4,5,7]。遗憾的是，由于组织和财政方面的不足，这些战略的实施迄今为止在很大程度上并不成功[4,5,7,34,57,58]。

对于不符合立即移植标准的肺，或由于器官分配的组织工作而需要延长保存时间的肺，集中的 EVLP 中心可以为移植中心安全地增加肺移植活动提供重要的价值。这种模式目前在美国正在增长，并且在未来很可能会扩展到其他国家。

## 6.6 总　结

由于对提高效率和降低与供体管理和器官获取相关的成本的日益关注，集中式器官管理和获取中心得以发展。SDCF 模式使用一个独立设施提供高效和成本效益的捐献护理。该模式可以增加器官产量，减少捐献器官的缺血时间。此外，SDCF 模式与减少获取器官的路程和减少夜间手术有关，其不仅可以改善治疗效果，还可以提高外科医生的生活质量，减少职业倦怠。EVLP 可以提高扩大标准供体肺的利用率，目前正在进行的临床试验正在评估专门的 EVLP 机构的作用。实际上，专用的 EVLP 设施有潜力集中与该模式相关的专业知识，并提高较小规模移植中心的器官利用率和手术量。这些模式越来越多地在美国应用，以解决持续的供体器官短缺问题并降低等待移植患者的死亡率。

**声明**

西佩尔是多伦多 XOR 实验室的创始人之一，也是肺生物工程公司的顾问。D. Kreisel 有一项专利正在申请，名为"检测 CCR2 受体的成分和方法"（申请号 15/611,577）。DK 获得美国国立卫生研究院拨款 1P01AI116501、R01HL094601、R01HL151078、囊性纤维化基金会和巴恩斯 - 犹太医院基金会的支持。AB 由美国国立卫生研究院拨款 5T32HL007317-44 资助。

## 参考文献

1. Valapour M, Lehr CJ, Skeans MA, et al. OPTN/SRTR 2019 annual data report: lung. Am J Transplant 2021;21(Suppl 2):441–520. https://doi.org/10.1111/ajt.16495.
2. United Network for Organ Sharing Transplant Trends. United network for organ sharing. https://unos.org/data/transplant-trends/. Accessed June 10, 2021.
3. Doyle MBM, Vachharajani N, Wellen JR, et al. A novel organ donor facility: a decade of experience with liver donors. Am J Transplant 2014;14(3):615–620. https://doi.org/10 1111/ajt.12607.
4. Doyle M, Subramanian V, Vachharajani N, et al. Organ donor recovery performed at an organ procurement organization-based facility is an effective way to minimize organ recovery costs and increase organ yield. J Am Coll Surg 2016;222(4):591–600. https://doi.org/10.1016/j. jamcollsurg. 2015. 12. 032.
5. Chang SH, Kreisel D, Marklin GF, et al. Lung focused resuscitation at a specialized donor care facility improves lung procurement rates. Ann ThoracSurg 2018;105(5):1531–1536. https://doi.org/10.1016/j. athoracsur. 2017. 12. 009.
6. Bollinger RR, Heinrichs DR, Seem DL, et al. UNOS Council for Organ Availability. United Network for Organ Sharing. Organ procurement organization (OPO), best practices. Clin Transplant 2001;15(Suppl 6):16–21. https://doi.org/10.1034/j.1399-0012. 2001. 00003. x.
7. Lynch RJ, Mathur AK, Hundley JC, et al. Improving organ procurement practices in Michigan. Am J Transplant 2009;9(10):2416–2423. https://doi.org/10.1111/j.1600-6143. 2009. 02784. x.
8. Jendrisak MD, Hruska K, Wagner J, et al. Cadavericdonor organ recovery at a hospital-independent facility. Transplantation 2002;74(7):978–982. https://doi.org/10.1097/00007890-200210150-00014.
9. Gauthier JM, Doyle MBM, Chapman WC, et al. Economic evaluation of the specialized donor care facility for thoracic organ donor management. J Thorac Dis 2020;12(10):5709–5717. https://doi.org/10.21037/jtd-20-1575.
10. Bery A, Marklin G, Itoh A, et al. The Specialized Donor Care Facility (SDCF) model and advances in management of thoracic organ donors. Ann ThoracSurg 2021. https://doi.org/10.1016/j.athoracsur. 2020. 12. 026.
11. Marklin GF, Klinkenberg WD, Helmers B, et al. A stroke volume-based fluid resuscitation protocol decreases vasopressor support and may increase organ yield in brain-dead donors. Clin Transplant 2020;34(2):e13784. https://doi.org/10.1111/ctr. 13784.
12. Dhar R, Cotton C, Coleman J, et al. Comparison of highand low-dose corticosteroid regimens for organ donor management. J Crit Care 2013;28(1):111. e1–7. https://doi.org/10.1016/j. jcrc. 2012. 04. 015.
13. Gauthier JM, Bierhals AJ, Liu J, et al. Chest computed tomography imaging improves potential lung donor assessment. J Thorac Cardiovasc Surg 2019;157(4):1711–1718. e1. https://doi.org/10.1016/j. jtcvs. 2018. 11. 038.
14. Marklin GF, O'Sullivan C, Dhar R. Ventilation in the prone position improves oxygenation and results in more lungs being transplanted from organ donors with hypoxemia and atelectasis. J Heart Lung Transplant 2021;40(2):120–127. https://doi.org/10.1016/j. healun. 2020. 11. 014.
15. Kotloff RM, Blosser S, Fulda GJ, et al. Management of the potential organ donor in the ICU: Society of Critical Care Medicine/American College of Chest Physicians/Association of Organ Procurement

16. Anwar ASMT, Lee J-M. Medical management of braindead organ donors. Acute Crit Care 2019;34(1):14–29. https://doi.org/10.4266/acc. 2019. 00430.

17. Avlonitis VS, Fisher AJ, Kirby JA, et al. Pulmonary transplantation: the role of brain death in donor lung injury. Transplantation 2003;75(12):1928–1933. https://doi.org/10.1097/01. TP. 0000066351. 87480. 9E.

18. Mascia L, Mastromauro I, Viberti S, et al. Management to optimize organ procurement in brain dead donors. Minerva Anestesiol 2009;75(3):125–133.

19. Venkateswaran RV, Patchell VB, Wilson IC, et al. Early donor management increases the retrieval rate of lungs for transplantation. Ann Thorac Surg 2008;85(1):278–286. https://doi.org/10.1016/j. athoracsur. 2007. 07. 092 [discussion 286].

20. Amado JA, López-Espadas F, Vázquez-Barquero A, et al. Blood levels of cytokines in brain-dead patients: relationship with circulating hormones and acutephase reactants. Metab Clin Exp 1995;44(6):812–816. https://doi.org/10.1016/0026-0495(95)90198-1.

21. Mascia L, Pasero D, Slutsky AS, et al. Effect of a lung protective strategy for organ donors on eligibility and availability of lungs for transplantation: a randomized controlled trial. JAMA 2010;304(23):2620–2627. https://doi.org/10.1001/jama. 2010. 1796.

22. Angel LF, Levine DJ, Restrepo MI, et al. Impact of a lung transplantation donor-management protocol on lung donation and recipient outcomes. Am J Respir Crit Care Med 2006;174(6):710–716. https://doi.org/10.1164/rccm. 200603-432OC.

23. Gabbay E, Williams TJ, Griffiths AP, et al. Maximizing the utilization of donor organs offered for lung transplantation. Am J Respir Crit Care Med 1999;160(1):265–271. https://doi.org/10.1164/ajrccm.160.1. 9811017.

24. Dhar R, Stahlschmidt E, Yan Y, et al. A randomized trial comparing triiodothyronine (T3) with thyroxine (T4) for hemodynamically unstable brain-dead organ donors. Clin Transplant 2019;33(3):e13486. https://doi.org/10.1111/ctr. 13486.

25. Dhar R, Stahlschmidt E, Marklin G. A randomized trial of intravenous thyroxine for brain-dead organ donors with impaired cardiac function. Prog Transplant 2020;30(1):48–55. https://doi.org/10.1177/1526924819893295.

26. Dhar R, Stahlschmidt E, Paramesh A, et al. A randomized controlled trial of naloxone for optimization of hypoxemia in lung donors after brain death. Transplantation 2019;103(7):1433–1438. https://doi.org/10.1097/TP. 0000000000002511.

27. Frye CC, Gauthier JM, Bery A, et al. Donor management using a specialized donor care facility is associated with higher organ utilization from drug overdose donors. Clin Transplant 2021;35(3):e14178. https://doi.org/10.1111/ctr. 14178.

28. Karasek R, Brisson C, Kawakami N, et al. The Job Content Questionnaire (JCQ): an instrument for internationally comparative assessments of psychosocial job characteristics. J Occup Health Psychol 1998;3(4): 322–355. https://doi.org/10.1037//1076-8998. 3. 4. 322.

29. Jesse MT, Abouljoud M, Eshelman A. Determinants of burnout among transplant surgeons: a national survey

in the United States. Am J Transplant 2015;15(3):772–778. https://doi.org/10.1111/ajt. 13056.

30. Bertges Yost W, Eshelman A, Raoufi M, et al. A national study of burnout among American transplant surgeons. Transplant Proc 2005;37(2):1399–401. https://doi.org/10.1016/j. transproceed. 2005. 01. 055.

31. Pondrom S. Has transplantation lost its luster? Am J Transplant 2011;11(6):1109–1110. https://doi.org/10.1111/j. 1600-6143. 2011. 03629. x.

32. Lindemann J, Dageforde LA, Brockmeier D, et al. Organ procurement center allows for daytime liver transplantation with less resource utilization: may address burnout, pipeline, and safety for field of transplantation. Am J Transplant 2019;19(5):1296–1304. https://doi.org/10.1111/ajt. 15129.

33. Englesbe MJ, Merion RM. The riskiest job in medicine: transplant surgeons and organ procurement travel. Am J Transplant 2009;9(10):2406–2415. https://doi.org/10.1111/j. 1600-6143. 2009. 02774. x.

34. Englesbe MJ, Shah S, Cutler JA, et al. Improving organ procurement travel practices in the United States: proceedings from the Michigan Donor Travel Forum. Am J Transplant 2010;10(3):458–463. https://doi.org/10.1111/j. 1600-6143. 2009. 02964. x.

35. Schenk AD, Washburn WK, Adams AB, et al. A survey of current procurement travel practices, accident frequency, and perceptions of safety. Transpl Direct 2019;5(10):e494. https://doi.org/10.1097/TXD. 0000000000000942.

36. Sugünes N, Bichmann A, Biernath N, et al. Analysis of the effects of day-time *vs.* night-time surgery on renal transplant patient outcomes. J Clin Med 2019;8(7). https://doi.org/10 3390/jcm8071051.

37. Ren S-S, Xu L-L, Wang P, et al. Circadian rhythms have effects on surgical outcomes of liver transplantation for patients with hepatocellular carcinoma: a retrospective analysis of 147 cases in a single center. Transplant Proc 2019;51(6):1913–1919. https://doi.org/10.1016/j. transproceed. 2019. 03. 033.

38. Hendrikx J, Van Raemdonck D, Pirenne J, et al. Outcome of transplantation performed outside the regular working hours: a systematic review and metaanalysis of the literature. Transpl Rev (Orlando) 2018;32(3):168–177. https://doi.org/10.1016/j. trre. 2018. 05. 001.

39. de Boer J, Van der Bogt K, Putter H, et al. Surgical quality in organ procurement during day and night: an analysis of quality forms. BMJ Open 2018;8(11):e022182. https://doi.org/10.1136/bmjopen-2018-022182.

40. Lonze BE, Parsikia A, Feyssa EL, et al. Operative start times and complications after liver transplantation. Am J Transplant 2010;10(8):1842–1849. https://doi.org/10.1111/j. 1600-6143. 2010. 03177. x.

41. George TJ, Arnaoutakis GJ, Merlo CA, et al. Association of operative time of day with outcomes after thoracic organ transplant. JAMA 2011;305(21):2193–2199. https://doi.org/10.1001/jama. 2011. 726.

42. Yang Z, Takahashi T, Gerull WD, et al. Impact of nighttime lung transplantation on outcomes and costs. Ann Thorac Surg 2021;112(1):206–213. https://doi.org/10.1016/j. athoracsur. 2020. 07. 060.

43. Cypel M, Yeung JC, Liu M, et al. Normothermic ex vivo lung perfusion in clinical lung transplantation. N Engl J Med 2011;364(15):1431–1440. https://doi.org/10.1056/NEJMoa1014597.

44. Aigner C, Slama A, Hötzenecker K, et al. Clinical ex vivo lung perfusion-pushing the limits: clinical ex vivo lung perfusion. Am J Transplant 2012;12(7):1839–1847. https://doi.org/10.1111/j. 1600-6143. 2012. 04027. x.

45. Slama A, Schillab L, Barta M, et al. Standard donor lung procurement with normothermic ex vivo lung perfusion: A prospective randomized clinical trial. J Heart Lung Transplant 2017;36(7):744–753. https://doi.org/10.1016/j. healun. 2017. 02. 011.

46. Sage E, Mussot S, Trebbia G, et al. Lung transplantation from initially rejected donors after ex vivo lung reconditioning: the French experience. Eur J Cardiothorac Surg 2014;46(5):794–799. https://doi.org/10.1093/ejcts/ezu245.
47. Valenza F, Citerio G, Palleschi A, et al. Successful transplantation of lungs from an uncontrolled donor after circulatory death preserved in situ by alveolar recruitment maneuvers and assessed by ex vivo lung perfusion. Am J Transplant 2016;16(4):1312–1318. https://doi.org/10.1111/ajt. 13612.
48. Wallinder A, Riise GC, Ricksten S-E, et al. Transplantation after ex vivo lung perfusion: a midterm follow-up. J Heart Lung Transplant 2016;35(11):1303–1310. https://doi.org/10.1016/j. healun. 2016. 05. 021.
49. Warnecke G, Moradiellos J, Tudorache I, et al. Normothermic perfusion of donor lungs for preservation and assessment with the Organ Care System Lung before bilateral transplantation: a pilot study of 12 patients. Lancet 2012;380(9856):1851–1858. https://doi.org/10.1016/S0140-6736(12)61344-0.
50. Boffini M, Ricci D, Bonato R, et al. Incidence and severity of primary graft dysfunction after lung transplantation using rejected grafts reconditioned with ex vivo lung perfusion. Eur J Cardiothorac Surg 2014; 46(5):789–793. https://doi.org/10.1093/ejcts/ezu239.
51. Zych B, Popov AF, Stavri G, et al. Early outcomes of bilateral sequential single lung transplantation after ex-vivo lung evaluation and reconditioning. J Heart Lung Transplant 2012;31(3):274–281. https://doi.org/10.1016/j. healun. 2011. 10. 008.
52. Henriksen ISI, Møller-Sørensen H, Møller CH, et al. First Danish experience with ex vivo lung perfusion of donor lungs before transplantation. Dan Med J 2014;61(3):A4809.
53. Zhang ZL, van Suylen V, van Zanden JE, et al. First experience with ex vivo lung perfusion for initially discarded donor lungs in the Netherlands: a single-centre study. Eur J Cardiothorac Surg 2019;55(5):920–926. https://doi.org/10.1093/ejcts/ezy373.
54. Khush KK, Cherikh WS, Chambers DC, et al. The international thoracic organ transplant registry of the international society for heart and lung transplantation: thirty-fifth adult heart transplantation report-2018; focus theme: Multiorgan transplantation. J Heart Lung Transplant 2018;37(10):1155–1168. https://doi.org/10.1016/j. healun. 2018. 07. 022.
55. Wigfield CH, Cypel M, Yeung J, et al. Successful emergent lung transplantation after remote ex vivo perfusion optimization and transportation of donor lungs: ex vivo lung perfusion transplantation after ECMO. Am J Transplant 2012;12(10):2838–2844. https://doi.org/10.1111/j. 1600-6143. 2012. 04175. x.
56. Yeung JC, Krueger T, Yasufuku K, et al. Outcomes after transplantation of lungs preserved for more than 12 h: a retrospective study. Lancet Respir Med 2017;5(2):119–124. https://doi.org/10.1016/S2213-2600(16)30323-X.
57. Abecassis M. Organ acquisition cost centers part I: medicare regulations–truth or consequence. Am J Transplant 2006;6(12):2830–2835. https://doi.org/10.1111/j. 1600-6143. 2006. 01582. x.
58. Abecassis M. Organ acquisition cost centers part II: reducing the burden of cost and inventory. Am J Transplant 2006;6(12):2836–2840. https://doi.org/10.1111/j. 1600-6143. 2006. 01583. x.

# 第 7 章 肺移植手术麻醉管理——2021 年新进展

Marek Brzezinski, Domagoj Mladinov, MD, Arne Neyrinck 著

孙树楷 译

周建平 校

【关键词】
- 肺移植
- 麻醉学
- 术中管理

【要点】
- 在高危患者生存率提高的推动下，计划接受肺移植的患者的风险稳步增加。
- 人们越来越认识到，许多术后并发症[如原发性移植物功能不全（PGD）或肺外器官衰竭]的病因源于内科因素，而非外科技术问题。
- 即使在需要围术期 ECMO 支持的高风险患者中，肺移植（LTx）也能提供极佳的结果。

## 7.1 引　言

目前，需要肺移植（LTx）患者的术中管理有 2 种趋势：①在高风险患者生存率提高的推动下，肺移植候选者的风险稳步增加[1-4]。其结果是临床表现的急性程度和移植桥接（BTT）支持的利用显著增加[2]。没有事先评估肺移植的患者，出现急性恶化性呼吸衰竭，并且需要体外膜肺氧合（ECMO）的移植桥接支持。肺移植（重新等待）的情况也有所增加[2,5]。总体而言，越来越多的 ECMO-BTT 患者使用边缘器官的需求可能会增加[6,7]，并且原发性移植物功能不全（PGD）的风险增加。②越来越多的人认识到，许多术后并发症，如原发性移植物功能不全或终末器官衰竭，都是由内科而非外科手术引起的[8-13]。因此，术中潜在危险因素的管理越来越受到重视。

本章的目标是总结最先进的肺移植术术中麻醉管理的关键概念，重点是血流动力学稳定、预防肺外并发症以及保存同种异体移植物功能。需要桥接移植的高风险患者群体

的规模和相关性不断增加，本章最后针对该群体的结局的最新文献进行了回顾。

## 7.2 术中同种异体移植物和肺外终末器官保护的关键概念

原发性移植物功能不全仍然是术后早期移植物的主要并发症[14-17]。目前，围手术期发生PGD的危险因素包括术中补液量、红细胞输注量、低血压、肺动脉压升高、血管阻力、体外循环［又称心肺转流术（cardiopulmonary bypass，CPB）］的使用、再灌注时吸入氧浓度（$FiO_2$）≥ 0.4、供体因素、缺血时间延长、吻合口并发症等[10,15,18-23]。这些危险因素也是许多围术期肺外终末器官并发症所共有的[11,24,25]。因此，麻醉医师可通过以下的方法积极保护移植物功能，预防肺外并发症的发生：①维持血流动力学稳定、最佳灌注和氧合，降低肺动脉压力和血管阻力；②采用肺保护性通气策略；③避免CPB；④减少手术并发症和缺血时间［如经食管超声心动图（transesophageal echocardiography，TEE）评价肺动脉（PA）和静脉吻合］。

## 7.3 术中关键时段维持血流动力学稳定

对于行肺移植手术的患者，应首先考虑低血压、急性右心室（right ventricular，RV）衰竭、缺氧和高碳酸血症的高风险[11,23-25]，且这种风险在诱导、肺动脉钳夹和异体移植物植入后最高。

在全身麻醉诱导和插管期间的管理。诱导的主要目标应该是维持血流动力学稳定，外科医生和灌注医生应立即提供紧急的心血管和肺部支持（如胸骨切开、导管置入、ECMO）。对于存在高危血流动力学衰竭风险的患者（例如，合并右心室功能降低的肺动脉高压患者，以及血流动力学不稳定的患者），应考虑进行术前ECMO导管置入[11,24,25]。鉴于目前缺乏支持特定麻醉诱导剂使用的临床证据，因此麻醉技术应根据患者的心血管和肺部风险特点来选择。诱导剂应缓慢和渐进地给予，并且需要高度的临床警惕性[11,24,25]。在对肺移植麻醉医师的最新调查中显示，异丙酚为最常用的麻醉诱导药物[26]。麻醉维持应根据患者的基础肺部疾病进行调整，可选择单独或联合使用吸入剂或全凭静脉麻醉（total intravenous anesthesia，TIVA）。例如，在有肺血流或通气不足风险的患者中，吸入麻醉药的摄取不可预测的情况下，强烈推荐使用TIVA。同样，TIVA也是需要ECMO患者的首选麻醉技术[11,24,25]。目前没有证据表明单侧肺通气时维持麻醉的方法会影响患者

## 第7章 肺移植手术麻醉管理——2021年新进展

结局（例如，通过影响肺血管张力、肺内分流或低氧血症）[27,28]。尽管有越来越多的肺隔离技术，但双腔管（double-lumen tubes，DLT）仍然是肺移植中最常见的选择，因为其易于使用、定位可靠、能够实现卓越的肺隔离，并可以在双侧肺进行支气管镜检查和黏液吸引。在双肺移植手术中，左侧DLT更常用，这是因为相对于右主支气管来说，左主支气管的长度较长。为了给支气管吻合留出足够的空间，导管应尽量靠近近端放置[11,13,24,25]。

在肺动脉夹闭、原生肺切除、同种异体肺移植过程中的管理。进行本体肺切除（即肺动脉夹闭）会导致肺动脉压力增加，可能会使原有肺动脉高压和右心室功能受损患者出现血流动力学不稳定[11,13,24,25]。对此类事件的预测，包括TEE在内的持续监测，以及及时使用正性肌力药物和血管活性药物进行血流动力学优化是管理成功的关键[11,13,24,25,29]。在供体肺的植入过程中，由于手术暴露和进入心房和肺门等结构的回缩，血流动力学不稳定也是可以预期的。在吻合术完成和移植物再灌注之后，可能会出现低血压，其原因可能是受到血管吻合处失血、缺血代谢产物的清除，以及移植物引起的肺麻痹，或是冠状动脉中进气的影响。在这些事件中可能需要高剂量的正性肌力药物和血管升压药。

总体而言，20%~40%的肺移植患者需要机械辅助循环支持（mechanical circulatory support，MCS）[26,30,31]。MCS可由CPB或静脉动脉（veno-arterial，VA）ECMO提供。静脉（venovenous，VV）ECMO虽然不提供循环支持，但也可以提供重要的呼吸支持，这部分将会在后面进行讨论（见后文）[26,30-32]。尽管MCS可以提供血流动力学稳定和气体交换，但它涉及引流和肝素化的操作，并可能引发全身和局部炎症反应，从而导致出现潜在的技术和医疗并发症。是否选择使用MCS通常取决于外科医生和医疗机构的偏好[26,30,31]。重度肺动脉高压和右心室功能显著降低的患者更可能需要MCS[11,13,24-26,30,31]。对于此类患者，应考虑在开始肺切除术前建立选择性MCS。术前需要桥接ECMO进行移植的患者，移植过程中也应进行MCS支持[2]。如果术中出现单侧肺通气时气体交换不充分、无法维持血压、进行纵隔结构手术操作时器官灌注不足或失血量大等情况，也可能需要使用MCS。

有的学者主张术中常规使用MCS，以便在第一肺植入后进行控制性再灌注并立即启动肺保护性通气[33,34]。在没有MCS时，第一肺植入后接受全心输出量，使肺动脉压力和静水压升高，可能会加重肺泡水肿和右心衰竭。机械辅助装置可将部分（或全部）心输出量从移植物中分流，以减少缺血再灌注损伤和原发性移植物功能不全的发生。一些研究表明，术中使用VA-ECMO可以提高患者的生存率。然而，对此目前的文献观点并不一致[35]。

## 肺移植：胸外科临床问题

CPB 与 ECMO 的优缺点一直是人们关注的话题。CPB 可以为失血性休克患者提供更好的血流动力学控制和复苏能力，这得益于储血器和右心吸引管的存在[36]。然而，CPB 需要充分的抗凝，可能会增加输血以及输血相关的肺损伤的发生率。此外，较大的预充量会导致血液稀释更多及凝血功能障碍。另一方面，与 CPB 相比，ECMO 的设置更简单，由于血气界面更小以及体外回路更短引起炎症反应也较小。ECMO 需要的肝素也更少：首先，对于术中启动的 ECMO 支持，通常在 ECMO 启动时静脉注射 5000 单位的肝素建立抗凝，将活化凝血时间（activated clotting time，ACT）维持在 180~210 秒范围内，而在 ECMO-BTT 患者中，肝素剂量应该根据其风险情况而进行调整。其次，ECMO 可以根据需要的支持系统在术后为心脏和（或）肺提供机械支持。近年来，越来越多的文献支持术中 ECMO 使用。研究表明，与 CPB 相比，ECMO 的使用更能够降低 PGD 发生率、减少术后出血和输血、减少再次手术、减少肾损伤和缩短重症监护病房（ICU）住院时间[37-39]。虽然一些移植中心报告常规使用 ECMO 具有良好的结果，但 2 种 MCS 模式之间的死亡率没有显著差异[38-40]。

当进行无机械循环支持的肺移植时，严重病变肺脏在术中单侧肺通气期间的管理会更加困难，因为低氧血症和高碳酸血症导致的酸中毒可能会增加肺血管阻力，并使右心室功能进一步恶化：

- 晚期原发性肺动脉高压患者常因右心室衰竭导致血流动力学不稳定[11,13,24,25]。在这种情况下，可能需要积极避免或治疗低氧血症和高碳酸血症，使用正性肌力药物以及严格（限制性）的液体治疗维持右心室功能。可加用吸入性肺血管扩张剂，吸入性一氧化氮或前列腺素[例如，通过喷射雾化器以 0.01~0.05 μg/（kg·min）的速度注射依前列醇][25,26,41,42]。

- 去甲肾上腺素和血管升压素是治疗肺动脉高压和右心室功能不全时低血压最常用的血管升压药物[26]，而血管升压素对肺血管阻力（pulmonary vascular resistance，PVR）的影响较小[43]。

- 对于有心力衰竭、右心室功能不全或终末器官低灌注证据的患者，应考虑使用正性肌力药物（肾上腺素、多巴酚丁胺或米力农）[44]，且尽可能地维持窦性心律。

- 在没有 MCS 的 LTx 期间，通常是在血管阻断前静脉使用 5000 单位的肝素进行抗凝治疗，然后在第二次肺移植前再次给药。

在异体移植物再灌注期间，应通过控制移植物的再灌注（低肺动脉压力，使用肺血管扩张剂）和低 $FiO_2$（< 0.3 最佳）来减少 PGD 的风险[23,25,45]。

## 7.4 肺移植过程中机械辅助循环支持的关键概念

尽管不同的 MCS 设备存在差异，但通常包括几个主要部件：一个将患者的血液从他们的静脉系统转移到设备中的进流导管，一个血液泵，一个氧合器，一个换热器，以及一个将血液返回给患者的出流导管。在肺移植期间通常使用的 MCS 包括 CPB、VA 或 VV-ECMO：

- 体外循环提供了充分的循环和呼吸支持。静脉血液的引流通常由重力和吸引辅助实现。根据不同的插管方式将血液通过主动脉或大动脉返回动脉系统。与其他 MCS 装置不同的是，CPB 含有吸引导管和储血器，可以在术中回收血液，以便快速输注大量血液。在手术过程的特定阶段，也可以通过减少患者（同时充盈 CPB 储血器）的血液回输，实现血流/压力的快速暂时性降低。CPB 除了持续输送氧气和清除血液中的二氧化碳外，还可输送挥发性麻醉药，在肺泡气体交换受损的情况下尤为重要。
- 与 CPB 类似，VA-ECMO 可以同时提供心脏和呼吸支持[46]。通常通过 1 根或 2 根大静脉将患者的血液从静脉系统中引出。与 CPB 不同的是，若血液引流不足可能会限制泵的前负荷，减少血流量。当使用中心静脉插管时，血液通常通过大动脉或主动脉返回。由于标准 ECMO 装置不具备储血器，因此体外回路不能用于容量复苏，也不能根据需要将患者的血液收集保存在体外回路中。静脉储血器的缺失也意味着静脉流入导管的任何阻塞或扭曲都会导致泵流量显著下降或完全停止。此外，ECMO 回路缺乏排气装置，增加了气体栓塞的风险，可能会导致灾难性的气体栓塞。
- VV-ECMO 仅用于呼吸支持[46]。将血液通过各种配置的静脉套管从静脉系统引流并返回静脉系统。装置泵维持体外回路的血液流动，而患者的自体心脏将血液输送到体内。
- MCS 插管可大致分为中央穿刺置管和外周穿刺置管。
- 中央穿刺置管需要行胸骨切开术，一般只在手术室中进行，并在全身麻醉后实施。使用 2 根套管时，需将动脉套管置入升主动脉，将静脉套管置入右心房和下腔静脉或上下腔静脉。中心置管常用于 CPB，然而，循环支持装置并不能决定插管部位，中央穿刺置管也经常用于 VA-ECMO。
- 外周穿刺置管可有以下入路：
  ○ 开放手术入路（切开法）或经股动脉或腋动脉穿刺入路。当行股动脉插管时，插管部位远端的血液供应可能会受阻，进而导致肢体缺血[47]。为降低灌注不良的风险，可在同侧股浅动脉放置顺行性远端灌注套管。与股动脉插管相关的另一个潜在并发症是上下肢体氧合不均的现象，即"南北综合征"或"Harlequin综合征"[48]。该现象常在肺功能严重受损时、心脏排出的低氧血液与股动脉导管输送的含氧血液在远端主动脉弓中混合时发生，可能导致心肌和脑组织缺氧，而由降主动脉灌注的身体部位的则优先氧合。

○ 外周 VV-ECMO 双部位置管可以通过左右股静脉，或者通过股静脉和颈内静脉进行。对于单部位 VV-ECMO 置管，通常将双腔导管置入颈内静脉（internal jugular，IJ）或锁骨下静脉。该方法通常用于清醒、行走的患者，作为桥接到移植手术的临时支持[49]。如果计划在肺移植手术中放置双腔 VV-ECMO 插管，则应避免在右侧颈内静脉放置标准的中心静脉导管。

### 7.4.1 机械通气

在气管插管后，通常使用低潮气量（4~6 mL/kg）、呼气末正压（PEEP）< 10 cm $H_2O$ 的通气模式，需调整呼吸频率（RR）和 $FiO_2$，以维持血氧饱和度在 92%~96% 之间，并保持术前基线水平的动脉血二氧化碳分压（$PaCO_2$）[23-26,44]。根据肺部病变情况，可以实施多种策略来改善氧合和通气[23,25,26]：

- 在有动态过度充气、气压伤和张力性气胸风险的阻塞性气道病变患者中（如慢性阻塞性肺疾病或肺气肿），可以通过小容量压力控制通气方法减少动态过度充气。相对于吸气时间，延长呼气时间（吸呼比 I∶E 为 1∶4 至 1∶3）可能减少内源性 PEEP（auto-PEEP），且不应使用外源性 PEEP 或应使用低水平 PEEP（3~4 cm $H_2O$）。
- 对于有大量分泌物或严重高碳酸血症，伴有囊性纤维化或支气管扩张的患者，可考虑先用单腔导管而不是双腔导管进行气管插管，以利于广泛的气道吸引，以及较高的气道压力和较高的外源性 PEEP。
- 以肺纤维化为特征的限制性肺疾病需要较高的驱动压，可以采用增加吸气时间（I∶E 为 1∶2 至 1∶1）和较高的外源性 PEEP（8~10 cm $H_2O$）的通气模式。

在移植肺植入完成且患者已脱离 MCS 后，建议术中机械通气的调整包括潮气量为 6 mL/kg 理想体重（当移植物体积过小时考虑使用供体体重），PEEP 为 6~8 cm $H_2O$，PIP < 30 cm $H_2O$，并使用尽可能低的 $FiO_2$ 维持 $PaO_2$ ≥ 70 mmHg[10,45,50-52]。频繁使用吸入性一氧化氮理论上可以舒张通气部位的肺血管，从而改善通气-灌注匹配和氧合。但

其在减轻移植肺损伤和改善预后方面的临床效果尚未得到明确证实[53,54]。最近在接受肺移植患者中进行的一项随机临床试验比较了吸入一氧化氮和吸入依前列醇的效果,发现两组患者发生严重3级原发性移植物功能不全(PGD-3)的风险与其他术后结果相似[55]。

### 7.4.2 液体管理

据报道,使用过多的液体量会增加肺水肿、肺损伤、术后机械通气时间延长以及PGD的风险[18-20]。因此,需要采用限制性液体策略。大多数机构使用晶体液进行液体维持,使用胶体液(如5%白蛋白)进行容量复苏[23],且必须与维持足够的心输出量和灌注压的目标相平衡。术中应尽量减少红细胞输注,因为其是PGD的危险因素,而且需根据临床标准(如混合/中心静脉氧饱和度)评估是否输注,而不是根据血红蛋白浓度。尽管没有报道称输注新鲜冰冻血浆(fresh frozen plasma,FFP)或血小板会增加PGD的风险,但在临床和实验室(现场检测)评估中有持续/失控出血和凝血功能障碍出现,因为认为采用限制性方法是合理的[10,20,21,56]。

对于存在液体超负荷或右心衰竭风险的患者,可以考虑使用凝血酶原复合物浓缩物(PCC)而非FFP。考虑到血栓事件的相关风险增加,应该避免使用或慎用小剂量的重组凝血因子Ⅶ。

### 7.4.3 经食管超声心动图

尽管TEE具有实用性和诊断相关性,但根据美国超声心动图学会,TEE仍然只是肺移植手术中监测的Ⅱb级指征[57]。此外,目前尚无统一的肺动脉瓣狭窄诊断标准[13,29,58]。尽管如此,因为它的临床实用性贯穿整个LTx手术过程,在一些高产量的机构,TEE经常进行(甚至在某些中心常规地进行)[13,23,26,29,58-62]。

- 起初,全面的经食管超声心动图检查可以明确术前的检验结果,并帮助检测间隔变化,特别是关于右心室功能和大小、三尖瓣反流以及存在的心内分流(如卵圆孔未闭、心房或心室间隔缺损),这些可能直接改变手术过程的进程(如需要体外膜肺氧合或手术闭合)。
- TEE可帮助连续监测左、右心大小和功能,评估其容量状态,指导血流动力学干预(如正性肌力药物)。这在肺动脉阻断、开放和移植肺再灌注时高度相关,因为这些信息可能决定是否需要启动CPB或ECMO。TEE还可以用于检测再灌注时左心房和心室中是否存在气体。

- 最后，TEE 在 LTx 手术中的一个重要作用是评估肺动脉（PA）和肺静脉（pulmonary venous，PV）的吻合情况[29,60]。

### 7.4.3.1 肺动脉吻合

目前，尚无共识指南对 PA 狭窄的诊断标准进行概述，提出的推荐意见也很少。但检查应包括测量 PA 直径，排除 PA 内血栓（二维 TEE），然后进行频谱和彩色多普勒。对于 PA 狭窄[健康男性志愿者 PA 平均直径：右侧 PA（16.6 ± 2.8）mm，左侧 PA（17.3 ± 2.5）mm][60,63-65]，通常采用小于同侧 PA 直径的 75% 作为临界值，以代替官方指南。PA 吻合口的湍流或显著的梯度也应引起对狭窄的关注。

### 7.4.3.2 肺静脉吻合

测量肺静脉直径，以及排除肺静脉内血栓（二维 TEE），并进行频谱和彩色多普勒检查。PV 直径 < 0.5 cm 且流速 > 1 m/s 时（S 波和 D 波的正常 PV 速度：30~60 cm/s）应引起对 PV 狭窄的关注。PV 直径小于 0.25 cm 提示移植可能失败[29,60,66-69]。最近的一项系统回顾指出了 LTx 手术中 PV 直径为（0.48 ± 0.02）cm 和 PV 速度为（1.59 ± 0.66）m/s 是 PV 功能障碍（狭窄或血栓形成）的预测因素，报告的死亡率为 32%[70]。PV 狭窄的诊断应基于多个特征的存在，因为在不平稳的 LTx 手术（如高动力循环、对侧肺动脉狭窄、供体静脉血管收缩、第二肺植入期等）中经常会出现假阳性[29]。

### 7.4.4 高风险患者肺移植的预后

随着手术技术、术中及术后管理的改进，LTx 术后患者的生存率有所提高，其中位生存期为 6.7 年，但仍落后于其他实质器官移植[71]。因此，移植中心在多个方面不断拓展，包括将年龄较大、健康状况较差和风险较高的候选人列入等待名单并进行移植手术。例如，65 岁以上的年龄曾为肺移植相对禁忌证[72]，目前在比利时依然如此。然而，今年早些时候发布的 ISHLT 肺移植候选人选择共识文件并未将年龄上限视为绝对禁忌证。目前，在美国 30% 的待移植者年龄超过 65 岁，而这一年龄组的候选人进行移植手术的速度最快[73]。在 2004—2016 年间，美国 65 岁以上的肺移植受者人数增加了 430%。在全球范围内，类似的趋势也有出现，但程度较轻[74]。然而，关于 60 岁以上肺移植受者生存结果的数据仍然存在矛盾[75-77]。Mosher 及其同事在移植受者科学登记处对接近 6000 例受者进行了回顾性调查，探讨 65 岁以上患者死亡的危险因素[78]。研究发现纳入研究的患

## 第7章 肺移植手术麻醉管理——2021年新进展

者的中位生存期为4.41年，且随着年龄的增加，生存期逐渐缩短。此外，在多因素分析中，他们还发现了其他与老年患者预后相关的危险因素：肌酐水平、胆红素水平、移植前病情急性加重入院、单肺移植、巨细胞病毒（cytomegalovirus，CMV）不匹配、供者糖尿病等。对于移植前住院治疗的患者，尤其是ICU患者，其短期生存状况明显差于65岁以上的门诊患者[78]。因此，尽管在围手术期护理方面取得了进展，但某些危险因素仍然可能阻碍高龄患者肺移植手术的成功。

既往研究显示，肺移植术前需要有创机械通气（invasive mechanical ventilation，IMV）的患者术后死亡率高于不需要IMV的患者[79-82]，因此IMV被列为LTx的相对禁忌证[83,84]。然而，Hamilton及其同事最近发表的一项研究表明，围手术期管理的进步显著改善了移植受者的生存率。在这项回顾性研究中，作者使用的数据来自器官共享联合网络的器官获取和移植网络登记处，2005—2018年期间，在21 375例接受LTx的患者中检查了LTx前IMV的安全性和结果[1]。研究通过倾向评分匹配和多变量建模，比较了2005—2011年和2011—2018年期间的结果，报告了2个主要发现：①尽管需要IMV的患者的严重程度和急性加重程度增加，但IMV受者的生存率随时间显著提高。与2005—2011年期间相比，2011—2018年期间移植的IMV受者在30天内的死亡风险降低了2.5倍，在14个月时降低了2倍，在3年时降低了1.4倍[1]；②与非IMV相比，在2011—2018年期间接受移植的IMV受者在30天内死亡率显著增加（$RR = 9.53$；$95\% CI$：$4.57 \sim 19.86$），而在随后的时间点没有显著差异[1]。研究者认为，该结果的改善归因于器官保存和ICU管理的进步。

同样，LTx前使用ECMO的历史生存率较低[79]。随着ECMO技术和围手术期管理的进步，目前ECMO-BTT的结果也有所改善[2,5,85,86]。据报道，ECMO-BTT的成功率高达89%[5,86,87]。即使在ILD高患病率的老年人群中，1年生存率范围高达86%~93%[2,5]（出院后1年生存率为88%[86]~97%[2]）。因此，在过去10年中，ECMO-BTT的使用增加了271%，而IMV-BTT的使用减少了38%[88]。随着ECMO-BTT使用者的增加，需要ECMO-BTT的患者的病情严重程度和年龄也随着时间的推移而增加[86,87,89]。

此外，研究者们还注意到，对于之前没有接受肺移植评估但因出现急性慢性呼吸衰竭而进入了待移植名单的患者，也需要机械支持[MV和（或）ECMO]作为BTT的患者的治疗[2,5]。这给医疗团队带来了关于最佳治疗的伦理道德问题。Kukreja及其同事最近在一项回顾性单中心研究中比较了2010—2018年间62名患者（其中紧急等待名单20名，主动等待名单42名）中紧急等待名单（emergently waitlisted，EWL）与ECMO部署后进行主动等待名单（actively waitlisted，AWL）的结果。研究者报告了2项主要发现：①AWL 和 EWL 的 BTT 成功率无统计学差异；②生存结果（出院生存率：EWL 组和 AWL 组分别为 100% 和 87%）无统计学差异[2]。EWL 组和 AWL 组出院时 1 年条件生存率分别为 91% 和 100%，无条件生存率分别为 91% 和 83%。

## 7.5 总　结

随着待移植患者的医疗复杂性稳步增加，需要 ECMO-BTT 支持的待移植患者数量稳步上升。人们逐渐意识到伴有潜在可变风险因素患者的术中管理对术后结果影响的重要性。同时确定了术中（麻醉）管理的多种干预措施可能可以减轻潜在可变的风险因素。

## 参考文献

1. Hamilton BCS, Dincheva GR, Matthay MA, et al. Improved survival after lung transplantation for adults requiring preoperative invasive mechanical ventilation: A national cohort study. J Thorac Cardiovasc Surg 2020;160(5):1385–1395 e1386.
2. Kukreja J, Tsou S, Chen J, et al. Risk Factors and Outcomes of Extracorporeal Membrane Oxygenation as a Bridge to Lung Transplantation. Semin Thorac Cardiovasc Surg 2020;32(4):772–785.
3. Stehlik J, Chambers DC, Zuckermann A, et al. Increasing complexity of thoracic transplantation and the rise of multiorgan transplantation around the world: Insights from the International Society for Heart and Lung Transplantation Registry. J Heart Lung Transplant 2018;37(10):1145–1154.
4. Chambers DC, Cherikh WS, Goldfarb SB, et al. The International Thoracic Organ Transplant Registry of the International Society for Heart and Lung Transplantation: Thirty-fifth adult lung and heart-lung transplant report-2018; Focus theme: Multiorgan Transplantation. J Heart Lung Transplant 2018; 37(10):1169–1183.
5. Banga A, Batchelor E, Mohanka M, et al. Predictors of outcome among patients on extracorporeal membrane oxygenation as a bridge to lung transplantation. Clin Transpl 2017;31(7).
6. Kukreja J, Chen J, Brzezinski M. Redefining marginality: donor lung criteria. Curr Opin Organ Transpl 2020;25(3):280–284.
7. Tsou S, Chen J, Brzezinski M, et al. Lung transplantation from swimming pool drowning victims: A case series. Am J Transplant 2021;21(6):2273–2278.
8. Kinaschuk K, Nagendran J. Improving long-term survival by preventing early complications after lung transplantation: Can we prevent ripples by keeping pebbles out of the water? J Thorac Cardiovasc Surg 2016;151(4):1181–1182.
9. Chan EG, Bianco V 3rd, Richards T, et al. The ripple effect of a complication in lung transplantation: Evidence for increased long-term survival risk. J Thorac Cardiovasc Surg 2016;151(4):1171–1179.

10. Diamond JM, Lee JC, Kawut SM, et al. Clinical risk factors for primary graft dysfunction after lung transplantation. Am J Respir Crit Care Med 2013;187(5): 527–534.
11. Kachulis B, Mitrev L, Jordan D. Intraoperative anesthetic management of lung transplantation patients. Best Pract Res Clin Anaesthesiol 2017;31(2): 261–272.
12. Marczin NKL, Wright IG, Simon AR. Anaesthesia for lung transplantation. In: R Peter Alston PSM, Ranucci Marco, editors. Oxford textbook of cardiac anaesthesia. Oxford University Press; 2015.
13. Sellers D, Cassar-Demajo W, Keshavjee S, et al. The Evolution of Anesthesia for Lung Transplantation. J Cardiothorac Vasc Anesth 2017;31(3):1071–1079.
14. Yusen RD, Edwards LB, Kucheryavaya AY, et al. The Registry of the International Society for Heart and Lung Transplantation: Thirty-second Official Adult Lung and Heart-Lung Transplantation Report–2015; Focus Theme: Early Graft Failure. J Heart Lung Transplant 2015;34(10):1264–1277.
15. Snell GI, Yusen RD, Weill D, et al. Report of the ISHLT Working Group on Primary Lung Graft Dysfunction, part I: Definition and grading-A 2016 Consensus Group statement of the International Society for Heart and Lung Transplantation. J Heart Lung Transplant 2017;36(10):1097–1103.
16. Gelman AE, Fisher AJ, Huang HJ, et al. Report of the ISHLT Working Group on Primary Lung Graft Dysfunction Part III: Mechanisms: A 2016 Consensus Group Statement of the International Society for Heart and Lung Transplantation. J Heart Lung Transplant 2017;36(10):1114–1120.
17. Van Raemdonck D, Hartwig MG, Hertz MI, et al. Report of the ISHLT Working Group on primary lung graft dysfunction Part IV: Prevention and treatment: A 2016 Consensus Group statement of the International Society for Heart and Lung Transplantation. J Heart Lung Transplant 2017; 36(10):1121–1136.
18. McIlroy DR, Pilcher DV, Snell GI. Does anaesthetic management affect early outcomes after lung transplant? An exploratory analysis. Br J Anaesth 2009; 102(4):506–514.
19. Assaad S, Kratzert WB, Perrino AC Jr. Extravascular lung water monitoring for thoracic and lung transplant surgeries. Curr Opin Anaesthesiol 2019; 32(1):29–38.
20. Geube MA, Perez-Protto SE, McGrath TL, et al. Increased Intraoperative Fluid Administration Is Associated with Severe Primary Graft Dysfunction After Lung Transplantation. Anesth Analg 2016; 122(4):1081–1088.
21. Cernak V, Oude Lansink-Hartgring A, van den Heuvel ER, et al. Incidence of Massive Transfusion and Overall Transfusion Requirements During Lung Transplantation Over a 25-Year Period. J Cardiothorac Vasc Anesth 2019;33(9):2478–2486.
22. Hamilton BCS, Dincheva GR, Zhuo H, et al. Elevated donor plasminogen activator inhibitor-1 levels and the risk of primary graft dysfunction. Clin Transpl 2018;32(4):e13210.
23. Gerlach RM. Lung transplantation: Anesthetic management. In: O'Connor MF, Marks JB, eds. UpToDate. Waltham, MA. 2021.
24. Buckwell E, Vickery B, Sidebotham D. Anaesthesia for lung transplantation. BJA Educ 2020;20(11):368–376.
25. Nicoara A, Anderson-Dam J. Anesthesia for Lung Transplantation. Anesthesiol Clin 2017;35(3): 473–489.
26. Tomasi R, Betz D, Schlager S, et al. Intraoperative Anesthetic Management of Lung Transplantation: Center-Specific Practices and Geographic and Centers Size Differences. J Cardiothorac Vasc Anesth 2018;32(1):62–69.

27. Pruszkowski O, Dalibon N, Moutafis M, et al. Effects of propofol vs sevoflurane on arterial oxygenation during one-lung ventilation. Br J Anaesth 2007; 98(4):539–544.
28. Modolo NS, Modolo MP, Marton MA, et al. Intravenous versus inhalation anaesthesia for one-lung ventilation. Cochrane Database Syst Rev 2013;(7): CD006313.
29. Abrams BA, Melnyk V, Allen WL, et al. TEE for Lung Transplantation: A Case Series and Discussion of Vascular Complications. J Cardiothorac Vasc Anesth 2020;34(3):733–740.
30. Moreno Garijo J, Cypel M, McRae K, et al. The Evolving Role of Extracorporeal Membrane Oxygenation in Lung Transplantation: Implications for Anesthetic Management. J Cardiothorac Vasc Anesth 2019;33(7):1995–2006.
31. Martin AK, Jayaraman AL, Nabzdyk CG, et al. Extracorporeal Membrane Oxygenation in Lung Transplantation: Analysis of Techniques and Outcomes. J Cardiothorac Vasc Anesth 2021;35(2):644–661.
32. Kiziltug H, Falter F. Circulatory support during lung transplantation. Curr Opin Anaesthesiol 2020;33(1): 37–42.
33. Marczin N, Royston D, Yacoub M. Pro: lung transplantation should be routinely performed with cardiopulmonary bypass. J Cardiothorac Vasc Anesth 2000;14(6):739–745.
34. Nazarnia S, Subramaniam K. Pro: Veno-arterial Extracorporeal Membrane Oxygenation (ECMO) Should Be Used Routinely for Bilateral Lung Transplantation. J Cardiothorac Vasc Anesth 2017;31(4):1505–1508.
35. Hoetzenecker K, Schwarz S, Muckenhuber M, et al. Intraoperative extracorporeal membrane oxygenation and the possibility of postoperative prolongation improve survival in bilateral lung transplantation. J Thorac Cardiovasc Surg 2018;155(5):2193–2206 e2193.
36. Bennett SCBE, Dumond CA, Preston T, et al. Mechanical circulatory support in lung transplantation: Cardiopulmonary bypass, extracorporeal life support, and ex-vivo lung perfusion. World J Respirol 2015;5(2):78–93.
37. Biscotti M, Yang J, Sonett J, et al. Comparison of extracorporeal membrane oxygenation versus cardiopulmonary bypass for lung transplantation. J Thorac Cardiovasc Surg 2014;148(5):2410–2415.
38. Machuca TN, Collaud S, Mercier O, et al. Outcomes of intraoperative extracorporeal membrane oxygenation versus cardiopulmonary bypass for lung transplantation. J Thorac Cardiovasc Surg 2015;149(4): 1152–1157.
39. Bermudez CA, Shiose A, Esper SA, et al. Outcomes of intraoperative venoarterial extracorporeal membrane oxygenation versus cardiopulmonary bypass during lung transplantation. Ann Thorac Surg 2014; 98(6):1936–1942.
40. Aigner C, Wisser W, Taghavi S, et al. Institutional experience with extracorporeal membrane oxygenation in lung transplantation. Eur J Cardiothorac Surg 2007;31(3):468–473.
41. Khan TA, Schnickel G, Ross D, et al. A prospective, randomized, crossover pilot study of inhaled nitric oxide versus inhaled prostacyclin in heart transplant and lung transplant recipients. J Thorac Cardiovasc Surg 2009;138(6):1417–1424.
42. Kim N, Lee SH, Joe Y, et al. Effects of Inhaled Iloprost on Lung Mechanics and Myocardial Function During One-Lung Ventilation in Chronic Obstructive Pulmonary Disease Patients Combined With Poor LungOxygenation. Anesth Analg 2020;130(5): 1407–1414.
43. Siehr SL, Feinstein JA, Yang W, et al. Hemodynamic Effects of Phenylephrine, Vasopressin, and Epinephrine

in Children With Pulmonary Hypertension: A Pilot Study. Pediatr Crit Care Med 2016;17(5):428–437.
44. Rana M, Yusuff H, Zochios V. The Right Ventricle During Selective Lung Ventilation for Thoracic Surgery. J Cardiothorac Vasc Anesth 2019;33(7): 2007–2016.
45. Barnes L, Reed RM, Parekh KR, et al. Mechanical Ventilation for the Lung Transplant Recipient. Curr Pulmonol Rep 2015;4(2):88–96.
46. Barry A, Brzezinski M. Adult Extracorporeal Membrane Oxygenation: An Update for Intensivists. ICU Director 2013;4(3):107–114.
47. Lamb KM, DiMuzio PJ, Johnson A, et al. Arterial protocol including prophylactic distal perfusion catheter decreases limb ischemia complications in patients undergoing extracorporeal membrane oxygenation. J Vasc Surg 2017;65(4):1074–1079.
48. St-Arnaud C, Theriault MM, Mayette M. North-south syndrome in veno-arterial extra-corporeal membrane oxygenator: the other Harlequin syndrome. Can J Anaesth 2020;67(2):262–263.
49. Biscotti M, Gannon WD, Agerstrand C, et al. Awake Extracorporeal Membrane Oxygenation as Bridge to Lung Transplantation: A 9-Year Experience. Ann Thorac Surg 2017;104(2):412–419.
50. Martin AK, Yalamuri SM, Wilkey BJ, et al. The Impact of Anesthetic Management on Perioperative Outcomes in Lung Transplantation. J Cardiothorac Vasc Anesth 2020;34(6):1669–1680.
51. Verbeek GL, Myles PS. Intraoperative protective ventilation strategies in lung transplantation. Transpl Rev (Orlando) 2013;27(1):30–35.
52. Diamond JM, Arcasoy S, Kennedy CC, et al. Report of the International Society for Heart and Lung Transplantation Working Group on Primary Lung Graft Dysfunction, part II: Epidemiology, risk factors, and outcomes-A 2016 Consensus Group statement of the International Society for Heart and Lung Transplantation. J Heart Lung Transplant 2017; 36(10):1104–1113.
53. Bhandary S, Stoicea N, Joseph N, et al. Pro: Inhaled Pulmonary Vasodilators Should Be Used Routinely in the Management of Patients Undergoing Lung Transplantation. J Cardiothorac Vasc Anesth 2017; 31(3):1123–1126.
54. Ramadan ME, Shabsigh M, Awad H. Con: Inhaled Pulmonary Vasodilators Are Not Indicated in Patients Undergoing Lung Transplantation. J Cardiothorac Vasc Anesth 2017;31(3):1127–1131.
55. Ghadimi K, Cappiello J, Cooter-Wright M, et al. Inhaled Pulmonary Vasodilator Therapy in Adult Lung Transplant: A Randomized Clinical Trial. JAMA Surg 2021;157(1):e215856.
56. Huddleston SJ, Jackson S, Kane K, et al. Separate Effect of Perioperative Recombinant Human Factor VIIa Administration and Packed Red Blood Cell Transfusions on Midterm Survival in Lung Transplantation Recipients. J Cardiothorac Vasc Anesth 2020; 34(11):3013–3020.
57. Ramadan ME, Shabsigh M, Awad H. Con: Inhaled Pulmonary Vasodilators Are Not Indicated in Patients Undergoing Lung Transplantation. J Cardiothorac Vasc Anesth. 2017 Jun;31(3):1127–31. https://doi.org/10.1053/j.jvca.2016.08.035. Epub 2016 Aug 31. PMID: 27856154.
58. Iyer MH, Bhatt A, Kumar N, et al. Transesophageal Echocardiography for Lung Transplantation: A New Standard of Care? J Cardiothorac Vasc Anesth 2020;34(3):741–743.
59. American Society of A, Society of Cardiovascular Anesthesiologists Task Force on Transesophageal E. Practice guidelines for perioperative transesophageal echocardiography. An updated report by the

American Society of Anesthesiologists and the Society of Cardiovascular Anesthesiologists Task Force on Transesophageal Echocardiography. Anesthesiology 2010;112(5):1084–1096.

60. Evans A, Dwarakanath S, Hogue C, et al. Intraoperative echocardiography for patients undergoing lung transplantation. Anesth Analg 2014;118(4):725–730.
61. Tan Z, Roscoe A, Rubino A. Transesophageal Echocardiography in Heart and Lung Transplantation. J Cardiothorac Vasc Anesth 2019;33(6):1548–1558.
62. Serra E, Feltracco P, Barbieri S, et al. Transesophageal echocardiography during lung transplantation. Transpl Proc 2007;39(6):1981–1982.
63. Hausmann D, Daniel WG, Mugge A, et al. Imaging of pulmonary artery and vein anastomoses by transesophageal echocardiography after lung transplantation. Circulation 1992;86(5 Suppl):II251–258.
64. Michel-Cherqui M, Brusset A, Liu N, et al. Intraoperative transesophageal echocardiographic assessment of vascular anastomoses in lung transplantation. A report on 18 cases. Chest 1997; 111(5):1229–1235.
65. Burman ED, Keegan J, Kilner PJ. Pulmonary artery diameters, cross sectional areas and area changes measured by cine cardiovascular magnetic resonance in healthy volunteers. J Cardiovasc Magn Reson 2016;18:12.
66. Huang YC, Cheng YJ, Lin YH, et al. Graft failure caused by pulmonary venous obstruction diagnosed by intraoperative transesophageal echocardiography during lung transplantation. Anesth Analg 2000;91(3):558–560.
67. Gentile F, Mantero A, Lippolis A, et al. Pulmonary venous flow velocity patterns in 143 normal subjects aged 20 to 80 years old. An echo 2D colour Doppler cooperative study. Eur Heart J 1997;18(1):148–164.
68. Gonzalez-Fernandez C, Gonzalez-Castro A, Rodriguez-Borregan JC, et al. Pulmonary venous obstruction after lung transplantation. Diagnostic advantages of transesophageal echocardiography. Clin Transpl 2009;23(6):975–980.
69. Cartwright BL, Jackson A, Cooper J. Intraoperative pulmonary vein examination by transesophageal echocardiography: an anatomic update and review of utility. J Cardiothorac Vasc Anesth 2013;27(1): 111–120.
70. Kumar N, Essandoh M, Bhatt A, et al. Pulmonary cuff dysfunction after lung transplant surgery: A systematic review of the evidence and analysis of its clinical implications. J Heart Lung Transplant 2019;38(5): 530–544.
71. Valapour M, Skeans MA, Heubner BM, et al. OPTN/SRTR 2012 Annual Data Report: lung. Am J Transplant 2014;14(Suppl 1):139–165.
72. Orens JB, Estenne M, Arcasoy S, et al. International guidelines for the selection of lung transplant candidates: 2006 update–a consensus report from the Pulmonary Scientific Council of the International Society for Heart and Lung Transplantation. J Heart Lung Transplant 2006;25(7):745–755.
73. Leard LE, Holm AM, Valapour M, et al. Consensus document for the selection of lung transplant candidates: An update from the International Society for Heart and Lung Transplantation. J Heart Lung Transpl 2021;40(11):1349–1379.
74. Courtwright A, Cantu E. Lung transplantation in elderly patients. J Thorac Dis 2017;9(9):3346–3351.
75. Ehrsam JP, Benden C, Seifert B, et al. Lung transplantation in the elderly: Influence of age, comorbidities,

underlying disease, and extended criteria donor lungs. J Thorac Cardiovasc Surg 2017;154(6):2135–2141.

76. Hayanga AJ, Aboagye JK, Hayanga HE, et al. Contemporary analysis of early outcomes after lung transplantation in the elderly using a national registry. J Heart Lung Transplant 2015;34(2):182–188.

77. McCarthy F, Savino D, Graves D, et al. Cost and Readmission of Single and Double Lung Transplantation in the U. S. Medicare Population. J Heart Lung Transplant 2017;36:S115.

78. Mosher CL, Weber JM, Frankel CW, et al. Risk factors for mortality in lung transplant recipients aged >/=65 years: A retrospective cohort study of 5, 815 patients in the scientific registry of transplant recipients. J Heart Lung Transplant 2021;40(1): 42–55.

79. Mason DP, Thuita L, Nowicki ER, et al. Should lung transplantation be performed for patients on mechanical respiratory support? The US experience. J Thorac Cardiovasc Surg 2010;139(3):765–773. e761.

80. Elizur A, Sweet SC, Huddleston CB, et al. Pre-transplant mechanical ventilation increases short-term morbidity and mortality in pediatric patients with cystic fibrosis. J Heart Lung Transplant 2007;26(2): 127–131.

81. O'Brien G, Criner GJ. Mechanical ventilation as a bridge to lung transplantation. J Heart Lung Transplant 1999;18(3):255–265.

82. Singer JP, Blanc PD, Hoopes C, et al. The impact of pretransplant mechanical ventilation on shortand long-term survival after lung transplantation. Am J Transplant 2011;11(10):2197–2204.

83. Maxwell BG, Mooney JJ, Lee PH, et al. Increased resource use in lung transplant admissions in the lung allocation score era. Am J Respir Crit Care Med 2015;191(3):302–308.

84. Weill D, Benden C, Corris PA, et al. A consensus document for the selection of lung transplant candidates: 2014–an update from the Pulmonary Transplantation Council of the International Society for Heart andLung Transplantation. J Heart Lung Transplant 2015;34(1):1–15.

85. Hoopes CW, Kukreja J, Golden J, et al. Extracorporeal membrane oxygenation as a bridge to pulmonary transplantation. J Thorac Cardiovasc Surg 2013;145(3):862–867.

86. Tipograf Y, Salna M, Minko E, et al. Outcomes of Extracorporeal Membrane Oxygenation as a Bridge to Lung Transplantation. Ann Thorac Surg 2019; 107(5):1456–1463.

87. Hoetzenecker K, Donahoe L, Yeung JC, et al. Extracorporeal life support as a bridge to lung transplantation-experience of a high-volume transplant center. J Thorac Cardiovasc Surg 2018; 155(3):1316–1328 e1311.

88. Hayanga JWA, Hayanga HK, Holmes SD, et al. Mechanical ventilation and extracorporeal membrane oxygenation as a bridge to lung transplantation: Closing the gap. J Heart Lung Transplant 2019; 38(10):1104–1111.

89. Benazzo A, Schwarz S, Frommlet F, et al. Twentyyear experience with extracorporeal life support as bridge to lung transplantation. J Thorac Cardiovasc Surg 2019;157(6):2515–2525 e2510.

# 第 8 章　肺移植受者术后的早期管理

Binh N. Trinh, Marek Brzezinski, Jasleen Kukreja　著

梁瑞茵　朱小冬　译

陈晓渝　校

【关键词】
- 重症监护管理　• 免疫抑制　• 感控预防　• 肺移植并发症
- 原发性移植物功能不全　• 体外膜肺氧合

【要点】
- 术后管理的重点是保持同种异体移植物功能的同时维持末端器官足够的灌注。
- 良好的疼痛管理有助于早期下床活动和肺部清洁，从而降低同种异体移植物肺炎的风险。
- 早期识别原发性移植物功能不全并选择性使用体外膜肺氧合是成功的关键。
- 心律失常很常见，主要目标是控制心率。
- 其他常见并发症包括感染、急性肾损伤和胸腔积液。

## 8.1　引　言

肺移植（LTx）已成为终末期肺疾病的标准治疗手段，根据 2019 年国际胸腔器官移植登记中心的报告显示，肺移植的病例数量已增加至每年 4000 多例[1]。尽管肺移植的长期生存率仍然很低，中位生存期为 6.7 年，但由于手术技术和围术期管理水平的提高，因此在过去 40 年里短期生存率有所提高[1,2]。

移植物衰竭和与巨细胞病毒（CMV）无关的感染是术后早期发病和死亡的主要原因。在较小程度上，心血管事件、多系统器官衰竭和技术原因会对生存率产生不利的影响[1]。多学科团队合作是确保成功移植的关键方法[3,4]。在本章中，作者对肺移植术后的管理策略进行了回顾。

## 8.2 患者选择

术后管理从肺移植受者的选择开始,并在很大程度上受到肺移植受者移植前医疗和身体状况优化的影响[5]。随着经验的积累,移植中心正在考虑既往有禁忌证的候选者。例如,患有并发症的老年患者[6]、既往接受过胸部手术的患者[6,8,9]或需要多器官移植的患者都可以接受肺移植手术[10]。此外,需要在机械通气和(或)体外膜肺氧合(ECMO)支持下的患者进行肺移植也越来越多[2,11,12]。这些患者的活动能力更差,身体更虚弱,其发病率和死亡率更高[13]。然而,越来越多的证据表明,即便是这些高风险候选者,通过谨慎选择受者、术前优化、手术计划和术后管理,也能获得良好的治疗结果[2,7,9,11,12]。

近期出现的严重急性呼吸综合征冠状病毒2(SARS-CoV-2)导致的呼吸衰竭,产生了一群前所未有的高风险受者群体。根据研究者所在中心的经验,这些患者通常在移植前的数周或数月需要依赖呼吸机和ECMO的支持[14,15]。尽管移植后的短期结果相对令人满意,但其长期生存率仍有待观察。需要强调的是,成功的治疗结果取决于营养优化[5,16]、肺康复[17,18]以及对可能构成挑战的生物因素的识别,如身材矮小、稀有血型和肺动脉高压等[12]。通过经胸超声心动图(transthoracic echocardiography,TTE)来管理肺动脉高压并密切监测右心室功能,有助于手术操作的优化[19]。

## 8.3 术中管理

术前计划和术中操作有助于为术后成功奠定基础[5,16]。研究者简要论述了他们的手术理念。关于供体的选择,一项对身高和体重进行匹配分析的研究发现,除因纤维化肺病而接受移植的群体外,供体偏小会导致生存率降低[1]。据推测,偏小的供体肺存在过度通气的风险,因此更容易发生原发性移植物功能不全(PGD)[20]。由于双侧肺移植具有更高的生存率[10],因此,研究者的做法是对70岁以下且无并发症的患者进行双肺移植。移植手术可以在ECMO、心肺转流术(CPB)或无体外支持的情况下进行[21]。由于使用CPB会增加输血需求和PGD的风险,因此在研究者中心和其他中心的双肺移植术中,凝血状况和移植结果更佳的ECMO支持基本上已取代了CPB[22-25]。目前仍有争论的是,是否所有的肺移植都应该在ECMO的支持下进行,而不考虑其潜在病因或病理生理因素。研究者选择性地对高危病例使用CPB。例如,在ECMO移植过渡期的粘连性肺病患者,这类患者在移植时预计会大量失血(>10单位的浓缩红细胞)。尽管新型冠状病毒肺炎

（COVID）成人呼吸窘迫综合征（adult respiratory distress syndrome，ARDS）的胸膜腔"环境恶劣"，但研究者仍在术中通过 ECMO 成功地对患者进行了管理[12,25]。在研究者所在的中心，通常是在没有体外支持的情况下对慢性阻塞性肺疾病（COPD）及无严重肺动脉高压的患者进行单肺移植术。

缺血时间过长会增加 PGD 的风险[8,26]，但也有缺血超过 6 小时仍可获得良好结果的报道[27]。研究者所在的中心在没有体外肺灌注的情况下，成功对缺血时间超过 11 小时的患者进行了肺移植术。建议在关闭胸腔前，密切监测是否存在明显的再灌注损伤。如果 $PaO_2/FiO_2$（PF 比值）< 150，应立即寻找可逆性的原因，并考虑使用 ECMO 支持。在严重的情况下，无论是否使用 ECMO，都应将胸腔部分开放以最大限度地减少气道压力和肺填塞的可能性，从而为同种异体移植物的改善争取时间[28-30]。临时性开胸策略有助于解决持续的凝血功能障碍和原发性移植物功能不全的问题，为后续的胸腔冲洗和最终闭合做好准备。

## 8.4 血流动力学术后管理

到达重症监护室后，建议使用小剂量升压药和正性肌力支持药物，并谨慎使用液体（晶体或胶体），旨在保持同种异体移植物干燥的同时也维持末端器官灌注[21]。出现大面积肺水肿时警惕严重再灌注损伤的出现，贫血伴不透明阴影可能提示血胸存在。床旁 TTE 可作为评估双心室功能和血容量状态以及排除心包填塞的有效辅助手段。

血流动力学术后管理的目标包括通过控制心率和每搏输出量来维持足够的前负荷和优化心输出量。由于代谢性酸中毒、低氧血症、低血压和电解质紊乱，移植后可能会出现心肌收缩力下降。TTE 评估有助于指导使用正性肌力支持药物，如多巴酚丁胺、肾上腺素、多巴胺和米力农。虽然米力农在改善心肌收缩力方面具有显著效果，但其对全身血管系统的广泛性舒张作用仍然存在一定的问题。因此，研究者在围术期很少使用米力农。鉴于许多间质性肺疾病患者已存在肺动脉高压和右心室功能障碍，因此需要特别注意避免 PGD[12,19]。联合一氧化氮吸入和前列环素可以改善血氧饱和度，但尚未证明其是否可以提高生存率或缩短住院时间[21,31,32]。

心律失常还会导致心输出量降低。Mason 及其同事[33]报告，心房颤动在肺移植术后的发生率为 20%，导致住院时间延长和死亡率增高[34]，高达 70% 的病例发生在前 4 天[33]。使用 β 受体阻滞剂和补充血清镁能有效控制心率。根据 2014 年美国胸外科协会指南，使用β受体阻滞剂、钙通道阻滞剂或胺碘酮有Ⅱ类证据支持[35]。目前的最佳实践旨在以控制心率为主要目标，以控制心律为次要目标[35]。静脉注射胺碘酮可用于药物心脏复律。血流动力学不稳定的患者需紧急进行R波直流电同步复律。Ⅰ类证据建议应逐渐减少或停用儿茶酚胺类正性肌力药物、优化电解质以及治疗应激事件，如疼痛、出血和感染[35]。最近一项针对心脏手术患者的多中心随机试验发现，在进行左心房闭塞术的同时采用抗凝治疗可使脑卒中发生率从7%降至4.8%[36]；然而，这在肺移植中目前尚未研究。

移植肺受益于避免容量超负荷。然而，由于术中出血、肺切除和血管麻痹会引起低血容量，术后早期通常会出现低心输出量状态。中心静脉压（CVP）、每搏量和肺毛细血管楔压（pulmonary capillary wedge pressures，PCWP）的降低，进一步证实了血容量低。实验室检测结果显示明显的代谢性酸中毒和血清乳酸水平升高，可通过胶体和晶体补液进行治疗[37,38]。

贫血、低血压、尿量减少、CVP低、PCWP低和混合静脉血氧饱和度（$SvO_2$）降低综合征均提示持续失血，通常需要输血复苏。据报道，9%~18%的病例会出现大出血[25,39,40]。胸膜外剥离术用于严重胸膜融合，使用需要抗凝的ECMO或CPB会加重出血，导致凝血功能障碍、低纤维蛋白原血症和血小板减少症的恶性循环[25]。应对输血引起的继发性低钙血症予以纠正，因为钙在心肌收缩中起核心作用。及早识别和治疗持续性失血对于预防过度输血、潜在的输血性相关急性肺损伤、肺水肿和同种异体免疫至关重要[41-43]。如果持续出现凝血功能障碍，低血压、血管升压药需求增加、肺顺应性降低和低氧血症可能会导致胸腔间隔综合征[28,29]。这是由肺水肿、肺体积过大以及持续性的胸腔出血造成的胸腔狭窄共同引发的。及早发现对于手术减压是必要的。难治性病例可能需要使用ECMO作为恢复过渡的支持[44]。

## 8.5 镇静和疼痛管理

研究者的方案是使用传统短效的丙泊酚进行镇静[45]。小剂量右美托咪定是一种有效的辅助药物，具有镇静和镇痛作用[45,46]。术后充分镇痛是围手术期管理的重要组成部分[47]。采用多模式方法进行疼痛控制，可以让患者能够活动、行走和参与肺部理疗，从而预防肺不张和肺炎。芬太尼和氢吗啡酮等阿片类药物可通过静脉注射或患者自控镇痛泵给药。另外，胸腔硬膜外麻醉（thoracic epidural anesthesia，TEA）可通过局部麻醉剂（如丁哌卡因）和阿片类药物联合使用来达到极好的镇痛效果，该方法可减少肺部并发症[47]。尽管围术期凝血功能障碍可能会延迟硬膜外导管的置入，TEA 仍可在拔管前进行。有用的非阿片类药物替代药包括静脉注射对乙酰氨基酚、加巴喷丁和利多卡因贴片。通常，研究者会添加软便剂来预防阿片类药物引起的便秘，必要时可口服纳洛酮或甲基纳曲酮。非必要时需避免使用非甾体抗炎药，以降低肾损伤的风险。最后，对漏斗胸修复术中的疼痛控制研究表明，肋间低温镇痛可有效减少阿片类药物和 TEA 的用量[48,49]。根据研究者的经验，这种方法基本上取代了 TEA，为肺移植受者提供了有效的镇痛，且无明显的并发症[50,51]。

## 8.6 移植物功能的管理

机械通气的目的是最大限度地降低高原气道压力，避免高潮气量以及预防缺氧[52]。通常基于供者体重进行潮气量的选择[20,52-54]。吸入一氧化氮可以缓解肺动脉高压引起的严重缺氧患者的灌注通气失调，但这种方法尚未被证实能预防 PGD[55,56]。大多数无明显 PGD 的患者可以在术后 72 小时内安全拔管[25]。临床实践表明，32% 的移植中心会在术后 24 小时内拔管，另有 32% 的移植中心会在术后 48 小时内拔管[52]。无创通气有助于减少呼吸耗氧量并支持现有的呼吸功能。预防肺不张和肺炎的措施包括肺活量测定、胸部理疗和进行早期活动。根据临床需要进行的支气管镜检查是评估气道健康状况的重要手段，有助于清除黏稠的分泌物[57]。插管时间延长的患者有可能会出现相关的并发症，如房性心律失常和气管切开[52]。

移植肺在早期会由于心脏、肺和胸腔等综合因素的影响而顺应性降低。主要的管理目标是提高肺顺应性的同时降低气道阻力，并尽可能避免液体超负荷。高 CVP 和 PCWP 提示容量超负荷，需要进行利尿[21]。黏液堵塞会增加呼吸道阻力，导致通气灌注失调和血氧饱和度较低。由于同种异体移植的气道因失去支气管动脉供应而相对缺血，易发生黏膜脱落，因此需要定期清理。在某些病例中，气道坏死、狭窄和裂开的发生率可高达 20%[58]。因此，支气管镜检查是诊断和治疗的重要手段[57]。由于肺泡表面活性物质功能受损、疼痛控制不佳以及气道分泌物增多，移植肺常出现早期肺不张和顺应性降低的现象[59]。胸膜腔并发症和膈肌功能障碍会限制胸腔，导致肺复张不全。出血、感染和淋巴引流丧失都可能会导致胸膜腔的并发症[60]。某些患者由于总肺活量和用力肺活量严重下降或膈肌功能障碍而导致胸腔受限，从而出现明显的压缩性肺不张。

PGD 是早晚期死亡的重要原因，并且与慢性肺同种异体移植物功能障碍（CLAD）的发展有关[8,26,61,62]，通常发生在术后 72 小时内，以低氧血症、肺水肿、顺应性降低以及其他无法解释原因的双侧放射学浸润为临床特征，其严重程度可从轻度到重度不等。国际心肺移植学会基于 PF 比值制定的标准化分级方案，从 1 级到 3 级严重程度依次递增[63]。PGD 的总体发生率约为 30%，其中 15%~20% 的受者在植入后的 48 小时和 72 小时出现 3 级 PGD[8]。除既往肺动脉高压是一个重要的危险因素，其他因素还包括缺血时间延长、肥胖、移植前诊断为结节病和特发性肺动脉高压以及供者的危险因素（如吸烟、年龄＞65 岁）[8,26,55]。早期识别 PGD 有助于制定降低风险的管理策略[64-66]。PGD 的管理主要是支持性治疗，预防措施主要包括最佳供者选择、适当的尺寸匹配和改善围术期管理。例如，使用最低的 $FiO_2$ 来支持血氧饱和度，因为高 $FiO_2$ 与移植物再灌注损伤有关[26]。同样，保持较低的 CVP 有助于最大限度地减少移植物水肿。延迟关胸已被用作管理 3 级 PGD 的策略[28,29]。有选择性地使用 ECMO 可以避免同种异体移植物受弥漫性肺泡损伤，并提高生存率[67]。早期预防性使用 ECMO 可改善预后[68]。对于血流动力学稳定、右心室功能正常且无明显肺动脉高压的患者可使用 VV-ECMO[67]。对于血流动力学不稳定且右心室功能障碍的患者，VA-ECMO 可以保护右心并减少持续性肺水肿[25,44]。ECMO 支持移植肺在潮气量低于 3 mL/kg 的超保护性通气条件下避免持续的呼吸性酸中毒。而在血流动力学稳定的患者中，选择 VV 还是 VA ECMO 存在一定的争议[66]。

作为特殊情况，单肺移植是 PGD 的独立危险因素[26]，并且与较差的生存率相关[10]。尽管选择单肺移植还是双肺移植仍存在争议[69-71]，但双侧肺移植是囊性纤维化和支气管扩张患者的首选手术方法，因为在这两种疾病中，既存的感染可能会污染新肺[69]。此外，单肺移植病例可能会出现严重的通气灌注失调[72]。在 COPD 患者中，正压通气期间可能会出现急性原生肺过度充气[71]，导致对侧纵隔移位、单肺异体移植物外压、低氧血症和血流动力学不稳定。在因间质性肺疾病而接受移植的患者中，仍可能会出现原生肺急性恶化的情况[73]。

## 8.7 免疫抑制

约 25% 的肺移植受者在第一年内至少经历过一次排斥反应[1]。关于肺同种异体移植排斥反应的讨论将在本书的其他章节展开。虽然各个移植项目的做法各有不同，但 2017 年的一项调查显示，80% 的移植项目纳入了诱导策略[1]。尽管没有强有力的证据支持某一特定策略，但在 75% 的移植项目中，淋巴细胞清除胸腺球蛋白和单克隆抗 CD52 阿仑妥珠单抗的使用率有所下降，而使用白细胞介素-2受体α链拮抗剂（即巴利昔单抗）有所增加[1]。这种趋势可能是由于患者的耐受性良好和不良反应较小[74]。诱导治疗会增加感染概率和淋巴组织增生性疾病的风险。胸腺球蛋白和阿仑妥珠单抗与严重的骨髓抑制有关，并可引起细胞因子释放反应[74]。在研究者的临床实践中，在每次同种异体移植灌注前给予静脉注射霉酚酸酯和巴利昔单抗以及甲泼尼龙冲击治疗。常规维持治疗使用皮质类固醇、钙调神经蛋白抑制剂（calcineurin inhibitor，CNI）（他克莫司或环孢素）和抗增殖剂（霉酚酸酯或硫唑嘌呤）。研究者更倾向于使用他克莫司联合霉酚酸酯，这种组合在国际上80%以上的移植病例中使用[74]。他克莫司因为其急性排斥反应和CLAD的发生率较低，已取代环孢素成为一线治疗药物[74,75]。CNI的不良反应包括高钾血症、高血压、高脂血症和神经毒性，其中肾毒性是最严重的不良反应之一。mTOR抑制剂西罗莫司和依维莫司是替代免疫抑制剂，有助于减少CNI剂量和降低肾毒性，但由于伤口愈合不良、蛋白尿和水肿等因素，致其使用受到限制[76,77]。至于霉酚酸酯与硫唑嘌呤的对比，研究并未支持某种特定的选择，但霉酚酸酯通常更受青睐，可能是因为患者对其耐受性更好且患皮肤癌的风险更低[74,78]，尽管其与骨髓抑制和胃肠道紊乱明显相关[79-81]。对于胃肠道症状严重的患者，研究者发现患者对霉酚酸的耐受性优于霉酚酸酯。而对于骨髓抑制的患者，由于白细胞减少，对霉酚酸酯的耐受性可能会因人而异[80]。

## 8.8 感染管理

感染是肺移植术后死亡的主要原因，也是导致肺移植术后生存率低于其他实质器官移植的主要原因[82]，常发生在移植后的前3~6个月内[83]。细菌感染通常以肺炎、胸膜腔和伤口感染的形式出现，但也可发生在泌尿道和胆道系统。根据感染发生时间和培养结果可对采取适当的治疗有所帮助。最好尽早使用广谱抗生素来应对医院感染，包括多重耐药菌[84]。供体的培养结果和支气管肺泡灌洗液培养结果以及药敏数据可帮助医疗服务提供者制定有针对性的抗菌治疗方案，从而以最窄的有效抗生素谱减少供体对宿主的传播[85]。众所周知，及时拔除留置的中心静脉导管和导尿管以及积极的肺部清洗是预防医院获得性感染的有效措施[86]。多重耐药微生物的出现可能会影响治疗方案，因此，万古霉素和碳青霉烯类分别是针对耐甲氧西林金黄色葡萄球菌和广谱β内酰胺酶的常用初始疗法[87]。耐万古霉素肠球菌可用利奈唑胺治疗。除厄他培南外，碳青霉烯类药物通常对假单胞菌株具有良好的经验性覆盖范围。对于鲍曼不动杆菌的感染可能具有挑战性，但可使用黏菌素和亚胺培南/西司他丁治疗[87]。诺卡菌、李斯特菌和红球菌等较罕见的感染较少遇到，而嗜麦芽窄食单胞菌的感染相较麻烦[88]。在患有囊性纤维化和支气管扩张的患者中，上呼吸道和下呼吸道中的多重耐药天然定植菌的感染治疗特别困难，因为单依靠肺移植无法消除所有潜在感染源[89-91]。

侵袭性真菌感染是发病的另一重要原因。侵袭性肺曲霉菌的死亡率可高达60%。一项针对约1700例病例的调查显示，移植后第一年的感染率接近9%[92]，其中曲霉菌占所有病例的70%以上[93]。缺血性吻合部位的曲霉菌定植和气管支气管炎导致的重度免疫抑制是造成严重感染的主要危险因素[94]。因此，以伏立康唑加或不加吸入两性霉素B脂质体的形式进行的真菌预防已成为许多项目的标准做法[95,96]。尽管这种做法得到广泛应用，但现有的数据并不支持使用抗真菌预防剂[97]。其他真菌来源包括酵母菌种，如念珠菌属、隐球菌属、肺孢菌属，以及非曲霉菌种，如丝孢菌属和镰刀菌属。研究者的方案提出，将预防性静脉注射伏立康唑，并把艾沙康唑作为预防治疗的替代药物。等肠内营养恢复后，再口服泊沙康唑以减少伏立康唑的已知不良反应[98,99]。泊沙康唑和艾沙康唑的肝毒性状况较好。30%的患者使用伏立康唑后会产生特有的幻觉、光敏感性和骨膜炎。伏立康唑还会抑制CNI的代谢，长期使用会增加患皮肤鳞状细胞癌的风险[100]。使用唑类药物会导致QTc延长和增加尖端扭转型室性心动过速的风险[99]。

最后，病毒感染与急性呼吸衰竭和闭塞性细支气管炎综合征（bronchiolitis obliterans syndrome，BOS）的发展有关。社区获得性呼吸道病毒（甲型和乙型流感病毒、偏肺病毒、鼻病毒、腺病毒和呼吸道合胞病毒）可导致严重的季节性发病[101]。受体和供体来源性病毒感染均可导致严重PGD。例如，研究者在第一次移植后30天对一例因供体源性偏肺病毒引起ARDS而导致同种异体移植受损的受者进行了再次移植。预防措施包括手卫生、避免接触患者和进行全面监测。治疗需针对特定的病原体及可使用的抗病毒药物。利巴韦林联合类固醇可用于治疗偏肺病毒和呼吸道合胞病毒[102]。腺病毒导致的肺炎和感染性疾病，尤其具有挑战性。西多福韦的使用已取得一些成效[103]。CMV感染是死亡的重要原因，并且与CLAD的发生有关。活动性CMV感染可通过血清和受累器官活检中的DNA来识别。由于供体受体CMV不匹配和严重的免疫抑制导致肺移植患者的发病率高于其他器官移植的患者。CMV感染的预防措施包括预防性使用抗病毒药物（通常为缬更昔洛韦）持续12个月或更长时间，并通过聚合酶链反应监测血清病毒载量[104]。

## 8.9 其他医疗并发症的管理

虽然保护肺功能是首要任务，但某些医疗并发症也会增加肺移植患者在住院期间的风险。免疫抑制剂会加重原有病情，包括骨质疏松症、糖尿病、高血压、冠状动脉疾病和胃食管反流病（gastroesophageal reflux disease，GERD）[3,74]。常见的代谢紊乱有高钾血症、高血糖和高脂血症。震颤、白细胞减少、贫血和腹泻是他克莫司、霉酚酸酯和缬更昔洛韦的常见不良反应[74,80]。

胃食管反流病在移植前的受者中发病率很高[105-107]。移植前测压和 pH 检测通常会显示相关的食管裂孔疝、食管运动障碍和 DeMeester 评分升高。移植后胃酸反流的情况可能会恶化[107,108]。BOS 与 GERD 有关[109]。因此，质子泵抑制剂可用于对抗胃酸反流，却无法治疗非胃酸反流引起的微吸入问题[106]。术后早期抗反流具有保护作用，并且可以提高生存率以及避免 BOS[108,110]。

急性肾损伤（acute kidney injury，AKI）是肺移植术后的常见并发症，也是影响长期结果的预后标志。Wehbe 等[111]的研究发现，65% 的患者在移植后 2 周内出现 AKI。出院时肾功能未恢复的患者，其慢性肾病发病率更高，12 个月的生存率更低。然而，与未发生 AKI 的患者相比，即使是肾功能恢复的患者其长期预后也相对较差。危险因素涉及多个方面，包括年龄偏大、糖尿病、高血压控制不佳、脓毒症、围术期低血压以及 CNI 的使用[111,112]。这强调了尽早识别危险因素并积极采取更多肾脏保护措施的重要性，包括控制高血压[113]、尽早转诊至肾病专科医生、尽量减少 CNI 的使用，同时平衡预防排斥反应的需求[112,114]。

胸膜并发症很常见，会对同种异体移植物的功能产生负面影响[115,116]。胸腔积液的特征会随时间变化，而过度引流则是继发于肺泡毛细血管通透性增加和肺淋巴管破坏[60]。事实上，研究者自己的观察结果与已发表的文献报道一致，即大量引流可持续 9~19 天[39,60]，因此，留置胸腔引流管会延长住院时间。Ferrer 等[39]观察到，在他们的队列中有 12 例患者胸腔引流管留置时间超过 30 天，研究者推测这可能是重建淋巴引流所需的时间。Tang 等[116]研究发现，在 1039 例患者中，近 200 例患者需要进行 300 多次胸腔穿刺和 200 多次的开胸术。有 140 例患者需要开胸手术进行冲洗，另有 88 例患者需要行胸膜剥脱术。在 Marom 等[117]的一项回顾性研究中，有 31 例胸腔积液患者接受了经皮小孔导管治疗，其中 16/31 例被归为感染性胸腔积液。引流时间中位数为 6 天，残留积液采用链激酶溶栓治疗。另外，9/31 例患者需要进行多次插管。在 3 个月的随访中，有 79% 的患者完全康复。然而，在16例脓胸患者中，有9例患者在引流干预后6个月内死亡。

最后，多份报告记录了移植人群中深静脉血栓形成（deep vein thrombosis，DVT）的高发病率[118]。一项单中心研究显示，常规下肢筛查在最初90天内识别出的DVT发生率为17%。Jorge等[119]的另一份报告指出，普及DVT筛查可能与1年生存率提高有关。由于DVT会对生存率产生负面影响[120]，研究者所在的项目会对住院患者皮下常规注射普通肝素进行DVT预防。

## 8.10 总　结

肺移植术后早期是关键阶段。及早识别和治疗PGD可以改变移植物的长期功能。心血管、胃肠道、肾脏、血液系统紊乱和感染性并发症很常见，需要进行密切管理以降低其不良后果。

### 利益声明

B.N. 特林：无利益声明。J. 库克雷亚：Trans-Medics（研究）；肺部生物工程（数据监测委员会）。M. 布热津斯基：Trevena和Grifols（研究）。

# 参考文献

1. Chambers, et al. The International Thoracic Organ Transplant Registry of the International Society for Heart and Lung Transplantation: thirty-sixth adult lung and heart-lung transplantation report-2019; focus theme: donor and recipient size match. J Heart Lung Transplant 2019;38(10):1042–1055.
2. Hamilton, et al. Improved survival after lung transplantation for adults requiring preoperative invasive mechanical ventilation: a national cohort study. J Thorac Cardiovasc Surg 2020;160(5):1385–1395. e6.
3. Sam, et al. Roles and impacts of the transplant pharmacist: a systematic review. Can J Hosp Pharm 2018;71(5):324–337.
4. Gordon, et al. Reducing length of stay after lung transplant through Implementation of multidisciplinary care coordination rounds. J Heart Lung Transplantation 2020;39(4):S209.
5. Allen, et al. The impact of recipient body mass index on survival after lung transplantation. J Heart Lung Transplant 2010;29(9):1026–1033.
6. Weill, et al. A consensus document for the selection of lung transplant candidates: 2014–an update from the Pulmonary Transplantation Council of the International Society for Heart and Lung Transplantation. J Heart

Lung Transplant 2015;34(1):1–15.

7. McKellar, et al. Lung transplantation following coronary artery bypass surgery-improved outcomes following single-lung transplant. J Heart Lung Transplant 2016;35(11):1289–1294.
8. Diamond, et al. Report of the International Society for Heart and Lung Transplantation Working Group on Primary Lung Graft Dysfunction, part II: epidemiology, risk factors, and outcomes-a 2016 consensus group statement of the International Society for Heart and Lung Transplantation. J Heart Lung Transplant 2017;36(10):1104–1113.
9. Wallinder, et al. Outcomes and long-term survival after pulmonary retransplantation: a single-center experience. Ann Thorac Surg 2019;108(4): 1037–1044.
10. Chambers, et al. The International Thoracic Organ Transplant Registry of the International Society for Heart and Lung Transplantation: thirty-fifth adult lung and heart-lung transplant report-2018; focus theme: multiorgan transplantation. J Heart Lung Transplant 2018;37(10):1169–1183.
11. Hoopes, et al. Extracorporeal membrane oxygenation as a bridge to pulmonary transplantation. J Thorac Cardiovasc Surg 2013;145(3):862–7 [discussion: 867–868].
12. Kukreja, et al. Risk factors and outcomes of extracorporeal membrane oxygenation as a bridge to lung transplantation. Semin Thorac Cardiovasc Surg 2020;32(4):772–785.
13. Singer, et al. Frailty phenotypes and mortality after lung transplantation: a prospective cohort study. Am J Transplant 2018;18(8):1995–2004.
14. Bharat, et al. Early outcomes after lung transplantation for severe COVID-19: a series of the first consecutive cases from four countries. Lancet Respir Med 2021;9(5):487–497.
15. Cypel, et al. When to consider lung transplantation for COVID-19. Lancet Respir Med 2020;8(10): 944–946.
16. Lederer, et al. Obesity and underweight are associated with an increased risk of death after lung transplantation. Am J Respir Crit Care Med 2009; 180(9):887–895.
17. Martinu, et al. Baseline 6-min walk distance predicts survival in lung transplant candidates. Am J Transplant 2008;8(7):1498–1505.
18. Rochester pulmonary rehabilitation for patients who undergo lung-volume-reduction surgery or lung transplantation. Respir Care 2008;53(9):1196–1202.
19. Chicotka, et al. Increasing opportunity for lung transplant in interstitial lung disease with pulmonary hypertension. Ann Thorac Surg 2018;106(6):1812–1819.
20. Eberlein, et al. Lung size mismatch and primary graft dysfunction after bilateral lung transplantation. J Heart Lung Transplant 2015;34(2):233–240.
21. Subramaniam, et al. Anesthetic management of lung transplantation: results from a multicenter, cross-sectional survey by the society for advancement of transplant anesthesia. Clin Transplant 2020;34(8):e13996.
22. Bermudez, et al. Outcomes of intraoperative venoarterial extracorporeal membrane oxygenation versus cardiopulmonary bypass during lung transplantation. Ann Thorac Surg 2014;98(6):1936–42 [discussion: 1942–1943].
23. Machuca, et al. Outcomes of intraoperative extracorporeal membrane oxygenation versus cardiopulmonary bypass for lung transplantation. J Thorac Cardiovasc Surg 2015;149(4):1152–1157.
24. Nagendran, et al. Should double lung transplant be performed with or without cardiopulmonary bypass?

Interact Cardiovasc Thorac Surg 2011; 12(5):799–804.

25. Hoetzenecker, et al. Bilateral lung transplantation on intraoperative extracorporeal membrane oxygenator: an observational study. J Thorac Cardiovasc Surg 2020;160(1):320–327 e1.
26. Diamond, et al. Clinical risk factors for primary graft dysfunction after lung transplantation. Am J Respir Crit Care Med 2013;187(5):527–534.
27. Grimm, et al. Association between prolonged graft ischemia and primary graft failure or survival following lung transplantation. JAMA Surg 2015; 150(6):547–553.
28. Force, et al. Outcomes of delayed chest closure after bilateral lung transplantation. Ann Thorac Surg 2006;81(6):2020–4 [discussion: 2024–2025].
29. Shigemura, et al. Delayed chest closure after lung transplantation: techniques, outcomes, and strategies. J Heart Lung Transplant 2014;33(7):741–748.
30. Tsou et al. Delayed chest closure following bilateral lung transplantation: risk factors and outcomes. Mar 2020 Present. . Mini-oral presentation at the 41st Annual Meeting & Scientific Sessions of the International Society for Heart and Lung Transplantation (ISHLT) April 24-28, 2021,
31. Yerebakan, et al. Effects of inhaled nitric oxide following lung transplantation. J Card Surg 2009; 24(3):269–274.
32. Khan, et al. A prospective, randomized, crossover pilot study of inhaled nitric oxide versus inhaled prostacyclin in heart transplant and lung transplant recipients. J Thorac Cardiovasc Surg 2009;138(6): 1417–1424.
33. Mason, et al. Atrial fibrillation after lung transplantation: timing, risk factors, and treatment. Ann Thorac Surg 2007;84(6):1878–1884.
34. Waldron, et al. Adverse outcomes associated with postoperative atrial arrhythmias after lung transplantation: a meta-analysis and systematic review of the literature. Clin Transplant 2017;31(4). https://doi.org/10.1111/ctr. 12926.
35. Frendl, et al. 2014 AATS guidelines for the prevention and management of perioperative atrial fibrillation and flutter for thoracic surgical procedures. J Thorac Cardiovasc Surg 2014 148(3):e153–193.
36. Whitlock, et al. Left atrial appendage occlusion during cardiac surgery to prevent stroke. N Engl J Med 2021;384(22):2081–2091.
37. Worrell, et al. Is lactic acidosis after lung transplantation associated with worse outcomes? Ann Thorac Surg 2020;110(2):434–440.
38. Xu, et al. The prognostic value of peak arterial lactate levels within 72 h of lung transplantation in identifying patient outcome. J Thorac Dis 2020;12(12):7365–7373.
39. Ferrer, et al. Acute and chronic pleural complications in lung transplantation. J Heart Lung Transplant 2003;22(11):1217–1225.
40. Navarro C, et al. [Complications after lung transplantation in chronic obstructive pulmonary disease]. Med Clin (Barc) 2013;140(9):385–389.
41. Zimring, et al. Current problems and future directions of transfusion-induced alloimmunization: summary of an NHLBI working group. Transfusion 2011;51(2):435–441.
42. Brand immunological complications of blood transfusions. Presse Med 2016;45(7–8 Pt 2):e313–324.

43. Bux, et al. The pathogenesis of transfusion-related acute lung injury (TRALI). Br J Haematol 2007; 136(6):788–799.
44. Fischer, et al. Extracorporeal membrane oxygenation for primary graft dysfunction after lung transplantation: analysis of the Extracorporeal Life Support Organization (ELSO) registry. J Heart Lung Transplant 2007;26(5):472–477.
45. King, et al. Early postoperative management after lung transplantation: results of an international survey. Clin Transplant 2017;31(7). https://doi.org/10.1111/ctr. 12985.
46. Schlichter Dexmedetomidine is an excellent agent for sedation status-post lung transplant. J Clin Anesth 2010;22(1):1–2.
47. Feltracco, et al. Thoracic epidural analgesia in lung transplantation. Transplant Proc 2010;42(4): 1265–1269.
48. Clemence, et al. Cryoablation of intercostal nerves decreased narcotic usage after thoracic or thoracoabdominal aortic aneurysm repair. Semin Thorac Cardiovasc Surg 2020;32(3):404–412.
49. Graves, et al. Intraoperative intercostal nerve cryoablation during the Nuss procedure reduces length of stay and opioid requirement: a randomized clinical trial. J Pediatr Surg 2019;54(11): 2250–2256.
50. Haro et al. Intercostal nerve cryoanalgesia versus thoracic epidural analgesia in lung transplantation. The Western Thoracic Surgical Association 2019 Abstract. 2019.
51. Parrado, et al. The use of cryoanalgesia in minimally invasive repair of pectus excavatum: lessons learned. J Laparoendosc Adv Surg Tech A 2019; 29(10):1244–1251.
52. Beer, et al. Mechanical ventilation after lung transplantation. An international survey of practices and preferences. Ann Am Thorac Soc 2014;11(4): 546–553.
53. Dezube, et al. The effect of lung-size mismatch on mechanical ventilation tidal volumes after bilateral lung transplantation. Interact Cardiovasc Thorac Surg 2013;16(3):275–281.
54. Mascia, et al. Effect of a lung protective strategy for organ donors on eligibility and availability of lungs for transplantation: a randomized controlled trial. JAMA 2010;304(23):2620–2627.
55. Liu, et al. Recipient-related clinical risk factors for primary graft dysfunction after lung transplantation: a systematic review and meta-analysis. PLoS One 2014;9(3):e92773.
56. Meade, et al. A randomized trial of inhaled nitric oxide to prevent ischemia-reperfusion injury after lung transplantation. Am J Respir Crit Care Med 2003;167(11):1483–1489.
57. Trulock. Flexible bronchoscopy in lung transplantation. Clin Chest Med 1999;20(1):77–87.
58. Machuzak, et al. Airway complications after lung transplantation. Thorac Surg Clin 2015;25(1): 55–75.
59. Amital, et al. Surfactant as salvage therapy in life threatening primary graft dysfunction in lung transplantation. Eur J Cardiothorac Surg 2009;35(2): 299–303.
60. Judson, et al. Pleural effusions following lung transplantation. Time course, characteristics, and clinical implications. Chest 1996;109(5):1190–1194.
61. Christie, et al. Primary graft failure following lung transplantation. Chest 1998;114(1):51–60.
62. Huang, et al. Late primary graft dysfunction after lung transplantation and bronchiolitis obliterans syndrome. Am J Transplant 2008;8(11):2454–2462.
63. Snell, et al. Report of the ISHLT Working Group on Primary Lung Graft Dysfunction, part I: definition and grading-a 2016 consensus group statement of the International Society for Heart and Lung Transplantation. J

Heart Lung Transplant 2017; 36(10):1097–1103.

64. de Perrot, et al. Report of the ISHLT Working Group on Primary Lung Graft Dysfunction part III: donor-related risk factors and markers. J Heart Lung Transplant 2005;24(10) 1460–1467.
65. Barr, et al. Report of the ISHLT Working Group on Primary Lung Graft Dysfunction part IV: recipient-related risk factors and markers. J Heart Lung Transplant 2005;24(10):1468–1482.
66. Van Raemdonck, et al. Report of the ISHLT Working Group on primary lung graft dysfunction part IV: prevention and treatment: a 2016 consensus group statement of the International Society for Heart and Lung Transplantation. J Heart Lung Transplant 2017;36(10):1121–1136.
67. Hartwig, et al. Improved survival but marginal allograft function in patients treated with extracorporeal membrane oxygenation after lung transplantation. Ann Thorac Surg 2012;93(2):366–371.
68. Wigfield, et al. Early institution of extracorporeal membrane oxygenation for primary graft dysfunction after lung transplantation improves outcome. J Heart Lung Transplant 2007;26(4):331–338.
69. Puri, et al. Single versus bilateral lung transplantation: do guidelines exist? Thorac Surg Clin 2015; 25(1):47–54.
70. Brown, et al. Outcomes after single lung transplantation in older patients with secondary pulmonary arterial hypertension. J Heart Lung Transplant 2013;32(1):134–136.
71. Siddiqui, et al. Lung transplantation for chronic obstructive pulmonary disease: past, present, and future directions. Curr Opin Pulm Med 2018; 24(2):199–204.
72. Stevens, et al. Regional ventilation and perfusion after lung transplantation in patients with emphysema. N Engl J Med 1970;282(5):245–249.
73. Marron, et al. Acute hypoxemic respiratory failure and native lung idiopathic pulmonary fibrosis exacerbation in single-lung transplant patients with cytomegalovirus disease: a case series. Transplant Proc 2019;51(10):3391–3394.
74. Chung, et al. Immunosuppressive strategies in lung transplantation. Ann Transl Med 2020;8(6): 409.
75. Treede, et al. Tacrolimus versus cyclosporine after lung transplantation: a prospective, open, randomized two-center trial comparing two different immunosuppressive protocols. J Heart Lung Transplant 2001;20(5):511–517.
76. Gottlieb, et al. A randomized trial of everolimus-based quadruple therapy vs standard triple therapy early after lung transplantation. Am J Transplant 2019;19(6):1759–1769.
77. Groetzner, et al. Airway anastomosis complications in de novo lung transplantation with sirolimus-based immunosuppression. J Heart Lung Transplant 2004;23(5):632–638.
78. Palmer, et al. Results of a randomized, prospective, multicenter trial of mycophenolate mofetil versus azathioprine in the prevention of acute lung allograft rejection. Transplantation 2001;71(12): 1772–1776.
79. Ceschi, et al. Acute mycophenolate overdose: case series and systematic literature analysis. Expert Opin Drug Saf 2014;13(5):525–534.
80. Tokman, et al. Clinical outcomes of lung transplant recipients with telomerase mutations. J Heart Lung Transplant 2015;34(10):1318–1324.
81. A blinded, randomized clinical trial of mycophenolate mofetil for the prevention of acute rejection in cadaveric renal transplantation. The Tricontinental Mycophenolate Mofetil Renal Transplantation Study

Group. Transplantation 1996;61(7):1029–1037.
82. Parada, et al. Early and late infections in lung transplantation patients. Transplant Proc 2010;42(1): 333–335.
83. Christie, et al. The registry of the International Society for Heart and Lung Transplantation: 29th adult lung and heart-lung transplant report-2012. J Heart Lung Transplant 2012;31(10):1073–1086.
84. Remund, et al. Infections relevant to lung transplantation. Proc Am Thorac Soc 2009;6(1):94–100.
85. Ruiz, et al. Donor-to-host transmission of bacterial and fungal infections in lung transplantation. Am J Transplant 2006;6(1):178–182.
86. Septimus, et al. Prevention of device-related healthcare-associated infections. F1000Res 2016;5. F1000 Faculty Rev-65.
87. Patel, et al. Carbapenem-resistant Enterobacteriaceae and Acinetobacter baumannii: assessing their impact on organ transplantation. Curr Opin Organ Transplant 2010;15(6):676–682.
88. Khan, et al. Nocardia infection in lung transplant recipients. Clin Transplant 2008;22(5):562–566.
89. Shteinberg, et al. The impact of fluoroquinolone resistance of Gram-negative bacteria in respiratory secretions on the outcome of lung transplant (noncystic fibrosis) recipients. Clin Transplant 2012; 26(6):884–890.
90. Hadjiliadis, et al. Survival of lung transplant patients with cystic fibrosis harboring panresistant bacteria other than Burkholderia cepacia, compared with patients harboring sensitive bacteria. J Heart Lung Transplant 2007;26(8):834–838.
91. Vital, et al. Impact of sinus surgery on pseudomonal airway colonization, bronchiolitis obliterans syndrome and survival in cystic fibrosis lung transplant recipients. Respiration 2013;86(1):25–31.
92. Pappas, et al. Invasive fungal infections among organ transplant recipients: results of the Transplant-Associated Infection Surveillance Network (TRANSNET). Clin Infect Dis 2010;50(8):1101–1111.
93. Doligalski, et al. Epidemiology of invasive mold infections in lung transplant recipients. Am J Transplant 2014;14(6):1328–1333.
94. Luong, et al. Pretransplant Aspergillus colonization of cystic fibrosis patients and the incidence of post-lung transplant invasive aspergillosis. Transplantation 2014;97(3):351–357.
95. Marino, et al. Prophylactic antifungal agents used after lung transplantation. Ann Pharmacother 2010;44(3):546–556.
96. Neoh, et al. Antifungal prophylaxis in lung transplantation–a world-wide survey. Am J Transplant 2011;11(2):361–366.
97. Pennington, et al. Antifungal prophylaxis in lung transplant recipients: a systematic review and meta-analysis. Transpl Infect Dis 2020;22(4): e13333.
98. Walsh, et al. Treatment of invasive aspergillosis with posaconazole in patients who are refractory to or intolerant of conventional therapy: an externally controlled trial. Clin Infect Dis 2007;44(1):2–12.
99. Klatt, et al. Review of pharmacologic considerations in the use of azole antifungals in lung transplant recipients. J Fungi (Basel) 2021;7(2):76.
100. Singer, et al. High cumulative dose exposure to voriconazole is associated with cutaneous squamous cell carcinoma in lung transplant recipients. J Heart Lung Transplant 2012;31(7):694–699.
101. Bailey, et al. A mini-review of adverse lung transplant outcomes associated with respiratory viruses. Front Immunol 2019;10:2861.

102. Li, et al. Oral versus inhaled ribavirin therapy for respiratory syncytial virus infection after lung transplantation. J Heart Lung Transplant 2012;31(8):839–844.
103. Sandkovsky, et al. Adenovirus: current epidemiology and emerging approaches to prevention and treatment. Curr Infect Dis Rep 2014;16(8):416.
104. Zuk, et al. An international survey of cytomegalovirus management practices in lung transplantation. Transplantation 2010;90(6):672–676.
105. Sweet, et al. The prevalence of distal and proximal gastroesophageal reflux in patients awaiting lung transplantation. Ann Surg 2006;244(4):491–497.
106. Blondeau, et al. Gastro-oesophageal reflux and gastric aspiration in lung transplant patients with or without chronic rejection. Eur Respir J 2008; 31(4):707–713.
107. Young, et al. Lung transplantation exacerbates gastroesophageal reflux disease. Chest 2003;124(5):1689–1693.
108. Hartwig, et al. Fundoplication after lung transplantation prevents the allograft dysfunction associated with reflux. Ann Thorac Surg 2011;92(2):462–8 [discussion; 468–468].
109. Davis, et al. Improved lung allograft function after fundoplication in patients with gastroesophageal reflux disease undergoing lung transplantation. J Thorac Cardiovasc Surg 2003;125(3):533–542.
110. Linden, et al. Laparoscopic fundoplication in patients with end-stage lung disease awaiting transplantation. J Thorac Cardiovasc Surg 2006; 131(2):438–446.
111. Wehbe, et al. Recovery from AKI and shortand long-term outcomes after lung transplantation. Clin J Am Soc Nephrol 2013;8(1):19–25.
112. Canales, et al. Predictors of chronic kidney disease in long-term survivors of lung and heart-lung transplantation. Am J Transplant 2006;6(9):2157–2163.
113. James, et al. 2014 evidence-based guideline for the management of high blood pressure in adults: report from the panel members appointed to the Eighth Joint National Committee (JNC 8). JAMA 2014;311(5):507–520.
114. Snell, et al. Sirolimus allows renal recovery in lung and heart transplant recipients with chronic renal impairment. J Heart Lung Transplant 2002;21(5): 540–546.
115. Rappaport, et al. Pleural space management after lung transplant: early and late outcomes of pleural decortication. J Heart Lung Transplant 2021;40(7): 623–630.
116. Tang, et al. Natural history of pleural complications after lung transplantation. Ann Thorac Surg 2021; 111(2):407–415.
117. Marom, et al. Pleural effusions in lung transplant recipients: image-guided small-bore catheter drainage. Radiology 2003;228(1):241–245.
118. Evans, et al. Venous thromboembolic complications of lung transplantation: a contemporary single-institution review. Ann Thorac Surg 2015; 100(6):2033–9 [discussion: 2039–2040].
119. Jorge, et al. Routine deep vein thrombosis screening after lung transplantation: incidence and risk factors. J Thorac Cardiovasc Surg 2020;159(3):1142–1150.
120. Neto R, et al. Venous thromboembolism after adult lung transplantation: a frequent event associated with lower survival. Transplantation 2018;102(4): 681–687.

# 第 9 章 肺移植的手术并发症

Gabriel Loor, Aladdein Mattar, Lara Schaheen, Ross M. Bremner 著

廖敏琪 袁金权 译

周建平 校

【关键词】
- 肺移植
- 伤口并发症
- 原发性移植物功能不全
- 气道缺血
- 血管并发症

【要点】
- 肺移植是终末期肺病患者挽救生命的干预措施。
- 尽管肺移植效果显著,但它是一项大手术,存在多种并发症的风险。
- 了解这些并发症有助于避免它们发生,并在它们发生时能够早发现、早治疗。

## 9.1 引　言

肺移植(LTx)是最具挑战性的外科专业之一,不仅是因为其技术要求高,也是因为外科医生必须预防、发现和处理许多并发症。外科医生能否做到这一点对患者的治疗效果有着深远的影响。在本章中,我们将对这些挑战进行讨论,以便移植外科医生、医学专家和移植项目能够发挥出最大的潜力。

## 9.2 伤口并发症

大约 15% 接受肺移植的患者会出现伤口并发症。伤口并发症的一般危险因素包括糖尿病、免疫抑制药物、受体疾病和肥胖[1-3]。而肺移植患者特有的危险因素包括高剂量的免疫抑制药物、进入气道的污染,以及有或无机械循环支持的广泛外科创伤。

感染性并发症通常由细菌性生物体引起,但也可能由真菌物种引起。特征性迹象包括红斑、发热、脓性分泌物和切口裂开,伴有伤口培养阳性。最初,患者使用针对最可

能致病菌的抗生素进行治疗。由于肺移植受者的免疫受到抑制，易受各种细菌生物体的感染，合理的方法是开始针对革兰阳性和革兰阴性细菌生物体使用广谱抗生素覆盖治疗，直到最终的培养结果返回。如果存在少量化脓，治疗轻微和浅表感染性伤口并发症可能需要打开切口。碘仿填塞或湿干纱布敷料更换可以实现局部清创和二次愈合。然而，如果怀疑伤口较深或邻近有异物（如手术线），外科医生应仔细在手术室中探索伤口（图9-1）。胸部计算机断层扫描有助于确定感染的程度。

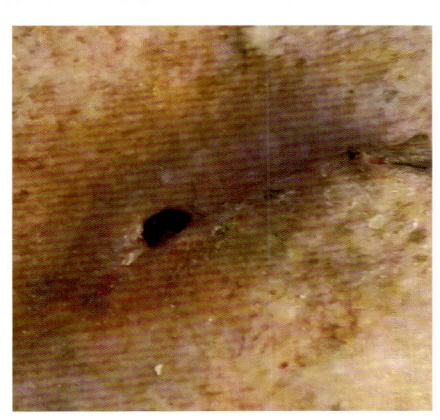

**图 9-1　患者因蚌壳式切口的伤口并发症出现红斑和裂开**
注：最初使用抗生素、局部切开、引流进行治疗。随后进行手术探查、清创、脉冲灌洗、移除胸骨和负压辅助闭合。整形外科医生通过使用带有部分肌肉组织的皮瓣来协助延迟闭合

如果感染性伤口并发症较深，伴有脓液积聚或异物，则需要进行手术探查。在这种情况下，外科医生会清除所有感染物质，只留下健康组织。其中涉及锐利解剖、用抗生素灌洗的脉冲冲洗以及应用临时湿干敷料，或更常见的负压辅助闭合装置[4,5]。通常，这种伤口通过负压辅助闭合治疗以次级愈合关闭，但另一个加速愈合的选择是主动闭合，肌肉瓣可能有可能没有[6]。如果在手术清创过程中，像线或缝合线这样的异物被清除，则应评估伤口的稳定性。如果胸骨或胸腔切口稳定，理想情况下应用负压辅助闭合装置，直到确认伤口感染源已被清除。如果移除线或缝合线使胸骨或胸腔切口不稳定，就会导致心脏或肺的损伤。一旦大部分感染消失，就需要使用缝合线、板、线、生物或人工网材料进行固定[7]。如果无法进行刚性固定，生物组织的推进，如肌肉或大网膜，可以根据情况为下方的肺或心脏提供一定的保护。

肺疝发生在大约2%的胸部手术切口中；然而，在肺移植中，由于免疫抑制，其发生率可能更高。对闭合技术的细致关注可以防止肺疝，但由于患者的活动性、体型或创伤愈合受损，这种并发症有时是不可避免的。在手术室中，治疗肺疝是通过从胸壁中分

离出疝出的肺部分，并主动闭合缺陷或缝合一层聚丙烯网以固定缺陷[8]。

外科医生可以通过使用多种技术来减少手术部位的感染，包括：①使用细致的闭合技术；②维持良好的血糖控制、出色的止血和正常体温；③治疗远处感染；④适当使用围手术期抗生素[3]。尽管对于最佳抗生素方案尚无共识，但许多中心会根据定植史来调整抗生素的使用[9]。大多数中心对于未显示先前定植的移植接受者最多使用 7 天革兰阳性和革兰阴性药物；对于有定植史的接受者使用至少 14 天[9]。在选择围术期抗微生物药物时，考虑先前耐药菌株十分重要。

外科暴露方式的选择可能会导致伤口并发症。双侧胸腔切开联合横向胸骨切开（也称为蚌壳式切口）是进行肺移植最常见的方法[10]。然而，这种方法会牺牲双侧乳腺动脉，从而影响愈合所需的血流。Elde 及其同事[11]的研究表明，如果可能的话，在进行体外循环（CPB）支持的肺移植时采用正中胸骨切口方法，主要伤口并发症的发生率为 0，而使用蚌壳式切口时 3 年内的发生率为 20%。另一个减少伤口感染发生率的选项是使用单独的胸腔切口而不采用横向胸骨切开。在我们看来，蚌壳式方法目前仍然是最具多功能性的切口。其出色的暴露度和灵活性允许移植进行，无需机械循环支持或只需限制性的体外膜肺氧合（ECMO）支持，便于中心插管操作。

## 9.3 原发性移植物功能不全

原发性移植物功能不全（PGD）是肺移植术后早期发病率和死亡率的最常见原因[12]。手术决策从选择和管理供体器官开始就极大地影响了 PGD 的发展。为了预防严重的 PGD，尽可能避免结合供体和受体的风险因素是一个合理的选择策略[13]。PGD 的受体风险因素（如身体质量指数增高、肺动脉高压、肉瘤病）和供体风险因素（如吸烟史）的结合可能增加严重 PGD 的风险，特别是增加与 PGD 相关的手术变量，如大量输血或使用 CPB。减少供体 PGD 风险的新型保存方法的使用是一个有潜力的研究领域。一项关于便携式体外肺灌注的随机对照研究证明，使用 Organ Care System Lung（TransMedics, Inc，安多弗，MA）可以将 PGD 的发生率降低 50%[14]。

此外，术中使用的体外生命支持策略会影响 PGD。Diamond 及其同事的研究[13]表明，在肺移植中使用 CPB 是 PGD 发展最重要的手术风险因素。然而，Hoetzenecker 及其同事[15]报告了在使用术中中央静脉动脉（VA）ECMO 的肺移植中，不论移植的适应证是什么，PGD 的发生率都很低。尽管移植界对使用 ECMO 表现出了高于 CPB 的热情，但 ECMO

是否应该优先于无泵支持策略作为减少 PGD 的支持策略仍不明确。最后，PGD 的发展可能受到术中血液制品的使用、再灌注时吸入氧分数以及夹闭释放实践的影响[13,16,17]。

当 PGD 发生时，会立即危及生命，并对长期移植物功能产生影响[12,18,19]。一旦发现 PGD，操作团队应提高警惕，确保足够的氧气输送，以支持终末器官功能。为了避免附带损害，外科医生应考虑将 ECMO 作为治疗严重 PGD 的主要手段[20]。通常，静脉-静脉 ECMO 提供充足的氧合，促进 $CO_2$ 清除，并通过显著减少呼吸机和血管升压要求使氧气输送正常化。然而，如果存在明显的右心室或左心室功能不全，则应考虑 VA-ECMO。

## 9.4 气道缺血

气道缺血是肺移植的潜在并发症，发生率为 15%~35%，具体取决于其定义[21-23]。气道缺血是由于吻合口水平的血液供应有限导致坏死，伴或不伴裂开。当气道愈合时，有过度颗粒化的倾向，导致狭窄。该手术固有的危险因素，包括供体缺血、缺血再灌注损伤、免疫抑制、支气管吻合处侧支血供稀缺以及细菌定植，使得某种程度的气道缺血几乎不可避免。

研究人员已经确定了供体和受体气道缺血的几个危险因素，其中一些是可变的。鲁汶肺移植小组于 2007 年发表的一项研究[23]表明，使用呼吸机 50~70 小时的捐献者出现气道并发症的风险最大，这归因于未经治疗的呼吸机相关性肺炎。在 Ruttmann 及其同事的一项研究中[24]，多因素分析发现移植物再灌注损伤是排斥反应的重要危险因素。因此，减少移植物功能障碍的策略可能会减少气道缺血。

供体气道和受体气道之间的大尺寸不匹配可能会导致气道并发症。如果受者的主支气管很大而供者的支气管很小，则径向张力可能会损害愈合。同样，如果较小的受者气道伸入较大的供体气道，则伸入的部分可能会出现缺血，可能与侧支血液供应受损有关[23]。Keshava 及其同事的一份报告[25]强调了儿科供体中的类似情况。

研究人员已经确定了可能导致气道缺血的供体保存因素。在 Necki 及其同事的一项研究中[22]，冷缺血时间延长是发生气道并发症的一个重要危险因素。相反，在 Li 及其同事的一项研究中[21]，使用便携式温血灌注的 Organ Care System Lung（TransMedics, Inc）保存的扩展标准供体肺的接受者比用冰以标准方式保存的肺的接受者更常发生气道缺血，特别是当吻合术采用连续缝合而非间断缝合技术时。

几位研究人员研究了外科技术在预防气道缺血中的重要性。Van Berkel 及其团队的

## 肺移植：胸外科临床问题

研究表明[26]，将供体气道修剪至次级隆突1个软骨环以内，可使气道并发症（吻合口裂开、阻塞或软化）的发生率从13%降至2%。同样，Fitz Sullivan及其同事[27]的研究显示，将气道修剪回次级隆突，并将中断的"八"字缝合技术纳入吻合的前软骨部分，可以将气道并发症的发生率从18%降至2%。

一项旨在减少气道缺血的潜在重要外科进展是支气管动脉再血管化。该技术要求将供体肺连同降主动脉一起获取，以便形成主支气管动脉或动脉的袖口，并将其缝合到接受者的左乳动脉或主动脉上[28,29]。该程序的技术挑战，加上与其使用相关的出血风险增加，限制了其广泛的应用。然而，我们认为这项技术值得进一步关注，并对其结果进行进一步分析。

从围术期的角度来看，有一些注意事项可能会降低气道缺血的风险。避免低血压、改善营养、维持良好的心输出量和混合静脉氧水平可能有助于减少缺血。虽然这些概念是直观的，但在文献中尚未得到很好的评估。医生还应小心限制有风险患者的激素使用，以防止气道缺血[24]。

根据2018年更新的国际心肺移植协会关于气道并发症的共识报告[30]，气道并发症的检测和分类有了改进。这些指南比以前的分级方案更为敏感，因其关注到影响吻合口不同部分的黏膜变化，而不仅仅是分离或狭窄[21]。外科医生通常会将所有评为B2级或更高级别的缺血，以及所有需要监测或干预的分离、狭窄或软骨病变，视为临床上重要的气道缺血（图9-2）。

气道缺血的治疗包括监测、受体优化以及必要时的支气管内干预。很少考虑外科干预或重新移植。大多数时候，外科医生或肺科医生使用监控支气管镜和必要时的温和清创术来监控无开裂的气道缺血。对于有限的开裂也是如此[31,32]。如果缺血因过度愈合而转变为狭窄，可能需要进行球囊扩张或放置支架[30,33]。如果开裂范围增大，放置支架可能有助于桥接间隙[31,32]并促进愈合。在严重的情况下，

| 缺血 | 类型 | A | 吻合口1 cm以内 |
|---|---|---|---|
|  |  | B | 离吻合口>1 cm |
|  |  | C | 延伸到远端气道 |
|  | 等级 | 1 | <50%周围性缺血 |
|  |  | 2 | >50%周围性缺血 |
| 狭窄 | 严重程度 | <50% | |
|  |  | >50% | |
| 开裂 | 所有均存在 | | |

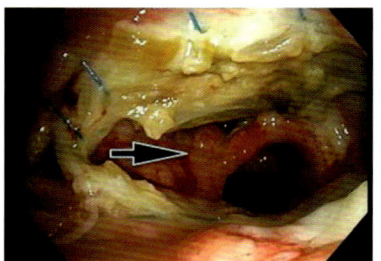

示例
右吻合口
缺血：C2
狭窄：无
开裂：是（箭头指示）

图9-2 国际心肺移植学会2018年气道缺血分级系统
注：图像显示一名患者周围性缺血超过50%，部分缺血延伸至远端气道并裂开。患者接受支架置入术，随着时间的推移，吻合口愈合（图像未显示）

如果支架未能提供足够的覆盖，外科医生可能需要考虑开放修复。根据我们的经验，这种修复很少是必要的，很少会成功，因为缺乏足够的组织来固定缝合线。此外，大网膜或心包组织可能由于免疫抑制和营养不良而受到限制。根据对侧肺的质量，外科医生可以考虑采用肺切除术作为一种替代方案。在这些需要手术干预的极端情况下，也应考虑挽救性的单肺移植的想法。

## 9.5 血管并发症

1%~3% 的病例会发生血管并发症，影响肺动脉或肺静脉[34,35]。任何肺血流阻塞都会损害同种异体移植物，其完全取决于肺动脉血流，但心肺阻滞及支气管动脉血运重建手术除外。肺动脉血流阻塞可导致实质坏死或气道缺血。肺静脉血流受阻可导致肺实质水肿。胸部 X 线检查结果显示单侧混浊增加，若无法用黏液堵塞或其他原因解释，应立即评估血管并发症。这是通过对比计算机断层扫描（动脉期和静脉期）、经食管超声心动图或核灌注扫描来完成的（图 9-3）。

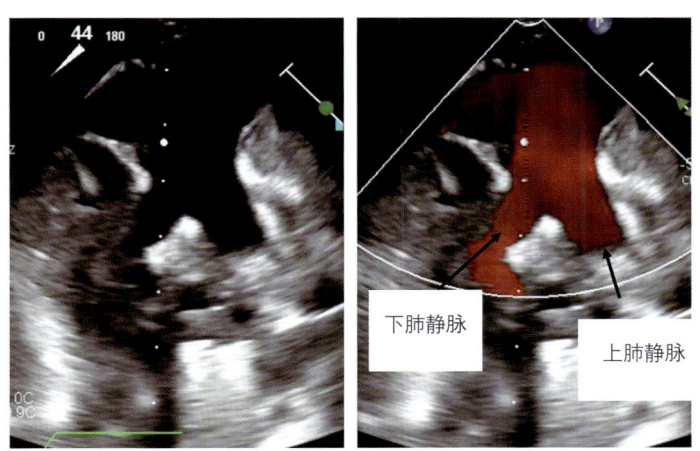

图 9-3　正常经食管超声心动图显示上、下肺静脉血流

接受肺移植的患者最常见的血管并发症是肺栓塞（图 9-4）。患者可能形成血栓的原因有多种，包括近期手术、肺动脉操作、活动受限、留置静脉导管和激素治疗。肺移植后肺栓塞的发生率为 6%~24%，该并发症的死亡率为 45%[36-38]。栓塞可以在主肺动脉中大量存在，也可以在较小的肺动脉分支中散布。后一种情况适合采用抗凝保守治疗，而前者则需要血管内或手术干预。使用或不使用溶栓剂的血管内血栓抽吸术是有效清除血栓的微创选择[39,40]。如果病情不稳定，出现严重右心衰竭，患者应立即进行 VA-ECMO[41,42]。虽然

## 肺移植：胸外科临床问题

移植后很少进行外科肺栓塞切除术，但其可用于适合手术的患者，以治疗主肺动脉中容易进入的大血栓。CPB 和通过栓塞切除术对肺动脉进行有限探查足以清除大部分血栓。

肺动脉的吻合并发症最常见的是由扭结、扭转、荷包效应、内膜增生或周围组织引起的狭窄（图 9-5）。手术后壁也可能发生。为了避免扭结的发生，外科医生应尽量避免肺动脉吻合口长度过长。

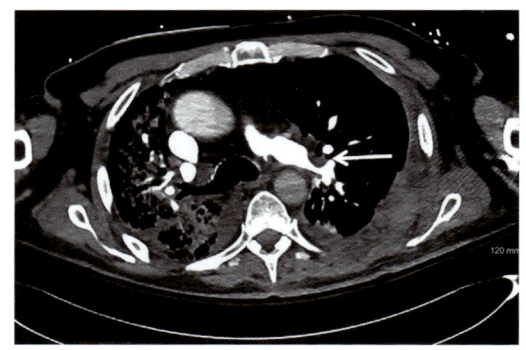

图 9-4　左主肺动脉（箭头）中的大血栓与超声心动图上相应的右心室变化有关

注：由于血流动力学不稳定，患者需要在床边紧急进行外周静脉动脉体外膜肺氧合插入术，并随后进行抽吸血栓切除术

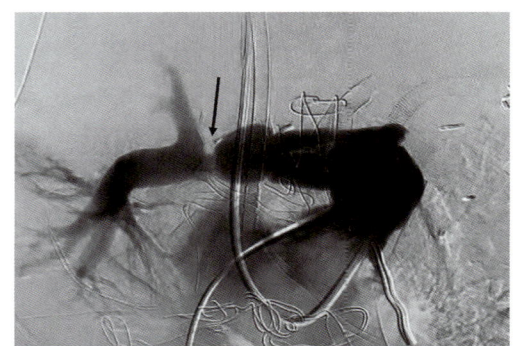

图 9-5　肺血管造影显示右肺主动脉吻合口狭窄（箭头）

注：压力梯度有 50% 的差异。这是保守治疗，因为患者缺氧的主要原因是对侧肺部的严重肺栓塞

精准的尺寸匹配有助于实现最理想的血流动力学流动模式。此外，缝合肺动脉时必须注意上下叶分支的方向，避免扭曲。如果存在明显的张力或角度不寻常，用牛心包或自体心包对前壁进行补片增强可能会有所帮助[43]。

如果发生血流动力学和症状性狭窄，可以选择包括再次手术或带或不带支架的球囊血管成形术。除非在移植后 1 周内，否则很少进行手术，并且人们担心球囊对缝合线的影响。在这种情况下，外科医生可以选择带或不带补片的手术修复。如果缝合线成熟，且狭窄很可能是由内膜增生或纤维化引起的，球囊和支架置入术则有所帮助[44]。

肺静脉阻塞是肺移植后一种罕见但可能致命的并发症，可能是由技术因素（如肺静脉扭曲或异常角度）而导致的。荷包效应或血管后壁也可能导致肺静脉阻塞。外科医生可以通过使用细致的技术轻松避免这些问题。由于套囊张力过大和孔口变平，可能会出现假性阻塞。此问题可能是由尺寸不匹配或供体袖带长度不足造成的。过度张力产生的压力会导致肺静脉高压及肺部充血。进行补片增强以降低左心房袖的压力是重要的预防解决方案（图 9-6）。其是通过首先缝合后壁，再估计接近前壁所需的面积，然后修剪一块心包以填充间隙来完成的。

肺静脉狭窄可由内膜增生引起，可通过使用带或不带支架的球囊血管成形术成功治疗[35]。幸运的是，这种并发症并不常见，因为肺静脉是通过使用大的广口心房缝合到受体上的，汇合处不易狭窄。

由于影响左心房闭合的技术因素，卒中是肺移植后可能发生的另一个重要并发症。左心房袖与中央动脉系统直接连通，因此，其可能是血栓栓塞物质的重要来源。肺移植后发生卒中应怀疑左心房可能存在栓塞（图9-7）。仔细冲洗心房的梳状肌侧以清除碎片，有助于减少栓塞事件。

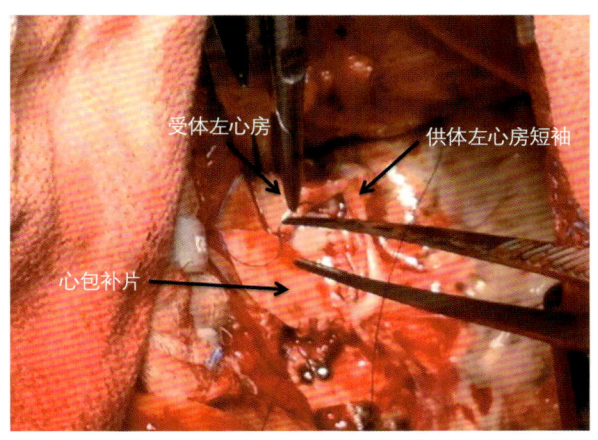

图9-6 使用肺静脉的一部分作为贴片，来补片增强被剪短的供体心房前端连接处

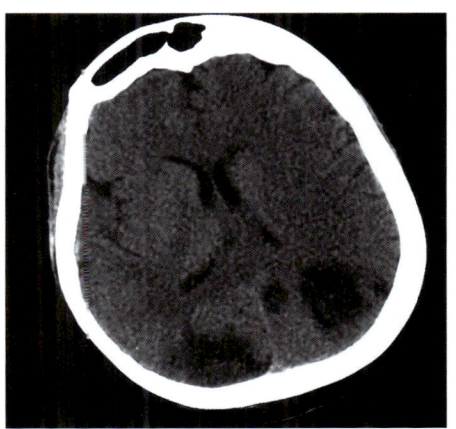

图9-7 肺移植后患者卒中

注：尽管肺静脉或左心房中没有发现血栓，但这是空气或栓塞碎片的潜在来源。通过使用叠瓦缝合技术并在完成吻合之前对袖带进行广泛冲洗，可以减少这种并发症

最后，扭转是肺移植的重要血管并发症，可影响静脉、动脉和支气管[45-49]。及时识别可以使外科医生在坏死发生前通过手术探查来纠正扭转。在有问题的情况下，再次观察可能有助于外科医生追踪肺实质的改善情况。对于明显的肺坏死，外科医生应准备进行全肺切除术或肺叶切除术。对于完全扭转伴肺坏死需要进行全肺切除术的，可以考虑重新移植。

## 9.6 出血并发症

肺移植经常在手术时或术后立即发生出血，偶尔在恢复后期也会发生出血。尽管手术技术和患者血液管理取得了进步，并且人们对血液制品输注的不良影响的认识有所提高，但出血仍然是肺移植后的常见并发症。

### 9.6.1 术中出血

对于任何肺移植手术，应预见到可能有血液损失和重大出血的风险。了解增加术中出血风险的因素，可能有助于移植外科医生和麻醉医生预先准备好手术中使用的血液制品。以往的胸部或心脏手术史、之前的胸膜干预治疗，以及化脓性肺病的存在，可能与原生肺与胸壁之间增加的血管粘连有关，通常会导致更多的围术期出血。Wang 及其同事[50]的研究显示，与单肺移植相比，在双肺移植中，血液制品的使用显著增多，这归因于手术复杂度的增加。艾森曼格综合征和囊性纤维化也被识别为肺移植期间血液损失和输血需求的风险因素[51,52]。

术中血液丢失、纤维蛋白原水平下降、血小板计数减少和同时进行的液体替代可能会导致凝血功能障碍。Adelmann 及其同事[53]发现，在 69% 的再次手术中，凝血功能障碍是术后出血的原因。同一组研究人员还发现，术后纤维蛋白原水平低，以及术前和术后使用 ECMO 是肺移植后出血的风险因素。

受体因素，如严重的肺动脉高压、解剖变异和重做移植，使许多主要血管结构在解剖过程中容易受伤。在进行困难的肺门解剖时，获得肺主动脉的近端控制，并确保有心肺支持和血液制品的可用性至关重要。

虽然许多肺移植手术是在没有心肺支持的情况下进行的，但那些表现出高肺动脉压力、难以控制的低氧血症和其他心肺不稳定情况的候选者，往往需要 ECMO 或 CPB 的支持。尽管 ECMO 具有较少的抗凝作用优点，但其对心脏减压和使用细胞保护剂进行血液挽救的能力有限。然而，体外循环的优点是在大出血时可以提供更好的心脏减压和泵心切开吸引术。Wang 及其同事[50]证明，接受 CPB 的患者会比不需要心肺支持的患者使用更多单位的血液制品（红细胞，8.28 $vs.$ 1.45；新鲜冰冻血浆，9.70 $vs.$ 0.73；血小板，1.86 $vs.$ 0.14；$P < 0.001$），与旁路时间相关。

### 9.6.2 术后出血

肺移植后早期出血是一种常见的并发症。Hong 及其同事[54]发现，通常在 48 小时后需要外科干预的血胸有 13% 的病例中会发生（图 9-8）。出血来源包括血管吻合口、分割的乳腺或支气管动脉、胸膜间隙的原始表面，以及胸壁切口。在需要大量血液制品的病例中，或在 CPB 下进行手术的病例中，通常需要积极纠正术后凝血功能缺陷。增加正压呼气末压可能有助于在胸膜粘连的情况下压迫胸壁出血。术后早期，密切注意胸管的引流情况，可能表明需要返回手术室进行探查。早期到达重症监护室后，如果出现快速血液引流，随后胸管引流量减少的情况，尽管患者需要增加肌力或血管升压支持，但更迫切需要进行胸部 X 线检查。显著血胸的存在以及无法获得充分胸管引流的情况通常需要手术清除。确定返回手术室的最佳时机十分复杂。必须考虑患者的稳定性、对持续或不断增加的支持需求，以及凝血状况。在急性临床失代偿情况下，如心包填塞和突然快速出血，可能需要进行床边探查。若干研究已经证明，输血会增加肺移植后的住院时间和死亡率[55]。

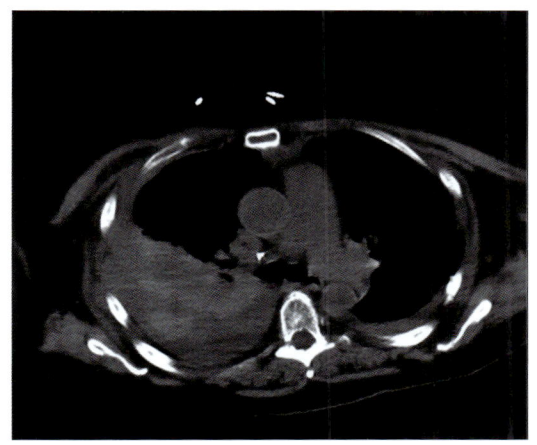

图 9-8　计算机断层扫描显示双侧肺移植后右侧血胸

Adelmann 及其同事[53]发现，严重的术后出血与 60 天生存率降低有关，迟发性血胸与抗凝治疗有关，术后血胸与 90 天生存率降低有关。此外，输血的经济费用不容低估，在美国，1 个单位浓缩红细胞的成本为 700~1200 美元[56]。

## 9.7 胸膜腔并发症

肺移植后胸膜腔并发症很常见，包括胸腔积液、气胸和脓胸。据 Kao 及其同事称[57]，22%~42%的肺移植受者会出现胸膜并发症。胸膜并发症的危险因素包括既往胸腔手术史、胸膜粘连、供受体尺寸不匹配[58,59]。肺移植后胸膜液量增加与同种异体移植物缺血再灌注引起的毛细血管渗漏、受体液体超负荷、出血和器官恢复时同种异体移植淋巴管的手术中断有关[58,59]。

### 肺移植：胸外科临床问题

移植后积液很麻烦，通常会导致住院时间延长和额外的手术干预。肺移植受者的胸腔积液较为复杂，如血胸、脓胸、乳糜胸等，需要仔细评估。胸水分析可能包括细菌、真菌和分枝杆菌培养、聚合酶链反应测定、细胞计数以及乳酸脱氢酶、蛋白质、葡萄糖和三酰甘油的测定[58,60]。

晚期胸腔积液（移植后＞2周）通常是感染、排斥、胸膜纤维化或恶性肿瘤的结果[61,62]。胸膜腔感染或脓胸使3%~7%的胸腔积液变得复杂。肺移植后90天内出现的胸腔积液中大约有1/4是感染引起的[59,63,64]。肺移植受者由于免疫抑制状态，可能会出现脓胸，因此，临床上需要对所有患者保持高度怀疑。复杂的胸腔积液与患者的不良预后相关，根据病情和严重程度，可采用一系列医疗和外科手术进行治疗。例如，乳糜胸可能需要手术结扎胸导管，以及血胸可能需要手术干预来识别和止血源或剥离肺组织。

移植患者的独特之处在于，他们不遵循胸膜腔问题的"规则"。高剂量激素会延迟愈合，并可能对胸膜粘连产生影响。此外，解剖和肺切除术所需的广泛暴露和大切口经常会导致壁层和脏层胸膜表面的复杂粘连和融合。因此，通过手术方法处理局限性积液（图9-9）具有挑战性，并且通常无法通过微创方法实现。导致固定空间和多重气漏的剥脱术可能难以长期管理，尤其是当该空间受到感染时。仔细考虑手术的好处对于避免这种情况很重要。通过仔细放置图像引导胸膜导管并尝试使用溶栓剂可以避免手术和剥脱术[65]。

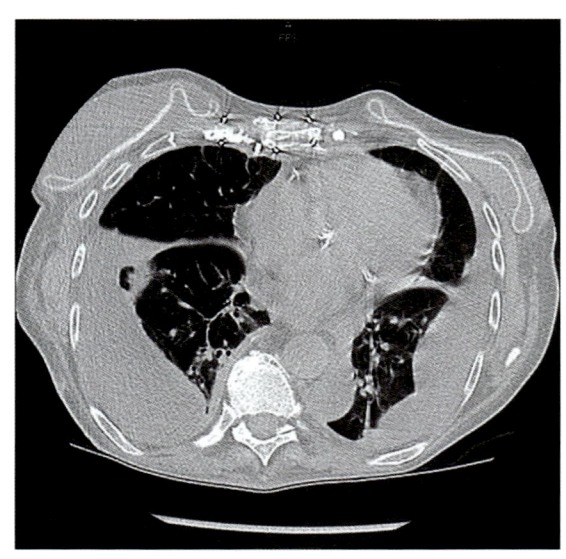

图9-9　计算机断层扫描显示双侧肺移植后出现局限性积液

Cleveland 小组[66]最近发表了他们关于肺移植后胸膜间隙问题的研究结果。研究者发现，在他们的研究中，有 45% 的肺移植接受者出现了胸膜并发症：26% 的受者出现积液，15% 的受者出现气胸，12% 的受者出现血胸，5% 的受者出现脓胸，1% 的受者出现乳糜胸。他们注意到，胸膜并发症的存在与更差的长期生存率相关[66]。Boffa 及其同事[67]研究了肺移植后进行剥脱术的需求和结果。结果提示，实现了完全的肺扩张的病例仅有 70%，清除了感染的病例仅有 64%，30 天的手术死亡率为 23%。剥脱术可能在一些患者中有用，但是决定进行这一手术应当考虑到巨大的手术风险[67]。

## 9.8 匹配供者和受者尺寸大小的挑战

尽管在确定供体器官与受体器官的大小时非常注意，但经常会出现供体与受体不匹配的情况（图 9-10）。供体肺与受体胸腔大小之间的不匹配可能导致肺移植后的机械性并发症。尺寸偏小的肺可能会导致胸膜间隙问题，如持续性积液，而过大的器官则会引起不同的问题，如持续的肺不张。一般认为供体肺与受体胸腔之间最多 25% 的尺寸差异是可以接受的[68]。

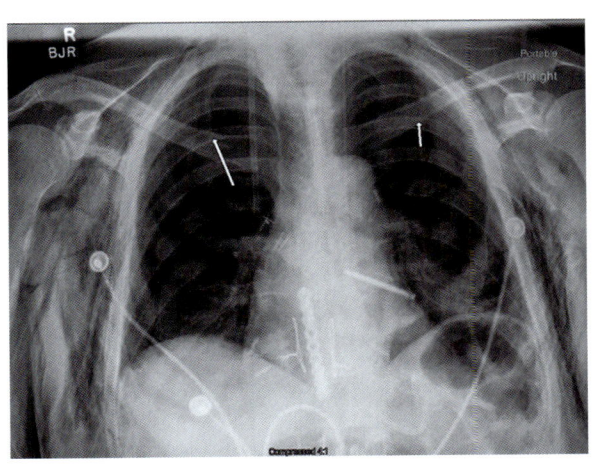

图 9-10 放射线照片显示供体受体尺寸不匹配（箭头所示的同种异体移植物尺寸过小）

### 9.8.1 尺寸过小的同种异体肺移植物

肺移植后发生气胸可能是由于手术损伤引起支气管胸膜瘘或实质性胸膜瘘。然而，当供体器官偏小时，支气管吻合口裂开或经支气管镜活检的并发症更为常见。肺移植后

### 肺移植：胸外科临床问题

稳定或小的气胸通常可以通过观察等待来管理，而较大或有症状的气胸可能需要胸腔引流管治疗。肺移植后持续性气胸并不常见，但当供体肺比受体胸腔小时，可能在胸腔引流管移除后发生。这种供体受体尺寸不匹配最常见于肺移植前有气肿和显著肺过度充气的肺气肿患者。在单侧肺移植的肺气肿或肺纤维化患者中，非移植的原生肺也可能发生气胸。此外，在因肺气肿进行单侧肺移植的患者中，将小的供体肺植入过大的胸腔可能导致过度膨胀的气肿性原生肺压迫异体移植肺。

#### 9.8.2 尺寸过大的肺移植物和减容手术

在严重肺纤维化患者中，胸膜空间通常十分受限，不一定与患者的身高相关。这些患者的膈肌通常非常高，但预计随着时间的推移和供体肺的适当尺寸，供体肺将扩张，膈肌将向下移动，使胸腔容积增加。然而，也有明显的情况表明供体器官对于受体胸腔来说太大了。在胸腔过小的情况下植入大的供体肺可能导致肺不张和通气受损。这些并发症在术后患者仍在接受正压通气时 X 线片上通常立即可见[68]。

在受者的胸腔中肺异体移植显著过大的情况下，可能需要通过减容手术闭合胸腔。Shigemura 及其同事[69]报告称，在肺过大的情况下，进行肺减容手术与早期及中期异体移植功能和总体并发症的改善相关联。可以通过肺叶切除术或连续楔形切除减少移植物体积。通常，切除右中叶和左肺舌叶足以调整大小，但可能需要进一步对下叶进行楔形切除。缝合线可能会漏气或导致肺在胸腔中的贴合度不佳，在术后可能会造成麻烦。因此，努力正确匹配供体器官与受体胸腔大小是最佳选择。

### 9.9 再移植

再移植带来独特的挑战，在本书其他章节有所讨论。这里强调几个重点。首先，仔细选择患者是关键。再移植通常保留给那些患有非限制性亚型的慢性肺异体移植功能障碍并且在第一次移植后至少存活了 2~3 年的患者[70-72]。其次，手术有几个方面需要讨论。重新进入时容易损伤心脏，解剖时容易损伤膈神经。体外生命支持策略通常十分必要。在再移植中，肺动脉解剖具有挑战性，常常迫切需要旁路。因此，建议考虑更近距离地控制心包内的肺动脉。在作者的实践中，预先在支气管和动脉吻合口之间放置一些附近的软组织（来自供者或受者），可以在患者后续需要第二次移植时便于解剖。如果遇到明显的粘连并且在解剖后留有显著的血管表面（特别是在需要体外循环支持的情况下），外科团队应考虑在手术结束时保持胸腔开放。在一些中心，经过精心筛选的患者进行再移植的结果接近初次移植的结果 [72,73]。

## 9.10 总　结

肺移植是一种挽救生命的干预措施，每年为全球数千名与不可逆转的终末期肺病作斗争的患者提供帮助。影响移植后结果的因素有很多，确保安全和积极的手术结果是朝着提供最佳长期结果迈出的重要一步。

> 【临床护理要点】
> - 肺移植后的气道缺血可能受到手术吻合技术的影响。
> - 肺栓塞是影响肺移植接受者的最常见血管并发症。
> - 肺移植后伤口并发症的发生率可能受到手术暴露选择的影响。
> - 原发性移植物功能不全的发生可能受到围术期因素的影响。

**致谢**

作者感谢得克萨斯心脏研究所科学出版部的 Nicole Stancel, PhD, ELS（D），以及诺顿胸腔研究所的 Kristine Nally, BS, ELS 对稿件的编辑审查。

**声明**

Loor 博士是 Abiomed Breethe 的顾问，他的机构（贝勒医学院）获得 Maquet 和 Transmedics 公司的资助，他们参与了与体外膜肺氧合和体外肺灌注相关的临床试验。

## 参考文献

1. Lemaignen A, Birgand G, Ghodhbane W, et al. Sternal wound infection after cardiac surgery: incidence and risk factors according to clinical presentation. Clin Microbiol Infect 2015;21(7):674 e11–18.
2. Ridderstolpe L, Gill H, Granfeldt H, et al. Superficial and deep sternal wound complications: incidence, risk factors and mortality. Eur J Cardiothorac Surg 2001;20(6):1168–1175.
3. Young PY, Khadaroo RG. Surgical site infections. Surg Clin North Am 2014;94(6):1245–1264.

4. Bakaeen FG, Haddad O, Ibrahim M, et al. Advances in managing the noninfected open chest after cardiacsurgery: negative-pressure wound therapy. J Thorac Cardiovasc Surg 2019;157(5):1891–18903 e9.

5. Seidel D, Diedrich S, Herrle F, et al. Negative pressure wound therapy vs conventional wound treatmentin subcutaneous abdominal wound healing impairment: the SAWHI randomized clinical trial. JAMA Surg 2020;155(6):469–478.

6. Nadir A, Kaptanoglu M, Sahin E, et al. Post-thoracotomy wound separation (DEHISCENCE): a disturbing complication. Clinics (Sao Paulo). 2013;68(1):1–4.

7. Pancholy B, Raman J. Chest wall reconstruction using sternal plating in patients with complex sternal dehiscence. Ann Thorac Surg 2015;99(6):2228–2230.

8. Athanassiadi K, Bagaev E, Simon A, et al. Lung herniation: a rare complication in minimally invasive cardiothoracic surgery. Eur J Cardiothorac Surg 2008;33(5):774–776.

9. Coiffard B, Prud'Homme E, Hraiech S, et al. World-wide clinical practices in perioperative antibiotic therapy for lung transplantation. BMCPulm Med 2020;20(1):109.

10. Ius F, Raemdonck D, Hartwig M, et al. Effect of surgical exposure on outcomes in lung transplantation: insight from the International Multicenter Extracorporeal Life Support (ECLS) in Lung Transplantation registry. J Heart Lung Transplant 2021;40:S164.

11. Elde S, Huddleston S, Jackson S, et al. Tailored approach to surgical exposure reduces surgical site complications after bilateral lung transplantation. Surg Infect (Larchmt) 2017;18(8):929–935.

12. Snell GI, Yusen RD, Weill D, et al. Report of the ISHLT working group on primary lung graft dysfunction, part I: definition and grading. A 2016 Consensus Group statement of the International Society for Heart and Lung Transplantation. J Heart Lung Transpl 2017;36(10):1097–1103.

13. Diamond JM, Lee JC, Kawut SM, et al. Clinical risk factors for primary graft dysfunction after lung transplantation. Am J Respir Crit Care Med 2013;187(5): 527–534.

14. Warnecke G, Van Raemdonck D, Smith MA, et al. Normothermic ex-vivo preservation with the portable Organ Care System Lung device for bilateral lung transplantation (INSPIRE): a randomised, open-label, non-inferiority, phase 3 study. Lancet Respir Med 2018;6(5):357–367.

15. Hoetzenecker K, Benazzo A, Stork T, et al. Bilateral lung transplantation on intraoperative extracorporeal membrane oxygenator: an observational study. J Thorac Cardiovasc Surg 2019;160(1):320–327. https://doi.org/10.1016/j. jtcvs. 2019. 10. 155.

16. Subramaniam K, Gabriel L, Bottiger B, et al. Intraoperative red blood cell transfusion is associated with primary graft dysfunction after lung transplantation. Am J Respir Crit Care Med 2021;203 .

17. Van Raemdonck D, Hartwig MG, Hertz MI, et al. Report of the ISHLT Working Group on primary lung graft dysfunction Part IV: prevention and treatment. A 2016 Consensus Group statement of the InternationalSociety for Heart and Lung Transplantation. J Heart Lung Transpl 2017;36(10):1121–1136.

18. DerHovanessian A, Weigt SS, Palchevskiy V, et al. The role of TGF-beta in the association between primary graft dysfunction and bronchiolitis obliterans syndrome. Am J Transplant 2016;16(2):640–649.

19. Whitson BA, Prekker ME, Herrington CS, et al. Primary graft dysfunction and long-term pulmonary function after lung transplantation. J Heart Lung Transpl 2007;26(10):1004–1011.

20. Hadaya J, Benharash P. Extracorporeal membrane oxygenation. JAMA 2020;323(24):2536.

21. Li G, Mankidy B, Liu Z, et al. A closer look at risk factors associated with airway complications in lung transplantation. J Heart Lung Transplant 2021;40.
22. Necki M, Antonczyk R, Pandel A, et al. Impact of cold ischemia time on frequency of airway complications among lung transplant recipients. Transpl Proc 2020;52(7):2160–2164.
23. Van De Wauwer C, Van Raemdonck D, Verleden GM, et al. Risk factors for airway complications within the first year after lung transplantation. Eur J Cardiothorac Surg 2007;31(4):703–710.
24. Ruttmann E, Ulmer H, Marchese M, et al. Evaluation of factors damaging the bronchial wall in lung transplantation. J Heart Lung Transpl 2005;24(3):275–281.
25. Keshava HB, Mason DP, Murthy SC, et al. Pediatric donor lungs for adult transplant recipients: feasibility and outcomes. Thorac Cardiovasc Surg 2012;60(4):275–279.
26. van Berkel V, Guthrie TJ, Puri V, et al. Impact of anastomotic techniques on airway complications after lung transplant. Ann Thorac Surg 2011;92(1):316–320.
27. FitzSullivan E, Gries CJ, Phelan P, et al. Reduction in airway complications after lung transplantation with novel anastomotic technique. Ann Thorac Surg 2011;92(1):309–315.
28. Guzman-Pruneda FA, Orr Y, Trost JG, et al. Bronchial artery revascularization and en bloc lung transplant in children. J Heart Lung Transpl 2016;35(1):122–129.
29. Pettersson GB, Karam K, Thuita L, et al. Comparative study of bronchial artery revascularization in lung transplantation. J Thorac Cardiovasc Surg 2013;146(4):894–900 e3.
30. Crespo MM, McCarthy DP, Hopkins PM, et al. ISHLT consensus statement on adult and pediatric airway complications after lung transplantation: definitions, grading system, and therapeutics. J Heart Lung Transpl 2018;37(5):548–563.
31. Machuzak M, Santacruz JF, Gildea T, et al. Airway complications after lung transplantation. Thorac Surg Clin 2015;25(1):55–75.
32. Santacruz JF, Mehta AC. Airway complications and management after lung transplantation: ischemia, dehiscence, and stenosis. Proc Am Thorac Soc 2009;6(1):79–93.
33. Mahajan AK, Folch E, Khandhar SJ, et al. The diagnosis and management of airway complications following lung transplantation. Chest 2017;152(3): 627–638.
34. de la Torre M, Fernandez R, Fieira E, et al. Post-operative surgical complications after lung transplantation. Rev Port Pneumol (2006) 2015;21(1): 36–40.
35. Loyalka P, Cevik C, Nathan S, et al. Percutaneous stenting to treat pulmonary vein stenosis after single-lung transplantation. Tex Heart Inst J 2012; 39(4):560–564.
36. Krivokuca I, van de Graaf EA, van Kessel DA, et al. Pulmonary embolism and pulmonary infarction after lung transplantation. Clin Appl Thromb Hemost 2011;17(4):421–424.
37. Kroshus TJ, Kshettry VR, Hertz MI, et al. Deep venous thrombosis and pulmonary embolism after lung transplantation. J Thorac Cardiovasc Surg 1995;110(2):540–544.
38. Saez-Gimenez B, Berastegui C, Loor K, et al. Deep vein thrombosis and pulmonary embolism after solid organ transplantation: anunresolved problem. Transpl Rev (Orlando) 2015;29(2):85–92.
39. Spratt JR, Shrestha P, Loor G, et al. Pulmonary transplant salvage using ultrasound-assisted thrombolysis of subacute occlusive main pulmonary artery embolus. Innovations (Phila). 2017;12(3):214–216.

40. Tu T, Toma C, Tapson VF, et al. A prospective, singlearm, multicenter trial of catheter-directed mechanical thrombectomy for intermediate-risk acute pulmonary embolism: the FLARE study. JACC Cardiovasc Interv 2019;12(9):859–869.
41. Ghoreishi M, Pasrija C, Kon Z. VA-ECMO for massive pulmonary embolism: when is the time to wean? Ann Thorac Surg 2020. https://doi.org/10.1016/j. athoracsur. 2020. 09. 047.
42. Thomas B, HassanI, Nobre C. Surgical embolec-tomy, ECMO, or thrombolytic therapy in massive pulmonary embolism. J Am Coll Cardiol 2020;76(23): 2797.
43. Alnajar A, Chen PC, Burt B, et al. Left pulmonary artery patch augmentation for lung transplant in a patient with situs inversus. Tex Heart Inst J 2021;48(1).
44. Sheikh MA, Chowdhury MA, Moukarbel GV. Safety and clinical outcomes of endovascular treatment of adult-onset pulmonary artery stenosis. J Invasive Cardiol 2016;28(5):202–208.
45. Cox CS, Decker SJ, Rolfe M, et al. Middle lobe torsion after unilateral lung transplant. J Radiol Case Rep 2016;10(5):15–21.
46. David A, Liberge R, Corne F, et al. Whole-lung torsion complicating double lung transplantation: CT features. Diagn Interv Imaging 2016;97(9):927–928.
47. Lin MW, Huang SC, Kuo SW, et al. Lobar torsion after lung transplantation. J Formos Med Assoc 2013; 112(2):105–108.
48. Nguyen JC, Maloney J, Kanne JP. Bilateral wholelung torsion after bilateral lung transplantation. J Thorac Imaging 2011;26(1):W17–19.
49. Stephens G, Bhagwat K, Pick A, et al. Lobar torsion following bilateral lung transplantation. J Cardiovasc Surg 2015;30(2):209–214.
50. Wang Y, Kurichi JE, Blumenthal NP, et al. Multiple variables affecting blood usage in lung transplantation. J Heart Lung Transpl 2006;25(5):533–538.
51. Hoechter DJ, von Dossow V, Winter H, et al. The Munich Lung Transplant Group: intraoperative extracorporeal circulation in lung transplantation. Thorac Cardiovasc Surg 2015;63(8):706–714.
52. Triulzi DJ, Griffith BP. Blood usage in lung transplantation. Transfusion 1998;38(1):12–15.
53. Adelmann D, Koch S, Menger J, et al. Risk factors for early bleeding complications after lung transplantation: a retrospective cohort study. Transpl Int 2019;32(12):1313–1321.
54. Hong A, King CS, Brown AW, et al. Hemothorax following lung transplantation: incidence, risk factors, and effect on morbidity and mortality. Multidiscip Respir Med 2016;11:40.
55. Weber D, Cottini SR, Locher P, et al. Association of intraoperative transfusion of blood products with mortality in lung transplant recipients. Perioper Med (Lond) 2013;2(1):20 .
56. Shander A, Hofmann A, Ozawa S, et al. Activity-based costs of blood transfusions in surgical pa-tients at four hospitals. Transfusion 2010;50(4): 753–765.
57. Kao CC, Cuevas JF, Tuthill S, et al. Pleural catheter placement and intrapleural fibrinolysis following lung transplantation. Clin Transpl 2019;33(6): e13592.
58. Arndt A, Boffa DJ. Pleural space complications associated with lung transplantation. Thorac Surg Clin 2015;25(1):87–95.
59. Ferrer J, Roldan J, Roman A, et al. Acute and chronic pleural complications in lung transplanta-tion. J Heart

Lung Transpl 2003;22(11):1217–1225.
60. Mills NL, Boyd AD, Gheranpong C. The significance of bronchial circulation in lung transplantation. J Thorac Cardiovasc Surg 1970;60(6):866–878.
61. Chhajed PN, Bubendorf L, Hirsch H, et al. Mesothelioma after lung transplantation. Thorax 2006;61(10): 916–917.
62. Judson MA, Handy JR, Sahn SA. Pleural effusion from acute lung rejection. Chest 1997;111(4):1128–1130.
63. Shields RK, Clancy CJ, Minces LR, et al. Epidemiology and outcomes of deep surgical site infections following lung transplantation. Am J Transplant 2013;13(8):2137–2145.
64. Wahidi MM, Willner DA, Snyder LD, et al. Diagnosis and outcome of early pleural space infection following lung transplantation. Chest 2009;135(2): 484–491.
65. Rahman NM, Maskell NA, West A, et al. Intrapleural use of tissue plasminogen activator and DNase in pleural infection. N Engl J Med 2011;365(6):518–526.
66. Tang A, Siddiqui HU, Thuita L, et al. Natural history of pleural complications after lung transplantation. Ann Thorac Surg 2021;111(2):407–415.
67. Boffa DJ, Mason DP, Su JW, et al. Decortication after lung transplantation. Ann Thorac Surg 2008;85(3): 1039–1043.
68. Frost AE. Donor criteria and evaluation. Clin Chest Med 1997;18(2):231–237.
69. Shigemura N, Bermudez C, Hattler BG, et al. Impact of graft volume reduction for oversized grafts after lung transplantation on outcome in recipients with end-stage restrictive pulmonary diseases. J Heart Lung Transpl 2009;28(2):130–134.
70. Halloran K, Aversa M, Tinckam K, et al. Comprehensive outcomes after lung retransplantation: a single-center review. Clin Transpl 2018;32(6):e13281.
71. Schaheen L, D'Cunha J. Re-do lung transplantation: keys to success. J Thorac Dis 2019;11(12):5691–5693.
72. Biswas Roy S, Panchanathan R, Walia R, et al. Lung retransplantation for chronic rejection: a single-center experience. Ann Thorac Surg 2018;105(1): 221–227.
73. Clausen ES, Weber JM, Neely ML, et al. Predicting survival for lung retransplantation patients at one and five years. J Heart Lung Transplant 2019; 38(4):S225–226.

# 第 10 章 肺移植受者的感染性并发症

Erika D. Lease, Marie M. Budev 著

谢哲凡 译

周建平 校

【关键词】
- 肺移植 • 感染 • 并发症 • 预防

【要点】
- 感染仍然是肺移植术后的常见死亡原因。
- 肺移植术后可使用抗生素预防多种不同的感染。
- 肺移植受者的感染性病原体包括细菌、病毒和真菌,这些病原体都有各自相关的危险因素、临床表现以及治疗方案。

## 10.1 引　言

肺移植(LTx)已成为终末期肺病患者挽救生命的选择,其长期生存率低于其他实质器官移植,部分是由于感染性并发症的直接和间接影响,部分是由于感染性并发症引起慢性同种异体肺移植物功能障碍(CLAD)。国际心肺移植学会(ISHLT)登记的数据显示,肺移植患者的术后中位生存期已提高至 6.7 年。然而,感染仍然是其常见的死亡原因,感染所致死亡人数占移植后第一年死亡人数的 35%,占移植后 1~3 年死亡人数的 21%[1]。因此,在肺移植患者的终生照护中,感染的治疗和预防至关重要。在本章中,我们将对围术期早期供体来源的感染以及随着时间的推移发展出现的后期感染风险的某些方面进行回顾。此外,我们将讨论移植后预防性抗细菌、抗真菌和抗病毒的基本原则,以及肺移植患者常见细菌、病毒和真菌感染后的治疗。

## 10.2 抗菌药物预防

肺移植术后经常使用抗微生物药物预防多种病原体感染(表 10-1)。预防性抗感染

第10章 肺移植受者的感染性并发症

可能是有针对性的（高危人群或已知既往感染/定植人群），也可能是无针对性的（所有肺移植受者），这取决于病原体类型、移植后时长以及其他临床因素。

**表 10-1 肺移植后的预防**

| | |
|---|---|
| 耶氏肺孢子菌 | • 磺胺噁唑-甲氧苄啶作为一线预防用药<br>• 考虑对非严重过敏者进行脱敏治疗<br>• 首选终身预防<br>• 磺胺甲噁唑-甲氧苄啶还可预防其他微生物的感染 |
| 抗真菌预防 | • 大多数肺移植中心常规进行预防性抗真菌治疗<br>• 预防性抗真菌治疗的获益、最佳药物和疗程尚不清楚<br>• 对于移植前真菌定植/感染的患者，可考虑针对性预防 |
| 抗病毒预防 | • 大多数肺移植中心常规给予 CMV 预防治疗<br>• 最佳预防用药疗程尚不清楚<br>• 对于未予预防性抗 CMV 治疗的受者，应考虑在移植后早期使用另一种抗病毒药物预防 HSV 和（或）VZV。最佳抗病毒疗程尚不清楚 |
| 抗细菌预防 | • 对于移植前存在细菌定植/感染的受者，应考虑使用针对性的预防治疗方案<br>• 抗菌药物的最佳使用时间尚不清楚 |

注：CMV，巨细胞病毒；HSV，单纯疱疹病毒；VZV，水痘带状疱疹病毒

耶氏肺孢子菌（以前也称为卡氏肺囊虫），是一种机会性致病真菌，可导致耶氏肺孢子菌肺炎（P. jirovecii pneumonia，PJP），尤其在具有免疫缺陷的宿主中[2]。在常规全面预防治疗之前，实质器官移植受者发生 PJP 的风险为 5%~15%，在移植后的前 6 个月患该病的风险最高[3]。一项荟萃分析显示，预防性使用磺胺甲噁唑-甲氧苄啶可使造血干细胞和实质器官移植受者的 PJP 发生率降低 91%[4]。肺移植受者是 PJP 的高危人群，一般建议终身预防用药[2]。可能起到预防性作用的治疗药物包括磺胺甲噁唑-甲氧苄啶、氨苯砜、阿托伐醌和吸入性喷他脒。一项荟萃分析显示，磺胺甲噁唑-甲氧苄啶效果较其他药更好，在适当的剂量下是罕见突破性病例的优势药物[2,4]。鉴于磺胺甲噁唑甲氧苄啶是进行预防性抗感染治疗的首选，在移植住院期间，可考虑对大部分对磺胺非严重过敏的受者进行成功脱敏治疗[5,6]。此外，磺胺甲噁唑-甲氧苄啶还具有可能同时预防其他感染的优势，如弓形虫、诺卡菌、单核球增多性李斯特菌感染以及其他常见的泌尿、呼吸道和胃肠道病原体感染[7,8]。

肺移植术后普遍会进行预防性抗真菌治疗，但由于缺乏相关数据，导致最佳治疗方案仍不确定。在对美国肺移植中心的调查中发现，90%的中心会使用普遍的预防性抗真

菌策略[9]。近 3/4 的受访者联合使用吸入型两性霉素和全身性抗真菌药，约 22% 的受访者单独使用全身性抗真菌药，约 6% 的受访者单独使用吸入型两性霉素。抗真菌药物预防的使用疗程也各不相同，约 89% 的受访者预防性抗真菌治疗的疗程超过了因移植住院的时间，近 70% 的受访者抗感染疗程持续至移植后 6 个月或更短。随后，一项针对现有数据进行的系统综述和荟萃分析发现，接受普遍预防性抗感染的肺移植受者和未接受预防性抗感染的受者相比，真菌感染的发生率并没有差异[10]。此外，吸入两性霉素的肺移植受者与全身使用三唑类药物的肺移植受者相比，移植术后第一年内真菌感染的发生率没有差异。预防性用药的疗程似乎也对肺移植术后短期或长期真菌感染的发生率没有影响。然而，研究者认为，由于各研究显著的异质性、高偏倚风险和现有研究汇总时缺乏准确性，没有足够的证据支持或否定预防性抗真菌治疗的益处。

预防性抗病毒治疗是肺移植术后的常规治疗措施。抗病毒预防的主要病原体是疱疹病毒，包括巨细胞病毒（CMV）、单纯疱疹病毒（herpes simplex virus，HSV）和水痘-带状疱疹病毒（varicella-zoster virus，VZV）。特别是 CMV，是肺移植术后发病率和死亡率的重要因素[10]。面对免疫抑制的情况，疱疹病毒可能在血清学阳性的受者（受者阳性，或 R+）中从潜伏形式重新激活。在 CMV 感染的情况下，也可能会出现以下情况：供者感染的 CMV 在血清学阳性的受者（供者阳性/受者阳性，或 D+/R+）中发生再激活，或在未感染的受者（供体阳性/受体阴性，或 D+/R-）中通过移植器官进行传播而发生原发感染。肺移植受者通常在移植术后前 6 个月发生 CMV 感染并且患病的风险更高[11,12]。虽然普遍首选口服更昔洛韦进行预防，但对于移植后早期或者对口服药物不耐受甚至无法服用口服药物的个体，也可以静脉注射（IV）更昔洛韦（ganciclovir，GCV）。尽管一项多中心随机研究发现，D+ 和（或）R+ 受者接受 12 个月的缬更昔洛韦预防治疗，其术后 1 年内 CMV 病发生率显著低于仅接受 3 个月该药预防治疗的受者，但最佳预防性治疗的疗程仍不确定[13]。在为期 12 个月的试验结束后的 6 个月中，2 个研究组的 CMV 发病率都很低。目前指南建议 CMV R+ 肺移植受者预防性用药 3 个月，D+/R 肺移植受者预防性用药 6~12 个月。许多中心的方案将预防性治疗的时间延长，有的中心甚至无限期地进行预防治疗[14,15]。

在未接受 CMV 预防性治疗的受者（CMV D-/R-）中，其与 HSV 和 VZV 相关的预防性治疗数据有限。然而，普遍共识是，HSV 或 VZV 血清学阳性的受者应在移植术后早期使用阿昔洛韦或伐昔洛韦进行抗病毒预防治疗[16,17]。尽管在心肺移植受者的治疗经验中发现，早期 HSV 感染发生在移植术后 2 个月内，但最佳用药疗程仍不清楚[18,19]。

但目前美国移植协会指南建议实质器官移植术后至少进行预防性抗感染 1 个月[16]。

一些拟行肺移植的患者，尤其是囊性纤维化（CF）患者，可能存在慢性呼吸道病原体定植或感染，包括细菌、真菌和分枝杆菌。可采用有针对性的预防方案对胸膜腔、吻合口、手术部位和移植肺的污染进行预防。对于 CF 的肺移植受者，当有毒性可接受的敏感抗生素供选择时，应给予具有敏感性的抗微生物治疗[20]。一项关于肺移植围术期抗生素治疗的全球调查发现，在进行移植前，所有受访者都对有慢性病原定植的受者使用敏感性驱动的治疗方案[21]。近 70% 的受访者表示，若在移植前存在多重耐药定植，他们会联合使用 2 种敏感抗生素。2/3 的受访者对移植后的受者的抗生素使用疗程为 7~21 天，大多数疗程为 14 天。总的来说，目前的数据并没有表明移植前存在多重耐药或泛耐药菌的受者移植后预后会更差，包括总生存率、急性排斥反应发生率或 CLAD 发生率[22,23]。

## 10.3 供体来源的感染

移植受者可能会发生供体来源的感染，供体来源的感染根据捐献前的评估可以分为"预期的"和"非预期的" 2 种情况。预期的病原传播可能来自于那些 CMV 血清学阳性或者患有活动性丙型肝炎的供者。预期的传播较为常见，可以使医疗团队在移植后进行规划和管理。例如，根据受者的 CMV 血清状态来确定适当的 CMV 预防策略。此外，肺移植受者可能有预期地感染捐献前的支气管镜检查和下呼吸道采样中发现的细菌。根据最近的研究报道，在捐献前的下呼吸道病原培养中发现潜在的致病细菌似乎很常见，比例为 48%~89%[24-26]。有研究发现，大约 5% 的细菌是多重耐药菌，而在移植后受者的呼吸道病原培养中并未发现这些多重耐药菌株[25]。

关于器官供者下呼吸道培养阳性结果对移植后受者预后的影响，不同的研究数据之间存在矛盾之处。一些研究发现，这些受者在移植后机械通气时间较长，并可能出现移植后肺炎。然而，大多数研究并未报道两组移植后初期的总体预后或生存率有差异[24-28]。目前，尚无数据支持在捐献前移植肺下呼吸道样本中发现的微生物应被视为真正的或潜在的病原体，也没有受者应接受治疗的最佳时间相关的数据。

非预期的供体疾病传播似乎不常见。美国最近的一项为期 10 年的数据显示，非预期的疾病传播发生在 0.18% 的受者中，0.23% 的供者将已确诊或可能的疾病传播给了至少 1 位受者[29]。在这些已确诊或可能的疾病传播中，近 73% 是感染性疾病，其中 31%

是病毒性感染，30% 是细菌性感染，22% 是真菌性感染，13% 是寄生虫感染，还有 4% 是结核分枝杆菌感染。大约 67% 的已确诊或可能的供体来源的感染在移植后 30 天内出现，而 88% 在移植后 90 天内出现。尽管非预期的供体来源的感染似乎很罕见，但这些感染可导致 15% 的受者死亡，其中寄生虫感染的死亡率最高，达到 35%。非预期的供体来源感染的高死亡率强调了以下内容的必要性：通过病史及社会史对供体进行风险分层，对供体及供体器官进行临床评估，以及在供者存在感染可能的情况下，进行除常规检测的额外实验室检查[30]。

## 10.4 细菌感染的管理

早期细菌感染可能由供体传播及受者本身的慢性感染和（或）定植引起，或与住院和（或）重症疾病相关的感染引起。肺移植受者术后早期感染的额外风险因素包括支气管吻合口处的坏死组织、同种异体肺移植物的去神经化导致黏液纤毛清除和咳嗽反射减弱，以及移植肺持续暴露于上呼吸道的环境和微生物中。肺移植接受者在其一生中可能会遇到的细菌感染范围很广，包括那些在免疫抑制宿主中占主导地位的感染，以及正常宿主会遇到的常规社区获得性感染。因此，本节将重点讨论移植后早期的细菌感染。

肺移植受者的手术部位感染主要为皮肤或软组织感染、胸膜腔或纵隔等肺外感染以及气道吻合口感染。在肺移植受者中，手术部位感染相对较为常见，发生率为 5%～19%[31]。一项研究发现，肺移植后的手术部位感染发生的中位时间为 25 天，其中脓胸最常见，占 42%；其次是手术切口感染占 29%，纵隔炎占 16%，胸骨骨髓炎占 6%，心包炎占 6%[32]。在这些感染中，41% 的受者体内同样发现了革兰阴性和革兰阳性的细菌病原体。在该研究中，由手术部位感染导致的 1 年死亡率较高，为 35%。鉴于死亡风险高且微生物学广泛，如果怀疑有手术部位感染，建议考虑先使用广谱抗生素，在明确病原体后进行针对性调整[31]。

## 10.5 随时间变化的感染风险

尽管根据最新的 ISHLT 注册数据来看，肺移植后的短期和长期生存率有所提高，但感染仍然是肺移植受者一生中死亡的重要原因[1]。与正常肺相比，移植肺更容易出现感染并发症，其原因有多种。与具有肺动脉和支气管动脉双重血供的原生肺不同，移植肺通常只有一个血供来源，除非进行了支气管动脉的血管重建[33]。这种有限的血供可能会导致远端上皮的破坏，从而影响愈合，并导致黏液清除障碍[34]。有证据表明，即使随着时间的推移，移植患者的黏液纤毛清除功能可能仍然受损[35]。此外，由于中央淋巴管在手术时未重新连接，因此移植后早期会出现淋巴引流受损。肺部直接暴露于环境中以及为了防止排斥所需的高水平免疫抑制都在移植后早期和晚期感染风险的增加中扮演了重要角色[36]。Fishman 和 Rubin 描述了实质器官移植后的 3 个感染期：①移植后的第一个月以医院获得性感染和供体来源的感染为特征；②接下来是与机会性感染相关的持续长达 6 个月的强化免疫抑制期；③随着免疫抑制的减弱，会出现社区获得性感染和较为罕见的病原体感染[8,37]。对这一时间线的认识改进了预防策略和经验性治疗方法。一些研究指出，细菌感染的风险在移植后第 1 年的第 1 个月（每 1000 个移植日发生 17.3 次感染）以及第 6~12 个月（每 1000 个移植日发生 2.6 次感染）最高[38,39]。在细菌感染中，最常见的是铜绿假单胞菌和肠杆菌科细菌引起的呼吸道感染[38]。

# 10.6 病毒感染的管理

## 10.6.1 巨细胞病毒

CMV 感染是肺移植受者中最常见的机会性感染，也是肺移植人群中仅次于细菌感染的第二常见感染[40]。与 CMV 感染相关的发病率和死亡率既是由于其对组织的直接损伤作用，也与急性细胞性排斥反应和 CLAD 的发展间接相关[41,42]。此外，CMV 可能通过免疫调节作用促进其他机会性细菌和真菌感染的发生[43]。CMV 感染性疾病定义为在组织、血液或其他体液中存在 CMV 复制，并伴有相应的临床症状和体征。CMV 疾病的临床表现有多样，包括病毒综合征、肺炎、结肠炎或肝炎[41]。在引入 GCV 之前，CMV 疾病的死亡率非常高。静脉注射 GCV 和口服缬更昔洛韦是治疗活动性 CMV 疾病的有效方法。这两种药物都需要根据肾功能进行剂量调整，但剂量不足也可能导致疗效降低和病毒耐药。此外，可以考虑谨慎降低免疫抑制的强度，并在可能的情况下给予 CMV 免疫球蛋白（注意：证据有限）[44]。应持续抗病毒治疗至少 2 周，直到症状和病毒血症消失，并且连续 2 次检测血清学阴性（每次间隔 1 周），随后使用口服缬更昔洛韦进行二次抑制，至少维持 1~3 个月。需对 CMV 病毒载量进行监测，以观察 CMV 是否产生耐药性。如果在持续抗病毒治疗的情况下，病毒载量依然持续上升或保持高位，应怀疑病毒出现耐药性。检测到病毒耐药性时，如检测到导致对 GCV 耐药的 UL97 磷酸转移酶基因突变，则可以选用其他替代药物，例如静脉注射的膦甲酸钠或西多福韦[45,46]。

### 10.6.2 社区获得性呼吸道病毒

社区获得性呼吸道病毒（community-acquired respiratory viruses，CARV）对肺移植后的死亡率有影响，包括增加急性排斥和 CLAD 的风险。CARV 会引起上呼吸道感染，包括流感、副流感病毒（parainfluenza，PIV）、在肺移植患者中最常见的人类鼻病毒（human rhinovirus，HRV），还有呼吸道合胞病毒（respiratory syncytial virus，RSV）、腺病毒（adenovirus，ADV）、冠状病毒（不包括 SARS CoV-2）、人类偏肺病毒（human metapneumovirus，hMPV）和博卡病毒（bocavirus，BCV）。CARV 感染的报告发病率在 7.7%~64% 之间，这种范围的波动是由诊断检测技术的多样性和病毒流行的季节性导致的[47,48]。目前，包括多重检测法在内的几种 PCR 检测方法，可以快速识别血清、拭子和支气管肺泡灌洗液（bronchoalveolar lavage，BAL）中的病毒[49]。对于大多数 CARV，除了支持性治疗外，还没有可用的有效治疗方法。对于那些有治疗方法的病毒，及时干预可以减少并发症，降低 ICU 住院率和死亡率。对于特定的 CARV，有特定的治疗方案可供选择。例如，奥司他韦或扎那米韦可以治疗甲流和乙流，口服利巴韦林可以治疗副流感病毒、呼吸道合胞病毒或人类偏肺病毒，西多福韦可以用于治疗腺病毒。对于其他常见的 CARV，包括鼻病毒、冠状病毒（不包括 SARS CoV-2）和博卡病毒，则建议进行支持性治疗[48]。高剂量皮质类固醇在治疗 CARV 感染中的作用仍然存在争议，但在 CARV 感染发生急性排斥反应时可以联用激素。但这种联用也有争议，Vu 及其同事对 34 项研究进行了系统评价，发现 CARV 感染与急性排斥反应之间的关系并不明确，仅在少数已发表的病例报告中出现[50]。然而，由于汇总的研究中缺乏对照组以及对急性排斥反应的定义存在差异，该系统评价的结果有一定局限性。因此，CARV 与急性排斥反应之间的关系尚无确切结论[50]。

### 10.6.3 EB 病毒

急性 EB 病毒（Epstein-Barr virus，EBV）感染会导致 B 细胞发生多克隆扩增，并表达病毒抗原，进而使 T 细胞对受感染的 B 细胞产生反应。当免疫抑制剂抑制 T 细胞免疫时，感染的 B 细胞可能会引发移植后淋巴增殖性疾病（posttransplant lymphoproliferative disorder，PTLD）。肺移植受者 PTLD 的发生率为 5%~15%[51]。通过 PCR 法常规监测血液的 EB 病毒载量有助于早期发现 PTLD[51]。对于存在原发性 EB 病毒感染（即供者 EB 病毒阳性而受者 EB 病毒阴性的情况）的高风险患者，一些移植中心提倡使用 ACV 或 GCV 等抗病毒药物，以预防 PTLD 的发生。然而，目前仍缺少足够的证据支持在 EBV 不匹配的受者中使用这些药物[51]。

### 10.6.4 水痘 - 带状疱疹病毒

肺移植受者发生 VZV 并发症的风险增加，如皮肤受累的带状疱疹（herpes zoster, HZ）到危及生命的终末器官受累，包括肺炎、脑炎和肝炎。VZV 和 HZ 可以进行抗病毒治疗，对于局部 HZ 感染，可以口服阿昔洛韦或伐昔洛韦，疗程通常为 7 天；对于播散性 HZ 或急性水痘，则需选择静脉给药并住院治疗[52,53]。人类疱疹病毒 6 型感染可在免疫受损宿主中引起脑炎。此外，人类疱疹病毒 8 型与器官移植受者口的播散型卡波西肉瘤相关[53]。

### 10.6.5 COVID-19

SARS CoV-2 病毒感染会对肺移植受者的发病率和死亡率产生深远的影响。COVID-19 检测阳性的肺移植受者感染的表现常常很严重，其中 80% 以上需要住院治疗，30% 需要重症监护。其中 COVID-19 引起的死亡率为 14%~39%[54-56]。根据美国传染病学会的建议考虑了几种治疗方案，包括针对高风险门诊患者的中和性单克隆抗体药物巴尼韦单抗和埃特司韦单抗，以及针对住院患者的地塞米松、托珠单抗和瑞德西韦[57]。而关于肺移植受者的免疫抑制管理，国际心肺移植学会在关于 SARS CoV-2 大流行期间的指导文件中建议，患有中、重度疾病的患者应停用霉酚酸酯、mTOR 抑制剂和硫唑嘌呤[58]。

## 10.7 真菌感染的管理

在实质器官移植的受者中，肺移植受者发生真菌感染的风险最高[52]。尽管其发病率可能会受多个因素的影响，但肺移植受者在 1 年内真菌感染的累积发病率约为 8.6%。真菌感染的类型和发生的时间会受到多种因素影响，包括移植前真菌定植、抗菌预防、免疫抑制强度和移植后时长[59-61]。其中中位发病时间约为移植后 11 个月，但有若干研究也注意到了晚期真菌感染。一项来自多伦多的研究表明，移植后 2~4 年内肺移植受者侵袭性曲霉菌病的发生率为 9%[62]。肺移植后的侵袭性真菌感染（Invasive fungal infections, IFIs）是导致肺移植受者死亡的主要原因。在一项单中心研究中，IFIs 被认为是肺移植

### 肺移植：胸外科临床问题

受者群体死亡的最强预测因素[63]。移植后最常见的 IFIs 报道是侵袭性霉菌病（invasive mold diseases，IMDs），最常见的是侵袭性曲霉菌所致的肺炎或气管支气管炎，其感染具有多器官播散的风险[61]。在术后初期（术后 30 天内）以念珠菌感染为主[61,63]。假丝酵母菌感染可能表现为纵隔炎、胸膜炎、脓胸或手术部位感染和假丝酵母菌血症，通常由留置管或导管引起。一些非曲霉类的真菌感染可在移植后的晚期发生，包括毛霉菌、链格孢菌、镰孢霉和赛多孢霉属，其发病率低于曲霉菌感染，但比侵袭性曲霉菌病的预后更差[59,64]。生活在高危地区的患者可感染地方性真菌病，病原包括荚膜组织胞质菌、皮炎芽生菌和球孢子菌。

诊断真菌感染的金标准为呼吸道病原培养识别真菌生长。可对培养阳性的真菌进行药敏试验，并且鉴定是否为非曲霉菌，而培养敏感性仅为 50%，限制了其在临床中的实用性[65,66]。真菌生物标志物包括最常检测的半乳甘露聚糖，用于识别曲霉菌细胞壁中的糖类残基。由于半乳甘露聚糖也存在于其他非曲霉菌的细胞壁中，如胞浆菌属、芽孢杆菌、镰孢霉属和青霉属，所以也有可能得到假阳性结果[67]。血清半乳甘露聚糖的敏感性较低，不应用于肺移植受者。相反，BAL 半乳甘露聚糖检测在实质器官移植受者中具有更高的诊断价值，其敏感性为 60%~82%，应被当作肺炎检查项目评估[68,69]。

肺移植后真菌感染的治疗是基于几个关键原则的多模式治疗，这些原则包括：首先，使用的抗真菌药物应针对特定的真菌病原体。其次，应对感染组织进行手术或支气管镜清创，同时移除受污染的管道和装置，以减少感染组织中的真菌负荷。最后应调整免疫抑制强度，使免疫系统能够攻克感染，并避免出现免疫排斥[70]。抗真菌治疗的选择取决于病原体的类型，表 10-2 提供了特定真菌感染抗真菌治疗的概述[70]。他克莫司和环孢霉素等唑类药物会增加钙调神经磷酸酶抑制剂的水平。可能需要对钙调磷酸酶抑制剂和唑类药物的浓度进行频繁监测，以观察药物吸收情况并避免毒性反应[70]。

## 第10章 肺移植受者的感染性并发症

**表 10-2　肺移植后常见真菌感染的治疗选择**

| 感染的真菌类型 | 抗真菌治疗的建议 |
|---|---|
| 曲霉菌 | 伏立康唑是侵袭性疾病的首选药物<br>替代药物：<br>　　三唑类：泊沙康唑、艾沙康唑<br>　　棘白菌素类：卡泊芬净、阿尼芬净、米卡芬净<br>可考虑联合治疗感染<br>吸入两性霉素 B 脂质体可用于治疗气管支气管炎 + 全身治疗 |
| 念珠菌属 | 念珠菌血症和侵袭性念珠菌病<br>初始经验性治疗：棘白菌素类药物，包括卡泊芬净、阿尼芬净、米卡芬净<br>基于药敏试验的针对性治疗<br>替代药物：<br>　　如果不考虑唑类药物耐药性问题，可使用氟康唑<br>　　两性霉素 B 脂质体 |
| 毛霉菌 | 侵袭性毛霉菌病<br>大剂量两性霉素 B 脂质体<br>替代药物：<br>　　三唑类药物：泊沙康唑、艾沙康唑 |
| 新生隐球菌 | 隐球菌脑膜炎<br>诱导治疗包括：<br>　　两性霉素 B 脂质体 +5- 氟胞嘧啶，持续 2~4 周<br>巩固阶段<br>　　氟康唑 400~800 mg，持续 8 周<br>维持阶段<br>　　氟康唑 200~400 mg，持续 12 个月<br>非中枢神经系统感染<br>　　重症：与脑膜炎相同的治疗方案<br>　　非重症：氟康唑 |
| 镰刀菌属 | 侵袭性镰刀菌病<br>　　最佳治疗方案目前尚不明确<br>　　药物选择包括两性霉素 B、伏立康唑、泊沙康唑、艾沙康唑 |
| 赛多孢子菌 | 侵袭性尖端赛多孢子菌病<br>伏立康唑是侵袭性疾病的治疗选择 |
| 卡氏肺囊虫 | 复方新诺明 ± 大剂量类固醇 |

注：根据以下资料改编：Kennedy CC, Razonable RR. Fungal Infections After Lung Transplantation. Clin Chest Med. 2017;38(3):511-520

## 10.8 人型支原体和解脲支原体感染

高氨血症是一种罕见但致命的情况，可发生在肺移植受者的围移植期的早期。人型支原体或解脲支原体全身感染可导致肺移植受者出现高氨血症[71,72]。在一项单中心研究中，807 例肺移植受者中只有 8 例患者确诊了高氨血症，但死亡率却高达 75%。高氨血症通常表现为嗜睡、精神状态改变、癫痫发作或昏迷，应对血清氨的水平进行监测，如果水平升高，应及时开始使用抗生素治疗。抗生素的选择包括大环内酯类、氟喹诺酮类或四环素类，同时要注意可能出现的耐药性情况。支气管肺泡灌洗液应被送去进行聚合酶链反应（PCR），并对这两种微生物进行特殊培养。

## 10.9 总 结

肺移植受者一生中对各种感染的易感性增加，这是由移植器官暴露于外部环境、黏液纤毛清除功能受损以及高水平的免疫抑制所致。与其他实质器官移植相比，肺移植受者的长期预后仍然较差，主要和感染及慢性移植器官功能障碍造成的死亡相关。移植后的第一个月感染的概率最大，但感染的风险会持续存在于患者的整个生命周期中。临床医生应始终对感染保持高度警惕，并对患者制定个体化预防和治疗方案，以确保移植器官的功能和患者的生存。

【临床护理要点】

- 感染仍然是肺移植术后常见的死亡原因。
- 与其他实质器官移植相比，肺移植受者的长期预后仍然较差，其主要原因是感染死亡和慢性移植物功能障碍。
- 针对肺移植后多种机会性感染，可进行预防性抗细菌、抗真菌和抗病毒治疗。
- 移植后第 1 个月主要是医院获得性感染和供体来源的感染。移植后第 1 个月至第 6 个月，是机会性感染的高发期。移植 1 年后，免疫抑制减轻，但感染风险仍然存在，最常见的是社区获得性感染和罕见病原体感染。
- 无论是细菌、真菌还是病毒，都有各自的危险因素、特定的临床表现和治疗方案的选择。
- 临床医生应在移植后各个阶段对感染保持警惕。

## 声明

作者没有相关的声明事项。

## 参考文献

1. Chambers DC, Cherikh WS, Harhay MO, et al. The International Thoracic Organ Transplant Registry of the International Society for Heart Lung Transplantation: Thirty –Fifth adult lung and heart lung report -2019; Focus theme donor and recipient size match. J Heart Lung Transplant 2019;38:1042–1055.
2. Fishman JA, Gans H. Pneumocystis jirovecii in solid organ transplantation: guidelines from the American Society of Transplantation Infectious Diseases Community of Practice. Clin Transplant 2019;33(9): e13587.
3. Iriart X, Challan Belval T, Fillaux J, et al. Risk factors of Pneumocystis Pneumonia in solid organ recipients in the era of the common use of posttransplant prophylaxis. Am J Transplant 2015;15:190–199.
4. Green H, Paul M, Vidal L, et al. Prophylaxis of Pneumocystis pneumonia in immunocompromised non-HIV-infected patients: Systematic review and meta-analysis of randomized controlled trials. Mayo Clin Proc 2007;82(9):1052–1059.
5. Ionnidis JP, Cappelleri JC, Sklnik PR, et al. A meta analysis of the relative efficacy and toxicity of pneumocystis carinii prophylactic regimens. Arch Intern Med 1996;156(2):177–188.
6. Pryor JB, Olyaei AJ, Kirsch D, et al. Sulfonamide desensitization in solid organ transplant recipients: a protocol-driven approach during the index transplant hospitalization. Transpl Infect Dis 2019;21(6): e13191.
7. Fishman JA, Issa NC. Infection in organ transplantation: risk factors and evolving patterns of infection. Infect Dis Clin North Am 2010;24(2):273–283.
8. Fishman JA. Infection in solid-organ transplant recipients. N Engl J Med 2007;357(25):2601–2614.
9. Pennington KM, Yost K, Escalante P, et al. Antifungal prophylaxis in lung transplant: a survey of United States' transplant centers. Clin Transpl 2019;33(7): e13630.
10. Pennington KM, Baqir M, Erwin PJ, et al. Antifungal prophylaxis in lung transplant recipients: a systematic review and meta-analysis. Transpl Infect Dis 2020;22(4):e13333.
11. Razonable RR, Humar A. Cytomegalovirus in solid organ transplant recipients – guidelines of the American Society of Transplantation Infectious Diseases Community of Practice. Clin Transpl 2019;33: e13512.
12. Humar A, Kumar D, Preiksaitis J, et al. A trial of valganciclovir prophylaxis for cytomegalovirus prevention in lung transplant recipients. Am J Transt 2005; 5(6):1462–1468.
13. Palmer SM, Limaye AP, Banks M, et al. Extended valganciclovir prophylaxis to prevent cytomegalovirus after lung transplantation: a randomized, controlled trial. Ann Intern Med 2010;152(12):761–769.
14. Kotton CN, Kumar D, Caliendo AM, et al. The third international consensus guidelines on the management of cytomegalovirus in solid-organ transplantation. Transplantation 2018;102(6):900–931.
15. Zuk DM, Humar A, Weinkauf JG, et al. An international survey of cytomegalovirus management practices in lung transplantation. Transplant 2010;90(6): 612–676.
16. Lee DH, Zuckerman RA. Herpes simplex virus infections in solid organ transplantation: guidelines

from the American Society of Transplantation Infectious Diseases Community of Practice. Clin Transpl 2019;33:e13526.

17. Pergam SA, Limaye AP. Varicella zoster virus in solid organ transplantation: guidelines from the American Society of Transplantation Infectious Diseases Community of Practice. Clin Transpl 2019;33:e13622.
18. Brooks RG, Hofflin JM, Jamieson SW, et al. Infectious Complications in Heart-Lung Transplant Recipients. Am J Med 1985;79(4):412–422.
19. Smyth RL, Higenbottam TW, Scott JP, et al. Herpes simplex virus infection in heart-lung transplant recipients. Transplantation 1990;49(4):735–739.
20. Shah P, Lowery E, Chapparro C, et al. Cystic fibrosis foundation consensus statements for the care of cystic fibrosis lung transplant recipients. J Heart Lung Transpl 2021;40(7):539–556.
21. Coiffard B, Prud'Homme E, Hraich S, et al. Worldwide clinical practices in perioperative antibiotic therapy for lung transplantation. BMC Pulm Med 2020;20(1):109–117.
22. Winstead RJ, Waldman G, Autry EB, et al. Outcome of lung transplantation for cystic fibrosis in the setting of extensively drug-resistant organisms. Prog Transplant 2019;29(3):220–224.
23. Lay C, Law N, Holm AM, et al. Outcomes in cystic fibrosis lung transplant recipients infected with organisms labeled as pan-resistant: An ISHLT Registry-based analysis. J Heart Lung Transpl 2019;38(5):545–552.
24. Ahmad O, Shafii AE, Mannino DM, et al. Impact of donor lung pathogenic bacteria on patient outcomes in the immediate post-transplant period. Transplantation 2018;20(6):e12986.
25. Bunsow E, Los-Arcos I, Martin-Gomez MT, et al. Donor-derived bacterial infections in lung transplant recipients in the era of multidrug resistance. J Infect 2020;80:190–196.
26. Bonde PN, Patel ND, Borja MC, et al. Impact of donor lung organisms on post-transplant pneumonia. J Heart Lung Transpl 2006;25(1):99–105.
27. Weill D, Dey GC, Hicks RA, et al. A positive donor gram stain does not predict outcome following lung transplantation. J Heart Lung Transpl 2002;21(5):555–558.
28. Avlonitis VS, Krause A, Luzzi L, et al. Bacterial colonization of the donor lower airways is a predictor of poor outcome in lung transplantation. Eur J Cardiothorac Surg 2003;24(4):601–607.
29. Kaul DR, Vece G, Blumberg E, et al. Ten years of donor-derived disease: a report of the disease transmission advisory committee. Am J Transpl 2021; 21(2):689–702.
30. Wolfe CR, Ison MG. Donor-derived infections: Guidelines from the American Society of Transplantation Infectious Diseases Community of Practice. Clin Transpl 2019;33:e13547.
31. Abb LM, Grossi PA. Surgical site infections: Guidelines from the American Society of Transplantation Infectious Diseases Community of Practice. Clin Transplant 2019;33(9):e13589.
32. Shields RK, Clancy CJ, Minces LR, et al. Epidemiology and outcomes of deep surgical site infections following lung transplantation. Am J Transpl 2013; 13(8):2137–2145.
33. Yun JJ, Unai S, Pettersson G. Lung transplant with bronchial arterial revascularization: review of surgical technique and clinical outcomes. J Thorac Dis 2019;11:S1821–1828.
34. Nørgaard MAB, Andersen CB, Pettersson G. Airway epithelium of transplanted lungs with and without direct bronchial artery revascularization. Eur J Cardiothorac Surg 1999;15(01):37–44.
35. Duarte AG, Myers AC. Cough reflex in lung transplant recipients. Lung 2012;190(01):23–27.

36. Rubin RH, Schaffner A, Speich R, et al. Introduction to the Immunocompromised Host Society Consensus Conference on epidemiology, prevention, diagnosis, and management of infections in solid organ transplant patients. Clin Infect Dis 2001;33:S1–4.
37. Fishman JA, Rubin RH. Infection in organ transplant recipients. N Engl J Med 1998;338:1741–1751.
38. Van Delden C, Stampf S, Hirsch HH, et al. Burden and timeline of infectious diseases in the first year after solid organ transplantation in the Swiss Transplant Cohort Study. Clin Infect Dis 2020;71:e159–169.
39. Gagliotti C, Morsillo F, Moro M, et al. Infections in liver and lung transplant recipients. A Natl Prospective Cohort 2018;37:399–407.
40. Fisher RA. Cytomegalovirus infection and disease in the new era of immunosuppression following solid organ transplantation. Transpl Infect Dis 2009;11: 195–202.
41. Zamora MR. Cytomegalovirus and lung transplantation. Am J Transpl 2004;4:1219–1226.
42. Ducan SR, Paradis IL, Yousem SA, et al. Sequelae of cytomeglovirus pulmonary infections in lung allograft recipients. Am Rev Respir Dis 1992;146: 1419–1425.
43. Razonable RR, Limaye RR. Cytomegalovirus infection after solid organ transplantation. In: Bowden RA, Ljungman P, Snydman DR, editors. Transplant infections. 3rd edition. Philadelphia (PA): Lippincott Williams and Wilkins; 2010. p. 328.
44. Kotton CN, Kumar D, Caliendo AM, et al. Updated international consensus guidelines on the management of cytomegalovirus in solid-organ transplantation. Transplantation 2013;96:333.
45. Piiparinen H, Hockerstedt K, Gronhagen-Riska C, et al. Comparison of two quantitative CMV PCR tests, Cobas Amplicor CMV Monitor and TaqMan assay, and pp65-antigenemia Assay in the Determination of Viral Loads from Peripheral Blood of Organ Transplant Patients. J Clin Virol 2004;30:258.
46. Hakki M, Chou S. The biology of cytomegalovirus drug resistance. Curr Opin Infect Dis 2011;24: 605–611.
47. Shalhoub S, Husain S. Community-acquired respiratory viral infections in lung transplant recipients. Curr Opin Infect Dis 2013;26:302–308.
48. Gottlieb J, Schulz TF, Welte T, et al. Community-acquired respiratory viral infections in lung transplant recipients: a single season cohort study. Transplantation 2009;87:1530–1537.
49. Mahony J, Chong S, Merante F, et al. Development of a respiratory virus panel test for detection of twenty human respiratory viruses by use of multiplex PCR and a fluid microbead-based assay. J Clin Microbiol 2007;45:2965–2970.
50. Vu DL, Bridevaux PO, Aubert JD, et al. Respiratory viruses in lung transplant recipients: a critical review and pooled analysis of clinical studies. Am J Transpl 2011;11:1071–1078.
51. Neuringer IP. Posttransplant lymphoproliferative disease after lung transplantation. Clin Dev Immunol 2013;2013:430209.
52. Nosotti M, Tarsia P, Morlacchi L. Infections after lung transplant. J Thorac Dis 2018;10:3849–3868.
53. Miller GG, Dummer JS. Herpes simplex and varicella zoster viruses: forgotten but not gone. Am J Transpl 2007;7:741–747.
54. Pereira MR, Mohan S, Cohen DJ, et al. COVID-19 in solid organ transplant recipients: initial report from the US epicenter. Am J Transpl 2020;20(07):1800–1808.
55. Saez-Giménez B, Berastegui C, Barrecheguren M, et al. COVID-19 in lung transplant recipients: a

multicenter study. Am J Transpl 2020. https://doi.org/10.1111/ajt. 16364.

56. Messika J, Eloy P, Roux A, et al, French Group of Lung Transplantation. COVID-19 in lung transplant recipients. Transplantation 2021;105(01):177–186.

57. Infectious Diseases Society of America Guidelines on the Treatment and Management of Patients with COVID-19. Available at: https://www. idsociety.org/practice-guideline/%20covid-19-guideline-treatmentand-management/. Accessed September 4, 2021.

58. Guidance from the International Society of Heart and Lung Transplantation regarding the SARS CoV-2 pandemic. Available at: https://ishlt.org/ishlt/media/documents/SARS-CoV-2_Guidance-for-Cardiothoracic-Transplant-and-VAD-center. pdf. Accessed September 4, 2021.

59. Doligalski CT, Benedict K, Cleveland AA, et al. Epidemiology of invasive mold infections in lung transplant recipients. Am J Transpl 2014;14: 1328–1333.

60. Vazquez R, Vazquez-Guillamet MC, Suarez J, et al. Invasive mold infections in lung and heart-lung transplant recipients: Stanford University experience. Transpl Infect Dis 2015;17:259–266.

61. Pappas PG, Alexander BD, Andres DR, et al. Invasive fungal infections among organ transplant recipients: results of the transplant –associated infection surveillance network (Transnet). Clin Infect Dis 2010;50:1101–1111.

62. Herrera S, Davoudi S, Farooq A, et al. Late onset invasive pulmonary aspergillosis in lung transplant recipients in the setting of targeted prophylaxis. Am J Transpl 2014;14:1328–1333.

63. Arthurs SK, Eid AJ, Deziel PJ, et al. The impact of invasive fungal disease on survival after lung transplantation. Clin Transpl 2010;24:341–348.

64. Koo S, Kubiak DW, Issa NC, et al. A targeted peri-transplant antifungal strategy for the prevention of invasive fungal disease after lung transplantation: a sequential cohort analysis. Transplantation 2012; 94:281–286.

65. Hoenigl M, Prattes J, Spiess B, et al. Performance of glactomannan, beta d-glucan, aspergillus lateral –flow device, conventional culture, pcr tests with bronchoalveolar lavage fluid for diagnosis of invasive pulmonary aspergillosis. J Clin Microbiol 2014; 52:2039–2045.

66. Geltner C, Lass-Florl C. Invasive pulmonary aspergillosis in organ transplantsfocus on lung transplants. Respir Investig 2016;54:76–84.

67. Patterson TF, Thompson GR, Denning DW, et al. Practice guidelines for the diagnosis and management of Aspergillosis: 2016 Update by the Infectious Disease Society of America. Clin Infect Dis 2016;63: e1–60.

68. Pfeiffer CD, Fine JP, Safdar N. Diagnosis of invasive aspergillosis using a galactomannan assay: metaanalysis. Clin Infect Dis 2006;42:1417–1427.

69. Husain S, Paterson DL, Studer SM, et al. Aspergillus galactomannan antigen in the bronchoalveolar lavage fluid for the diagnosis of invasive aspergillosis in lung transplant recipients. Transplantation 2007;83:1330–1336.

70. Kennedy CC, Pennington KM, Bean E, et al. Fungal infection in lung transplantation. Sem Respir Crit Care Med 2021;42:471–482.

71. Lichtenstein GR, Yang YX, Nunes FA, et al. Fatal hyperammonemia after orthotopic lung transplantation. Ann Intern Med 2000;132:283–287.

72. Chen C, Bain KB, Iuppa JA, et al. Hyperammonemia syndrome after lung transplantation: a single center experience. Transplantation 2016;100:678–684.

# 第11章 同种异体肺移植排斥反应

Deborah J. Levine, Ramsey R. Hachem 著

方年新 译

周建平 校

【关键词】
- 肺移植
- 抗体介导的排斥反应
- 急性细胞性排斥反应
- 供体特异性抗体

【要点】
- 尽管免疫抑制的治疗方面取得了进展,但同种异体肺移植排斥反应仍很常见。
- 急性细胞性排斥反应和抗体介导的排斥反应是肺排斥反应的常见形式。
- 同种异体肺移植排斥反应是肺移植术后长期预后不良的主要原因。

## 11.1 引　言

肺移植(LTx)是多数终末期肺疾病的最佳治疗手段。根据2019年国际心肺移植学会(ISHLT)的登记显示,肺移植的中位生存期为6.7年[1],显著低于其他实质器官移植。排斥反应是导致同种异体肺移植失败的主要原因,也是影响长期生存的阻碍。相较于其他器官移植,肺异体移植又因其长期与外界环境相通,更容易受到损伤和感染,因此发生排斥反应的风险更大[2]。

慢性肺同种异体移植物功能障碍(CLAD)是移植后第一年死亡的主要原因。CLAD的发生常常出现在移植后早期,包括免疫介导的和非免疫介导的过程,同时也是影响移植后器官远期功能的高危因素。急性排斥反应是发生CLAD的主要危险因素之一[3]。急性排斥反应可通过T细胞[急性细胞性排斥反应(acute cellular rejection,ACR)]或B细胞[抗体介导的排斥反应(antibody-mediated rejection,AMR)]介导。CLAD的风险随着急性排斥反应发作的严重程度和频率的增加而增加。然而,即使是一次轻微的ACR也可能会造成CLAD[4,5]。

急性排斥反应的早期识别和及时治疗对保护移植物功能和受体存活非常重要。对肺

功能测试（pulmonary function tests，PFTs）、抗体评估、影像学和组织学进行综合评估是目前用于发现急性排斥反应的主要工具[2]。

## 11.2 急性细胞性排斥反应

### 11.2.1 机制

ACR 是移植后最常见的急性排斥反应类型，其会影响血管和小气道，可能会导致移植器官发生不可逆性损伤。ACR 主要由 T 细胞识别外来的主要组织相容性复合体蛋白[人白细胞抗原（human leukocyte antigens，HLAs）]和其他供体抗原[6]。供体抗原的识别会激活先天性免疫系统，触发适应性免疫反应，从而产生促炎症反应。ACR 的共同通路包括募集并激活 T 细胞，导致同种异体移植物损伤和功能丧失[7]。

### 11.2.2 诊断

患有 ACR 的移植受者可能无症状，也可出现非特异性症状，如呼吸困难、发热、咳嗽或咳痰[8,9]。ACR 临床表现无特异性，故其诊断具有挑战性，并可能延误治疗。应通过对肺活检、影像学和实验室检查来提高诊断的准确性[9]。

动态的 PFT 检查是目前识别 ACR 风险患者的最佳筛查工具。肺活量可以作为初步评估方法来识别早期同种异体移植器官功能障碍，并有助于进一步研究[10]。但对无症状且 PTF 检查结果稳定的患者进行活检后仍然可能发现 ACR 的存在[11]。

影像学检查可为 ACR 的发现提供线索，但其鉴别的准确性是有限的[12,13]，活检证实只有 50% 的 ACR 在影像学上有异常表现。鉴于 PFTs 临床诊断的特异性较差，影像学检查和经支气管镜肺活检组织检查（transbronchial biopsies，TBBs）已成为诊断 ACR 最可靠的工具。

目前，对于检测活检的效用、方案或意义还没有统一的标准；然而，通过可视支气管镜是最常用的方法。但 TBB 仍存在很大争议，因为存在一定的风险（如发生气胸、出血、呼吸衰竭和肺炎），而且不同研究中心的方案也不尽相同。一项 2020 年的国际调查报告显示，87% 的研究中心会在不同阶段进行可视性 TBB[14]。其余中心仅在出现可疑临床问题时才进行 TBB。

2007 年，ISHLT 病理学委员会工作组对 ACR 诊断相关的肺移植病理学术语表进行了

# 第11章 同种异体肺移植排斥反应

修订，并制定了一套标准[15]。检查是以血管周围单核细胞浸润为基础的表现，结果非常具有特征性。其中就包括以小血管（动脉/小静脉）为中心或者在细支气管周围的散在淋巴组织细胞炎性浸润。ACR 的分级是根据炎症的严重程度和所涉及的结构而定的。血管成分分级为 A0 级（无排斥反应）至 A4 级（严重排斥反应），大多数病例为 A1 级或 A2 级。对于气道成分来说，气道淋巴细胞性支气管炎（lymphocytic bronchiolitis，LB）的特点是不明原因的气道炎症反应，严重程度为 B0（无气道炎症）至 B2R（高级别）。对于没有足够气道组织来进行分级的活检样本，还有一个无法分级的类别（BX）[15]。急性血管排斥反应和气道排斥反应可分别出现，也可同时出现在同一患者身上（表 11-1 和表 11-2）。

表 11-1 急性细胞性排斥反应的病理分级

| 等级 | 严重程度 | 特征描述 |
|---|---|---|
| A0 | 无排斥反应 | 正常实质 |
| A1 | 轻微排斥反应 | 散在的、少见的血管周围 2~3 层的单核细胞浸润 |
| A2 | 轻度排斥反应 | 低倍镜下即可见多处血管周围单核细胞浸润，浸润的细胞可能包括淋巴细胞、巨噬细胞和嗜酸性粒细胞 |
| A3 | 中度排斥反应 | 血管周围密集的单核细胞浸润，形成明显的内皮血管炎；炎性细胞常浸润至肺泡间隔及肺泡腔；常常有嗜酸粒细胞甚至是中性粒细胞浸润 |
| A4 | 重度排斥反应 | 血管周围、肺间质和肺泡内弥漫性的单核细胞浸润；肺泡细胞损伤和血管内皮炎 |

注：数据来自于 Stewart S, Fishbein MC, Snell GI, Berry GJ, Boehler A, Burke MM Glanville A, Gould FK, Magro C, Marboe CC, McNeil KD, Reed EF, Reinsmoen NL, Scott JP, Studer SM, Tazelaar HD, Wallwork JL, Westall G, Zamora MR, Zeevi A, Yousem SA. Revision of the 1996 working formulation for the standardization of nomenclature in the diagnosis of lung rejection. J Heart Lung Transplant. 2007 Dec;26(12):1229-42

表 11-2 淋巴细胞性细支气管炎病理分级

| 级别 | 严重性 | 描述 |
|---|---|---|
| B0 | 无气道炎症 | 无细支气管炎症 |
| B1R | 低级别的气道炎症 | 支气管黏膜下可见单核细胞浸润，偶可见嗜酸性粒细胞 |
| B2R | 高级别的气道炎症 | 支气管黏膜下可见大量活化的单核细胞、嗜酸性粒细胞和浆细胞样细胞；黏膜上皮损伤的依据，包括坏死、化生和淋巴细胞浸润 |
| BX | 无法分级的 | 未见细支气管组织 |

注：数据来自 Stewart S, Fishbein MC, Snell GI, Berry GJ, Boehler A, Burke MM Glanville A, Gould FK, Magro C, Marboe CC, McNeil KD, Reed EF, Reinsmoen NL, Scott JP, Studer SM, Tazelaar HD, Wallwork JL, Westall G, Zamora MR, Zeevi A, Yousem SA. Revision of the 1996 working formulation for the standardization of nomenclature in the diagnosis of lung rejection. J Heart Lung Transplant. 2007 Dec;26(12):1229-42

在诊断和解释 ACR 的病理标本时，观察者之间存在很大的差异，尤其是在低级排斥反应中，对患者管理以及多中心试验的标准化产生极大的挑战。ISHLT 建议获取至少 5 份"足够的"肺泡实质样本，以助于获得最佳解释[15]。与 A0 或 A1 级患者相比，A2 级或更高级别排斥反应患者出现症状更为常见[10]。等级小于 A2 的患者通常无症状，PFT 值也通常稳定或呈上升趋势。另一方面，一项研究表明，第一秒用力呼气容积（$FEV_1$）较排斥前值平均下降 10.4%，这对于发现 A2 级的 ACR 或者感染有 60% 以上的敏感性。但是，其无法区分这两者[11]。

### 11.2.3 流行病学

ACR 最常见于移植后的第 1~2 年，且最大概率是在最初的 3~6 个月内[11]。约有 3.5% 的死亡病例发生在移植后的前 30 天内[5]。30% 的成年受体在移植后第一年内至少发生一次 ACR[1]。然而报道的 ACR 发生率并不一致，其主要原因是监测方案不同读片者之间的组织读片差异[11]。Glanville 及其同事[16]报告称，移植后第一年 ACR 的发生率为 46%。而 Hachem 及其同事[17]发现，49% 的受体在移植后的第一年内至少出现过一次 A2 级排斥反应。2018 年，在一项多中心研究中，Hachem 及其同事[18]报告称 64% 的患者至少发生过一次 ACR。Todd 及其同事[19]指出，在 400 例受者中，超过 50% 的人至少发作过一次 ACR，其中大多数发作发生在受体移植后 3 个月内。

### 11.2.4 风险因素

识别 ACR 的早期风险因素非常重要，可以帮助对患者进行风险分层，并在发现危险因素时对其进行额外监测。一些移植前和移植后的受体和供体因素已被评估为潜在的危险因素，但其中许多因素还需要更多的验证[20,21]。目前已发现一些与 ACR 相关的特征。受体年龄与 ACR 事件有关。不同年龄组的患者会因为免疫功能与年龄相关而对该治疗产生不同的反应。患者对治疗产生的反应与年龄段相关。据报道，非常年轻的受体（1 岁以下）的排斥率较低，而处于青少年和青年期的受者的排斥率则最高[22]。多篇文献报道反映，抗 HLA 抗体和 HLA 错配的数量都与 ACR 事件发生倾向的增加有关[23-26]。进行的移植类型与 ACR 有关，单肺移植的 ACR 发生率高于双肺移植[22]。移植后第一年内发生 ACR 的风险最高。既往有严重排斥反应的患者发生周期性 ACR 的风险增高[23]。免疫抑制不足是 ACR 的重要危险因素，因此必须保持足够的免疫抑制水平并对其进行监测[27]。巨细胞病毒感染与肺移植后的 ACR 密切相关。大多数研究采用预防性抗病毒疗法，从而降低患者的风险[28,29]。除此之外，胃肠道反流与CLAD之间的关联研究最为深入，研究发现，反流患者发生ACR的风险也会增加[30,31]。存在的供体特异性抗体（donor-specific antibodies，DSAs）通常与AMR患者有关，但它也是ACR的一个重要风险因素[32]。

### 11.2.5 管理

ACR的治疗方案因移植中心和ACR分级而异。各中心普遍认为A2级及以上的患者需要治疗。具体的治疗方案通常取决于具体患者以及是否有症状。Gordon及其同事发现[8]，治疗LB的中心只有少数（50%），会治疗无症状的A1 ACR的中心甚至更少（35%）。所有的治疗方案都需要增加免疫抑制剂的使用，通常以一个疗程的皮质类固醇激素静脉冲击治疗作为一线方案。大多数中心使用静脉注射甲泼尼龙，剂量为每日10~15 mg/kg或每日500~1000 mg，连续3天，随后口服泼尼松并逐渐减少剂量。在严重（A3或A4）或难治性ACR的情况下，要给予额外治疗。则常将钙调磷酸酶抑制剂由环孢素改为他克莫司[33]和（或）硫唑嘌呤改为霉酚酸酯。重症患者还应使用抗胸腺细胞球蛋白（antithymocyte globulin，ATG）、阿仑单抗[34]、总淋巴细胞放疗[35]、体外光疗[36]、吸入环孢素[37]等治疗。在过去10年中，我们对ACR的发病机制、识别、监测和管理的认识有所提高。然而，我们现有诊断工具的灵敏度和特异度低反映了我们需要持续与中心之间的合作，以改进当前的治疗，并评估开展新的诊断工具，以便我们可以更容易地识别这些排斥反应，以延迟或预防慢性移植物损伤。

## 11.3 抗体介导的排斥反应（AMR）

### 11.3.1 历史观点和超急性排斥反应

虽然AMR早已在其他实质器官移植中确立，但我们对肺部AMR的认识仍在不断发展。直到大约15年前，对肺移植后AMR的认识仅限于超急性排斥反应[38-40]。超急性排斥反应是肺排斥反应的暴发性形式，由预先形成的DSAs与不匹配的HLAs引起，通常会导致同种异体移植失败[38-40]。

超急性排斥反应在再灌注后很早期即表现为严重的同种异体移植物功能障碍。临床上可能很难将其与严重的原发性移植物功能不全（PGD）区分开来。预先形成的DSAs会导致超急性排斥反应，导致直接供体-受体交叉配型阳性。因此，预先形成的DSAs

和阳性交叉配型的存在是超急性排斥反应和 PGD 之间的区别特征。超急性排斥反应的发病机制是基于内皮细胞上预先形成的 DSA 与 HLA 分子的结合。随后补体级联激活，骨髓细胞浸润同种异体移植物，导致内皮细胞坏死，基底膜暴露，随后激活凝血级联[41]。其特征性病理表现为透明膜形成、肺泡水肿、肺泡内纤维蛋白和血管损伤，伴小动脉纤维蛋白样坏死、血管内血小板和纤维蛋白血栓，常伴有明显的中性粒细胞毛细血管损伤[42]。HLA 抗体检测方法的进步和特异性的提高使得即使是低水平的 HLA 抗体也能被精确地识别，从而避免潜在供体中的反应性 HLA[43,44]。这种做法被称为"虚拟交叉配型"，可以在接受供体器官前预测阳性的直接交叉配型和超急性排斥反应，从而改善供体选择以及移植后的结果。因此，目前超急性排斥反应十分罕见。然而，这表明抗体可导致肺移植失败，而毛细血管内皮是初始损伤的焦点。

## 11.3.2 抗体介导的排斥反应

在过去的 10 年里，人们对肺部 AMR 的认识越来越多。迄今为止，AMR 主要是存在于同种异体移植物功能障碍的背景下，尽管其亚临床形式也可能存在于细胞排斥反应中。AMR 的发病机制与超急性排斥反应相似，但 DSAs 则是从头发展而不是预先形成的。AMR 的诊断十分困难，需要临床高度的怀疑。与 ACR 不同，其没有特定的组织学特征，需要多学科方法诊断。2016 年，ISHLT 明确了 AMR 的定义，以标准化命名法并促进多中心研究[45]。在这个框架中，需要多个标准进行诊断，临床确定性的程度基于现有标准的数量。如果符合以下所有标准，则可以诊断为 AMR：

- 同种异体移植物功能障碍；
- 循环 DSAs；
- 出现肺组织病理异常；
- C4d 在毛细血管内皮上沉积；
- 排除同种异体移植物功能障碍的其他潜在原因。

上述诊断标准符合 4 项时诊断为拟诊 AMR，符合 3 项标准时诊断为疑诊 AMR[45]。然而，工作组指出，在没有 C4d 沉积的情况下，可以对 AMR 作出"可靠"的诊断。C4d 沉积可以对补体级联激活和抗体对同种异体移植物的影响提供直接证据。的确，C4d 沉积是肾移植后 AMR 鉴定的突破性进展[46,47]。然而，C4d 沉积在肺移植中一直存在问题。事实上，许多来自多个中心的 AMR 病例 C4d 都是阴性的[48,49]。同样，一项关于 C4d 沉积在 AMR 诊断中的作用的回顾性研究指出，大多数病例均为 C4d 阴性[50]。此外，C4d 阴性病例的临床表现、组织学发现和临床结果与 C4d 阳性病例相似[50]。所有 C4d 阳性病例都与补体结合的 DSAs（C1q 阳性）有关，而一些 C4d 阴性病例的 C1q 也为阴性，这表明 AMR 可能会在没有激活补体级联的情况下发生，而且 AMR 表型可能有所不同。事实上，C4d 阴性 AMR 现已在肾移植中得到广泛认可[51,52]，其发病机制是由自然杀伤细胞与结合在内皮细胞上的 DSAs 相互作用介导的[53,54]。如果考虑使用补体抑制剂，补体激活在 AMR 发病机制中的作用对治疗具有重要意义。

最新进展表明，供体来源的细胞游离 DNA（cell-free DNA，cfDNA）是一种敏感的异体移植物损伤标志物，循环中的 cfDNA 水平与损伤的严重程度和发生 AMR 的可能性密切相关[55,56]。此外，AMR 确诊前约 3 个月，外周血中就可检测到 cfDNA 水平升高[55]，因此该检测方法是一种十分具有吸引力的 AMR 非侵入性筛查工具。尽管 cfDNA 水平升高是异体移植物损伤的非特异性标志，但在出现 DSA 和异体移植物功能障碍且无明显其他临床原因的情况下，高水平的 cfDNA 可提示 AMR 的存在。

### 11.3.3 AMR 的一般管理

指导肺移植中 AMR 管理的数据非常有限。研究主要集中在描述 AMR 的特征，如特征性组织学和相关的 DSA。虽然治疗和结果都很详细，但在没有对照组的情况下，很难对治疗或治疗方案的疗效得出结论。目前暂无随机对照试验（randomized controlled trials，RCT），也无不同治疗方案的正面比较。此外，治疗方案通常是根据异体移植功能障碍的严重程度和对一线治疗的临床反应量身定制的。目前还没有专门针对 AMR 的治疗方法，所有治疗方法都是从肿瘤学和风湿病学领域借鉴而来的。

AMR 的治疗目标是清除 DSA、抑制额外的 DSA 产生，并改善同种异体移植物损伤。血浆置换虽能清除血液循环中的抗体，但不能抑制抗体的产生，因此还需要其他抑制 B 细胞或浆细胞增殖和活性的治疗方法。虽然尚无关于肺部 AMR 的随机对照临床试验，但有 4 项关于肾移植中血浆置换的小型随机对照临床试验，然而其结果存在矛盾[57-60]。不过，目前尚不清楚这些较早研究中是否所有患者都患有目前定义的 AMR。此外，这些研究均未使用静脉注射免疫球蛋白（intravenous immunoglobulin，IVIG）（如今通常与血浆置换联合使用）以及其他抑制 B 细胞或浆细胞的治疗方法。

一项 RCT 研究了利妥昔单抗在肾脏 AMR 中的应用[61]。利妥昔单抗是针对 CD20 的单克隆抗体，CD20 是成熟 B 细胞上的细胞表面分子，而不是浆细胞。使用利妥昔单抗治疗会延长外周 B 细胞的耗竭时间。该研究将患有 AMR 的肾移植受者随机分配到"标准治疗加上血浆置换、IVIG、大剂量皮质类固醇激素"和"标准治疗加利妥昔单抗"两个治疗组中。两组患者在异体移植功能丧失或肾功能改善不足的主要复合终点方面没有显著差异。然而，在随机分配到对照组的患者中，有超过 40% 的患者接受了利妥昔单抗挽救治疗。除了这种高交叉率之外，法国 21 个中心在 3 年时间内只招募到 38 例患者，说明在 AMR 中开展临床试验面临的挑战。在另一项针对肾移植后晚期 AMR 患者的 RCT 中，对照组与接受硼替佐米（一种蛋白酶体抑制剂，可促进浆细胞凋亡）治疗的患者在肾功能、DSA 或异体移植生存率方面没有显著差异[62]，这些 RCT 的研究结果与以往回顾性单组临床试验的结果不同[63-65]。虽然这些随机对照试验的规模较小，没有足够的说服力，但没有对照组的研究是偏差更大，无法确定其治疗效果。显然，需要在 AMR 领域开展更多严谨设计、充分验证的对照试验，在肺移植领域尤其如此。

### 11.3.4 肺部 AMR 的管理及结局

多项回顾性研究报告了肺移植后关于抗体介导性排斥反应不同治疗方案的单中心实验结果。在一项研究中，10 例 AMR 患者接受了血浆置换、IVIG、大剂量皮质类固醇、利妥昔单抗和硼替佐米等不同组合治疗，其中 5 例患者死于难治性 AMR，2 例患者死于治疗后的脓毒血症[48]。在另一项研究中，9 例患者接受了血浆置换、IVIG、大剂量皮质类固醇和利妥昔单抗治疗，其中 6 例患者死于进展性慢性肺移植功能障碍[49]。另一项针对 21 例 AMR 患者的研究中也报告了类似的结果[66]，治疗包括 IVIG、血浆置换、利妥昔单抗、硼替佐米、抗胸腺细胞球蛋白和依库珠单抗等各种组合[66]。15 例患者有初步的临床疗效，但其很快在后续的研究中死于难治性 AMR 或者慢性肺移植功能障碍[66]。在该研究中，持续存在供者特异性抗体的患者的生存率明显更差[66]。在另一项研究中，22 例 AMR 患者接受了血浆交换、IVIG 和利妥昔单抗治疗，其中 12 例在研究期间死亡[67]。在该研究中，经治疗后供者特异性抗体清除率与更好的生存率相关[67]。卡菲佐米（Carfilzomib）是第二代蛋白酶抑制剂，以不可逆的结合方式持续抑制蛋白酶的活性并诱发浆细胞凋亡。在一项研究中，有 14 例 AMR 患者接受了卡菲佐米、血浆置换和 IVIG 的治疗[68]，注射卡菲佐米后表现为 C1q 结合活性丧失的称为应答者，其中 10 例患者被认为是应答者。应答者发生闭塞性毛细支气管炎的可能性比无应答者低，但两组之间在限制性移植物综合征的发生率及生存率间没有显著差异[68]。表明即使是经过积极治疗的 AMR 患者预后非常差，虽然有些患者初期可能会有临床疗效，但还是会发生进展性的慢性肺移植功能障碍甚至死亡。很显然，我们需要更好的治疗方案，但是目前缺乏足够的证据，因此最佳治疗方案尚不明确。

## 11.4 总　结

尽管在免疫抑制治疗方面取得了进展，但肺移植后的非斥反应仍然是一个常见的问题。急性排斥反应及抗体介导的排斥反应在慢性肺移植功能障碍的进展中是导致移植后1年后死亡的主要危险因素，也是改善长期预后的主要阻得。机制研究学显示，同种异体肺移植比其他实质器官更容易发生排斥反应，并可以在改进临床治疗方面提供更好的见解。我们需要新的免疫抑制方案来降低排斥反应的风险，同时兼并毒性小的优点，并且最好可以开展随机对照实验来验证结果。

【临床护理要点】

- 急性排斥反应的最佳筛查工具是肺活量测定。当 $FEV_1$ 下降10%或更多时，应启动全面评估以判断肺活量下降是否继发于排斥反应、感染、呼吸道问题或其他临床诊断。
- 如果/当建立支气管镜检查监测计划时，应将支气管镜检查主要安排在移植后的第一年，因为在此期间急性排斥反应的发生率最高，建议至少活检5片肺泡肺实质用于急性排斥反应的评估。
- 普遍认为，患者发生A2级或更高级别的急性排斥反时应需要接受强化的免疫抑制治疗，尽管其与慢性肺移植功能障碍的发生有关，但对无急性排斥反应症状A1级的处理仍然存在争议。对于个别患者，仔细考虑治疗与密切随访（包括可能的需要进行的支气管镜检查）的风险/收益比是当务之急。
- 在发生急性同种异体移植功能障碍的情况下，应考虑AMR的可能性。初步评估应包括对供体特异性抗体的检测，并根据评估结果进一步进行支气管镜检查和经支气管镜肺活检。

**声明**

R.R.哈赫姆有以下财务关系需要声明：来自百时美施贵宝的赠款资金，来自 Mallinckrodt 制药公司的赠款资金，为 TransMedics 提供咨询，为 Natera 提供咨询，为 CareDx 提供咨询。D.J.莱文有以下财务关系需要声明：CareDx 的赠款资金，为 Natera 提供咨询，为 CareDx 提供咨询。

## 参考文献

1. Chambers DC, Cherikh WS, Harhay MO, et al. International Society for Heart and Lung Transplantation. J Heart Lung Transplant 2019;38(10):1042–1055.
2. Benjamin R, Koutsokera A, Cabanero M, et al. Acute rejection in the modern lung transplant era. Semin Respir Crit Care Med 2021;42:411–427.
3. Girgis RE, Tu I, Berry GJ, et al. Risk factors for the development of obliterative bronchiolitis after lung transplantation. J Heart Lung Transplant 1996; 15(12):1200–1208.
4. Hachem RR, Khalifah AP, Chakinala MM, et al. The significance of a single episode of minimal acute rejection after lung transplantation. Transplantation 2005;80(10):1406.
5. Burton CM, Iversen M, Carlsen J, et al. Acute cellular rejection is a risk factor for bronchiolitis obliterans syndrome independent of post-transplant baseline FEV1. J Heart Lung Transplant 2009;28(09):888–893.
6. Hsiao HM, Scozzi D, Gauthier JM, et al. Mechanisms of graft rejection after lung transplantation. Curr Opin Organ Transplant 2017;22(01):29–35.
7. Snyder LD, Palmer SM. Immune mechanisms of lung allograft rejection. Semin Respir Crit Care Med 2006;27(5):534–543.
8. Gordon I, Bhorade VW, Vigneswaran WT, et al. SaLUTaRy: a survey of lung transplant rejection. J Heart Lung Transplant 2012;31(09):972–979.
9. De Vito Dabbs A, Hoffman LA, Iacono AT, et al. Are symptom reports useful for differentiating between acute rejection and pulmonary infection after lung transplantation? Heart Lung 2004;33:372–380.
10. Van Muylem A, Melot C, Antoine M, et al. Role of pulmonary function in the detection of allograft dysfunction after heart–lung transplantation. Thorax 1997; 52(7):643–647.
11. Martinu T, Pavlisko EN, Chen DF, et al. Acute allograft rejection: cellular and humoral processes. Clnics Chest Med 2011;32(2):295.
12. Park CH, Paik H, Haam S, et al. HRCT features of acute rejection in patients with bilateral lung transplantation: the usefulness of lesion distribution. Transplant Proc 2014;46(05):1511–1416.
13. Kundu S, Herman S, Larhs A, et al. Correlation of chest radiographic findings with biopsy proven acute lung rejection. J Thorac Imaging 1999; 14(03):178–184.
14. Martinu T, Koutsokera A, Benden C, et al. Bronchoalveolar lavage standardization workgroup. ISHLT consensus statement for the standardization of bronchoalveolar lavage in lung transplant. J Heart Lung Transplant 2020;39(11):1171–1190.
15. Stewart S, Fishbein MC, Snell GI, et al. Revision of the 1996 working formulation for the standardization of nomenclature in the diagnosis of lung rejection. J Heart Lung Transplant 2007;26(12): 1229–1242.
16. Glanville AR, Aboyoun C, Klepetko W, et al. Three-year results of an investigator-driven multicenter, international, randomized open-label de novo trial to prevent BOS after lung transplantation. J Heart Lung Transplant 2015;34:16–25.
17. Hachem RR, Yusen RD, Chakinala MM, et al. A randomized controlled trial of tacrolimus versus cyclosporine after lung transplantation. J Heart Lung Transplant 2007;26:1012–1018.
18. Hachem RR, Kamoun M, Budev MM, et al. Human leukocyte antigens antibodies. Primary results of the HALT study. Am J Transplant 2018;18(9): 2285–2294.

19. Todd J, Neely M, Kopetskie H, et al. Risk factors for acute rejection in the first year after lung transplant. A multicenter study. Am J Respir Crit Care Med 2020;202(4):576–585.
20. Martinu T, Chen DF, Palmer SM. Acute rejection and humoral sensitization in lung transplant recipients. Proc Am Thorac Soc 2009;6(1):54–65.
21. Bando K, Paradis IL, Komatsu K, et al. Analysis of time-dependent risks for infection, rejection, and death after pulmonary transplantation. J Thorac Cardiovasc Surg 1995;109(01):49–57 [discussion 57–59].
22. Mangi AA, Mason DP, Nowicki ER, et al. Predictors of acute rejection after lung transplantation. Ann Thorac Surg 2011;91(06):1754–1762.
23. Smith JD, Ibrahim MW, Newell H, et al. Pre-transplant donor HLA-specific antibodies: characteristics causing detrimental effects on survival after lung transplantation. J Heart Lung Transplant 2014; 33(10):1074–1108.
24. Snell GI, Levy BJ, Paraskeva M, et al. The influence of clinical donor factors on acute rejection among lung and kidney recipients from the same multiorgan donor. Ann Transplant 2013;18:358–367.
25. Gammie JS, Pham SM, Colson YL, et al. Influence of panel-reactive antibody on survival and rejection after lung transplantation. J Heart Lung Transplant 1997;16(04):408–415.
26. Peltz M, Edwards LB, Jessen ME, et al. HLA mismatches influence lung transplant recipient survival, bronchiolitis obliterans and rejection: implications for donor lung allocation. J Heart Lung Transplant 2011; 30(04):426–434.
27. Glanville AR, Aboyoun CL, Morton JM, et al. Cyclosporine C2 target levels and acute cellular rejection after lung transplantation. J Heart Lung Transplant 2006;25(08):928–934.
28. Johansson I, Martensson G, Nyström U, et al. Lower incidence of CMV infection and acute rejections with valganciclovir prophylaxis in lung transplant recipients. BMC Infect Dis 2013;13:582.
29. Roux A, Mourin G, Fastenackels S, et al. CMV driven CD8(þ) T-cell activation is associated with acute rejection in lung transplantation. Clin Immunol 2013;148(01):16–26.
30. Hathorn KE, Chan WW, Lo W-K. Role of gastroesophageal reflux disease in lung transplantation. World J Transplant 2017;7(02):103–116.
31. Shah N, Force SD, Mitchell PO, et al. Gastroesophageal reflux disease is associated with an increased rate of acute rejection in lung transplant allografts. Transplant Proc 2010;42(07):2702–2706.
32. Girnita AL, McCurry KR, Iacono AT, et al. HLA-specific antibodies are associated with high-grade and persistent-recurrent lung allograft acute rejection. J Heart Lung Transplant 2004;23(10):1135–1141.
33. Sarahrudi K, Carretta A, Wisser W, et al. The value of switching from cyclosporine to tacrolimus in the treatment of refractory acute rejection and obliterative bronchiolitis after lung transplantation. Transpl Int 2002;15(01):24–28. Lung Allograft Rejection 227
34. Ensor CR, Rihtarchik LC, Morrell MR, et al. Rescue alemtuzumab for refractory acute cellular rejection and bronchiolitis obliterans syndrome after lung transplantation. Clin Transplant 2017;31(04).
35. Valentine VG, Robbins RC, Wehner JH, et al. Total lymphoid irradiation for refractory acute rejection in heart-lung and lung allografts. Chest 1996;109(05): 1184–1189.
36. Isenring B, Robinson C, Buergi U, et al. Lung transplant recipients on long-term extracorporeal photopheresis. Clin Transplant 2017;31(10).

37. Keenan RJ, Iacono A, Dauber JH, et al. Treatment of refractory acute allograft rejection with aerosolized cyclosporine in lung transplant recipients. J Thorac Cardiovasc Surg 1997;113(02):335–340 [discussion 340–341].

38. Frost AE, Jammal CT, Cagle PT. Hyperacute rejection following lung transplantation. Chest 1996;110: 559–562.

39. Bittner HB, Dunitz J, Hertz M, et al. Hyperacute rejection in single lung transplantation – case report of successful management by means of plasmapheresis and antithymocyte globulin treatment. Transplantation 2001;71:649–651.

40. Masson E, Stern M, Chabod J, et al. Hyperacute rejection after lung transplantation caused by undetected low-titer anti-HLA antibodies. J Heart Lung Transplant 2007;26:642–645.

41. Valenzuela NM, Reed EF. Antibody-mediated rejection across solid organ transplants: manifestations, mechanisms, and therapies. J Clin Invest 2017; 127:2492–2504.

42. Berry G, Burke M, Andersen C, et al. Pathology of pulmonary antibody-mediated rejection: 2012 update from the Pathology Council of the ISHLT. J Heart Lung Transplant 2013;32:14–21.

43. Tait BD, Süsal C, Gebel HM, et al. Consensus guidelines on the testing and clinical management issues associated with HLA and non-HLA antibodies in transplantation. Transplantation 2013;95:19–47.

44. Tambour AR, Campbell P, Claas FH, et al. Sensitization in transplantation: assessment of risk (STAR) 2017 working group meeting report. Am J Transplant 2018;18:1604–1614.

45. Levine DJ, Glanville AR, Aboyoun C, et al. Antibody-mediated rejection of the lung: a consensus report of the International Society for Heart and Lung Transplantation. J Heart Lung Transplant 2016;35: 397–406.

46. Feucht HE, Felber E, Gokel MJ, et al. Vascular deposition of complement-splint products in kidney allografts with cell-mediated rejection. Clin Exp Immunol 1991;86:464–470.

47. Feucht HE, Schneeberger H, Hillebrand H, et al. Capillary deposition of C4d complement fragment and early renal graft loss. Kidney Int 1993;43: 1333–1338.

48. Lobo LJ, Aris RM, Schmitz J, et al. Donor-specific antibodies are associated with antibody-mediated rejection, acute cellular rejection, bronchiolitis obliterans syndrome, and cystic fibrosis after lung transplantation. J Heart Lung Transplant 2013;32: 70–77.

49. Otani S, Davis AK, Cantwell L, et al. Evolving experience of treating antibody-mediated rejection following lung transplantation. Transpl Immunol 2014;31:75–80.

50. Aguilar PR, Carpenter D, Ritter J, et al. The role of C4d deposition in the diagnosis of antibody-mediated rejection after lung transplantation. Am J Transplant 2018;18:936–944.

51. Haas M, Sis B, Racusen LC, et al. Banff 2013 meeting report: Inclusion of C4d-negative antibody-mediated rejection and antibody-associated arterial lesions. Am J Transplant 2014;14:272–283.

52. Orandi BJ, Alachkar N, Kraus ES, et al. Presentation and outcomes of C4d-negative antibody-mediated rejection after kidney transplantation. Am J Transplant 2016;16:213–220.

53. Hidalgo LG, Sis B, Sellarés J, et al. NK cell transcripts and NK cells in kidney biopsies from patients with donor-specific antibodies: evidence for NK cell involvement in antibody mediated rejection. Am J Transplant 2010;10:1812–1822.

54. Sellarés J, Reeve J, Loupy A, et al. Molecular diagnosis of antibody-mediated rejection in human kidney

transplants. Am J Transplant 2013;13:971–983.

55. Agbor-Enoh S, Jackson AM, Tunc I, et al. Late manifestation of alloantibody-associated injury and clinical pulmonary antibody-mediated rejection: evidence from cell-free DNA analysis. J Heart Lung Transplant 2018;37:925–932.

56. Agbor-Enoh S, Wang Y, Tunc I, et al. Donor-derived cell-free DNA predicts allograft failure and mortality after lung transplantation. EBioMedicine 2019;40: 541–553.

57. Bonomini V, Vangelista A, Frasca GM, et al. Effects of plasmapheresis in renal transplant rejection: a controlled study. Trans Am Soc Artif Intern Organs 1985;31:698–703.

58. Blake P, Sutton D, Cardella CJ. Plasma exchange in acute renal transplant rejection. Prog Clin Biol Res 1990;337:249–252.

59. Allen NH, Dyer P, Geoghegan T, et al. Plasma exchange in acute renal allograft rejection: a controlled trial. Transplantation 1983;35:425–428.

60. Kirubakaran MG, Disney AP, Norman J, et al. A controlled trial of plasmapheresis in the treatment of renal allograft rejection. Transplantation 1981;32: 164–165.

61. Sautenet B, Blancho G, Büchler M, et al. One-year results of the effects of rituximab on acute antibody-mediated rejection in renal transplantation: RITUX ERAH, a multicenter double-blind 228 Levine & Hachem randomized placebo-controlled trial. Transplantation 2016;100:391–399.

62. Eskandary F, Regele H, Baumann L, et al. A randomized trial of bortezomib in late antibody-mediated kidney transplant rejection. J Am Soc Nephrol 2018;29:591–605.

63. Faguer S, Kamar N, Guilbeaud-Frugier C, et al. Rituximab therapy for acute humoral rejection after kidney transplantation. Transplantation 2007;83: 1277–1280.

64. Everly MJ, Everly JJ, Susskind B, et al. Bortezomib provides effective therapy for antibody and cell0mediated acute rejection. Transplantation 2008;86: 1754–1761.

65. Mulley WR, Hudson FJ, Tait BD, et al. A single lowfixed dose of rituximab to salvage renal transplants from refractory antibody-mediated rejection. Transplantation 2009;87:286–289.

66. Witt CA, Gaut JP, Yusen RD, et al. Acute antibody-mediated rejection after lung transplantation. J Heart Lung Transplant 2013;32:1034–1040.

67. Roux A, Bendib Le Lan I, Holifanjaniaina S, et al. Antibody-mediated rejection in lung transplantation: clinical outcomes and donor-specific antibody characteristics. Am J Transplant 2016;16:1216–1228.

68. Ensor CR, Yousem SA, Marrai M, et al. Proteasome inhibitor carfilzomib-based therapy for antibody-mediated rejection of the pulmonary allograft: use and short-term findings. Am J Transplant 2017;17: 1380–1388.

# 第 12 章　慢性移植肺功能障碍

Aida Venado, Jasleen Kukreja, John R. Greenland　著

黎昱江　译

周建平　校

【关键词】
- 慢性移植肺功能障碍
- 限制性同种异体移植综合征
- 毛细支气管炎闭塞综合征
- 胸膜弹力纤维增生综合征

【要点】
- 慢性肺同种异体移植物功能障碍（CLAD）是肺移植后进行性肺功能下降的一种综合征。
- CLAD 可发展为一种毛细支气管炎闭塞综合征（BOS），一种限制性同种异体移植综合征（RAS），或具有这 2 种特征的混合表型。RAS 通常比 BOS 进展得更快，生存率也更低。
- CLAD 的治疗方法包括增强免疫抑制、免疫调节和抗纤维化药物。由于其整体无效，再移植是目前唯一的可延长进展性 CLAD 患者生存期的治疗方法。

## 12.1 慢性移植肺功能障碍定义

慢性肺同种异体移植物功能障碍（CLAD）是以肺移植（LTx）后进行性肺功能下降为表现的综合征，主要归因于慢性排异反应，可表现为阻塞性和(或)限制性功能障碍。随着时间的推移，我们对 CLAD 及其定义的理解有着不同的改进。1993 年，国际心肺移植协会（ISHTL）发起了慢性移植肺功能障碍的命名标准化的工作，该方案发现第一秒用力呼气容积（$FEV_1$）是最可靠、最一致的移植物功能指标。

毛细支气管炎闭塞综合征（BOS）被定义为继发于进行性气道疾病的不明原因的移植物功能恶化，可能是慢性排斥反应的表现。根据 $FEV_1$ 下降程度，可将 BOS 分为 4 类，并将病理性闭塞性毛细支气管炎分别划分为 "a" 和 "b"[1]。"a" 和 "b" 亚型很少被使用，

# 第12章 慢性移植肺功能障碍

因为经支气管活检检测闭塞性细支气管炎的敏感性较低[2]。2001年，增加了一个潜在的BOS阶段（BOS 0-p），其中包括呼气中流速（FEF 25~75）下降低于75%基线[3]，后来由于预测效用不足而被删除[4]。

约在2010年，CLAD一词被引入[5]，限制性同种异体移植综合征（restrictive allograft syndrome，RAS）被认为是与BOS不同的亚型[6]。2014年，国际心肺移植协会将CLAD定义为$FEV_1$或用力肺活量（FVC）下降至基线的80%或更低，并对阻塞性和限制性这2种形式表示认可[7]。引入术语急性移植肺功能障碍，是指$FEV_1$下降10%，同时需对感染、排斥或其他可逆原因的调查。

2019年，国际心肺移植学会对CLAD的定义如下：

- "可能的CLAD"：$FEV_1$为基线的80%，这是移植后至少间隔3周进行的2次最佳$FEV_1$测量的平均值；
- "很可能的CLAD"：$FEV_1$在3周后持续下降；
- "确定CLAD"：$FEV_1$下降持续3个月[8]。

基于$FEV_1$下降（表12-1），CLAD有4个阶段。不认为导致$FEV_1$持续下降的机械因素和其他因素是CLAD综合征的一部分，包括胸腔积液、气道狭窄、膈肌功能障碍和体重增加。当$FEV_1$的下降归因于不太可能与慢性排斥有关反应的病理因素时，一旦$FEV_1$保持稳定6个月，就可以建立新的基线水平。

尽管在定义上存在一些争议，仍可将CLAD细分为BOS、RAS、混合或未定义模式（表12-2）[8]。

表 12-1 慢性移植肺功能障碍分级

| 分级 | $FEV_1$与基线的百分比 |
| --- | --- |
| CLAD 0 级 | >80% |
| CLAD 1 级 | >65%~80% |
| CLAD 2 级 | >50%~65% |
| CLAD 3 级 | >35%~50% |
| CLAD 4 级 | ≤35% |

注：改编自 Verleden GM, Glanville AR, Lease ED, et al. Chronic lung allograft dysfunction: Definition, diagnostic criteria, and approaches to treatment-A consensus report from the Pulmonary Council of the ISHLT. J Heart Lung Transplant. May 2019;38(5):493-503

### 表 12-2　慢性移植肺功能障碍表型的关键特征

| CLAD 表型 | 肺功能损失 | 胸部 CT 检查结果 |
| --- | --- | --- |
| BOS | 阻塞性 | 存在空气潴留但没有持续的肺部模糊影 |
| RAS | 限制性 | 与肺和（或）胸膜纤维化相一致的持续性模糊影 |
| 混合 | 阻塞性和限制性 | 与肺和（或）胸膜纤维化相一致的持续性模糊影。可能存在空气潴留现象 |
| 未定义 | 阻塞性 | 与肺和（或）胸膜纤维化相一致的持续性模糊影。可能存在空气潴留现象 |
| 未定义 | 阻塞性和限制性 | 存在空气潴留但没有持续的肺部模糊影 |

注：所有 CLAD 表型的 $FEV_1$ 从基线持续下降到 80%，这是移植后 2 个最佳 $FEV_1$ 值的平均值，间隔 3 周或更长时间
阻塞是指 $FEV_1/FVC$ 小于 0.7
限制是指小于基线 TLC 的 90%，是移植后 2 个最佳 TLC 值的平均值或接近 2 个最佳 $FEV_1$ 值。"可能的 RAS"一词用于当 TLC 不可用和 FVC 小于基线的 80% 和 $FEV_1/FVC$ 大于 0.7 时。但需注意，闭塞性细支气管炎综合征（BOS）引起的气体潴留可导致用力肺活量（FVC）下降。基线 FVC 是 FVC 值与移植后 2 个最佳 $FEV_1$ 值配对的平均值
持续性模糊影是指持续 3 个月或以上
改编自文献 [7-9]

- 如果有气流阻塞，且 $FEV_1/FVC$ 小于 70%，且没有持续的影像学改变，则可以诊断为 BOS；
- 如果总肺活量（total lung capacity，TLC）较基线下降 90%，且胸部影像学显示出持续的实质性阴影则诊断为 RAS，需同时进行的 2 次最佳 TLC 测量的平均值或非常接近最佳 $FEV_1$ 数值进行相应的评估。由于并非所有中心都会例行性进行 TLC 测量，当 FVC 低于基线的 80% 从而怀疑为限制性时（使用移植后最佳 $FEV_1$ 值时 2 次 FVC 测量的平均值），可以使用术语"可能的 RAS"。RAS 的典型影像学[9]表现包括斑片、纤维化和蜂窝样变，尤其是在上叶和（或）胸膜附近，与胸膜弹力纤维增生综合征（pleuroparenchymal fibroelastosis，PPFE）的病理特征相对应。

RAS 占 CLAD 病例的 25%~35%，预后较差，诊断后的中位生存期为 8~10 个月，而 BOS 诊断后的中位生存期为 35 个月[10,11]。虽然 BOS 是主要的 CLAD 表型，但 10% 的 BOS 病例演变为 RAS，该混合表型的生存率高于 RAS，但低于 BOS[12]。

## 12.2　CLAD 的病理生理学

对 CLAD 病理的研究可以追溯到 20 世纪 80 年代，在当时第一次成功的肺移植的尸

检中发现。可以观察到肺部进行性梗阻性病变，以及一些受体存在叠加限制性缺陷[13]。尸检结果一致显示为缩窄性细支气管炎，少数患者还出现明显的胸膜纤维化，与现在的 BOS 和 RAS 一致[14]。

CLAD 发病机制可能反映出超过肺细胞再生能力的同种免疫损伤的后遗症，但其全面的机制理解仍尚未有阐述。CLAD 综合征的生理和病理表现可能有多种原因。事实上，即使在缺乏同种免疫的情况下，也可以观察到缩窄性细支气管炎和 PPFE。我们对 CLAD 发病机制的理解主要集中在导致这些病理性疾病的机制上。

### 12.2.1 闭塞性细支气管炎

细支气管是直径 1~10 mm，连接支气管和肺泡的非软骨性气道。考虑到外周气道的大横截面积，必须有显著的损伤发生才能诱发阻塞性生理疾病。正如 CLAD 所示，狭窄性或闭塞性细支气管炎的特征是黏膜下和细支气管周围纤维化导致的气道管腔受压。由于小气道受累不均匀，即使邻近的气道已经完全塌陷，仍有一些气道看起来是正常的[15]。闭塞性细支气管炎是不可逆的，且不同于炎症性细支气管炎（后者常发生于病毒感染后）以及增殖性细支气管炎（亦称机化性肺炎，其由明确病因或隐源性病因导致的细支气管损伤），可引发跨管腔成纤维组织沉积（即 Masson 小体）。

PPFE 是同时存在于脏层胸膜纤维化和胸膜下实质纤维弹性改变。在肺移植之外，PPFE 是一种典型的与特发性肺纤维化（IPF）相关的间质性肺疾病，并与端粒功能障碍有关[16]。尽管 PPFE 是与 RAS 有关的最常见的疾病，但也能观察到非特异性间质性肺炎、渗出性纤维化和急性纤维蛋白样机化性肺炎[17]。

### 12.2.2 同种免疫激活

在同种异体干细胞移植后以及肺移植中主要组织相容性复合体（major histocompatibility complex，MHC）抗原不匹配的情况下，可以观察到类似 CLAD 的病理和生理现象[15]。尽管供体受体 HLA 不匹配数量的增加只是人类 CLAD 的风险因素之一[18]，但即使是单一抗原不匹配也足以在 CLAD 小鼠模型中诱发闭塞性气道疾病[19]。急性细胞性排斥反应（ACR）可以反映同种免疫激活。血管周围淋巴细胞炎症和淋巴细胞性支气管炎、ISHLT A 级和 B 级急性排斥反应以及大气道急性炎症都是 CLAD 的危险因素[20-22]。然而，少量的 ACR 可能不会增加 CLAD 的风险，并且在没有 ACR 的情况下 CLAD 也可能会发生[22-24]。这些发现可能反映了经支气管活检的不敏感性，因为对同种免疫反应的观察先于支气管活检组织的病理学检查[2,25]。

尽管 1 型免疫反应被认为是慢性肺同种异体移植物功能障碍（CLAD）的主要机制，但 2 型和 17 型同种免疫反应也被证实参与其中[26]。17 型免疫反应可以驱动中性粒细胞炎症。BAL 中中性粒细胞超过 15% 和 $FEV_1$ 下降 10% 的综合征被称为中性粒细胞可逆性同种异体移植功能障碍（neutrophilic reversible allograft dysfunction，NRAD），除通过阿奇霉素治疗逆转，否则会导致 CLAD[27]。从机制上讲，阿奇霉素阻断了这一过程是因为 NRAD 可以通过钙调神经磷酸酶抑制剂增强气道上皮细胞中 IL-17 依赖的中性粒细胞趋化性来解释[28]。

### 12.2.3 体液免疫反应

同种免疫 CD4+ T 细胞可以驱动 B 细胞和浆细胞产生针对供体 MHC 抗原的抗体，称为供体特异性抗体（DSA）。抗体介导的排斥综合征，包括同种异体移植物功能障碍、DSA、补体（C4d）沉积、肺组织学相容性并排除其他病因，进展为 CLAD（特别是 RAS）的风险显著增加[29-31]。DSA 可激活补体级联反应，导致中性粒细胞、单核细胞和 T 细胞的 C5a 介导的趋化并激活膜攻击复合物，导致直接细胞裂解[32]。DSA 还可刺激自然杀伤（natural killer，NK）细胞，诱导抗体依赖性细胞介导的细胞毒性（antibody-dependent cell mediated cytotoxicity，ADCC）[33]。因此，能与 DSA 结合更多 Fc- 受体基因型的受试者更快发展为 CLAD，可能是因为其更易产生 ADCC[34]。DSA 还可直接刺激气道上皮细胞，产生可驱动 CLAD 独立于其他免疫细胞的增殖信号[35]。总体而言，DSA 会增加 CLAD 的风险，对其进行妥善处理是预后良好的信号[36]。由于清除 DSA 的干预措施不一定会改善预后，因此 DSA 可能是直接致病因素，也可能是更广泛的同种免疫生物标志物[37,38]。

### 12.2.4 其他免疫反应

自体免疫性抗体（如 V 型胶原蛋白和 K-α1 微管蛋白）可在肺移植后产生，并且是发展为 CLAD 的风险因素[39]。先天免疫基因多态性通过直接免疫激活或通过增加对感染的易感性与不同的 CLAD 风险相关[40-42]。

NK 细胞可根据被激活的特定细胞受体产生多种影响。在杀伤细胞免疫球蛋白样受体（killer-cell immunoglobulin-like receptor，KIR）MHC 不匹配的情况下，NK 细胞可以靶向受体抗原呈递细胞，从而降低 CLAD 的风险[43]。但是，NK 细胞通过 NKG2C 激活同种异体移植物中的巨细胞病毒、通过 NKG2D 激活应激分子或通过 FcR 激活抗体会增加 CLAD 的风险[33,44]。

### 12.2.5 上皮细胞的损伤与再生

CLAD 病理可观察到直接上皮损伤的结果[45]。原发性移植物功能不全（PGD）[46]、空气污染[47]、胃食管反流[48]和感染[45,49,50]增加了 CLAD 的风险。虽然这些损伤可能在一定程度上可以增强免疫激活，但它们也会驱动上皮细胞的损伤和逆转。

气道上皮细胞的恢复需要来自上皮细胞前体细胞的再生。Club 细胞既可以保护肺上皮细胞，也可以通过分化为细支气管芽和纤毛细胞来再生细支气管，Club 细胞丢失是 CLAD 的标志之一[51]。在同种免疫不相容的小鼠肺移植模型中，Club 细胞的耗竭会导致闭塞性毛细支气管炎病理的产生[52]。若气道上皮细胞更新速率超过 Club 细胞的修复能力，则可能成为慢性肺同种异体移植物功能障碍（CLAD）的重要驱动因素。同种异体移植物中的端粒功能障碍可以解释 Club 细胞为什么不能跟上慢性同种免疫损伤的转换。在端粒酶缺乏的小鼠 Club 细胞中导致闭塞性毛细支气管炎病理中缺乏同种免疫反应[53]。此外，短端粒供体同种异体移植物发生 CLAD 的风险增加[54]。在机制上，上皮细胞会主动发出信号以防止间充质增殖，这解释了它们的丢失是如何导致闭塞性毛细支气管炎的[55]。

## 12.3 CLAD 的治疗

有几种疗法已被用于治疗 CLAD，但结果各不相同。类固醇（泼尼松）、嘌呤抑制剂（霉酚酸酯或硫唑嘌呤）和钙调神经磷酸酶抑制剂（CNI）（他克莫司或环孢霉素）的三联免疫抑制是肺移植后的标准药物。在缺乏强有力的证据指导管理的情况下，治疗 CLAD 的常见方法是增加属于免疫调节类别的治疗方法，如阿奇霉素、孟鲁司特、体外光疗（extracorporeal photopheresis，ECP）、免疫抑制增强剂［mTOR 抑制剂、阿仑单抗、抗胸腺细胞球蛋白（antithymocyte globulin，ATG）、吸入环孢霉素］，以及最近的抗纤维化药物（吡非尼酮、尼达尼布）。由于药物治疗对逆转或阻止 CLAD 进展总体无效，因此目前再移植是唯一一种能延长生存期的治疗方法（表 12-3）。

## 肺移植：胸外科临床问题

**表 12-3　慢性移植肺功能障碍目前的药物治疗**

| 治疗 | 潜在作用机制 | 潜在的不良事件 | 参考文献 |
|---|---|---|---|
| 阿奇霉素系 | 大环内酯类抗生素可减少气道中性粒细胞增多和 IL-8 信使 RNA 的表达 | 腹泻、恶心、呕吐、QT 延长、心律失常、听力损失 | [56-61] |
| 孟鲁司特 | 白三烯受体拮抗剂，可减少气道嗜酸性炎症 | 恶心 | [62,63] |
| 体外光化学疗法 | 可促进效应淋巴细胞凋亡和（或）稳定调节性 T 细胞 | 置管后感染、短暂性低血压 | [64-73] |
| 西罗莫司和依维莫司 | mTOR 抑制剂可降低 B 细胞和 T 细胞、NK 细胞和成纤维细胞的增殖。与调节性 T 细胞的增加有关 | 水肿、高血压、高三酰甘油血症、贫血、白细胞减少、伤口裂开、肺炎 | [75-79] |
| 吸入环孢霉素 | 钙调神经磷酸酶抑制剂，通过阻止细胞因子的转录来降低 T 细胞的活性 | 结膜炎、咽炎、咳痰 | [80-82] |
| 阿仑单抗 | 抗 CD52 抗体通过补体介导的细胞裂解、抗体介导的细胞毒性和凋亡诱导 B 细胞和 T 细胞消耗 | 淋巴细胞减少、感染 | [83-87] |
| 抗胸腺细胞球蛋白 | 抗体来自家兔和马抗人胸腺细胞，具有针对 B 细胞和 T 细胞的多个靶点，通过补体介导的裂解、调理导致淋巴细胞耗竭、吞噬作用和凋亡 | 淋巴细胞减少、感染 | [88,89] |
| 全淋巴照射 | 靶向照射膈上和膈下血管周围淋巴结、脾脏和胸腺，导致 T 细胞衰竭、功能受损和异常成熟 | 骨髓抑制、血小板减少、白细胞减少、感染 | [90-92] |
| 吡非尼酮 | 通过阻断 TGF-β 信号通路来抑制肺成纤维细胞的增殖及其向肌成纤维细胞分化的小分子 | 恶心、呕吐、腹泻、体重减轻、光敏性、肝毒性 | [93-97] |
| 尼达尼布 | 酪氨酸激酶抑制剂，可抑制肺成纤维细胞、肌成纤维细胞分化、纤维连接蛋白和胶原蛋白 1 表达中的 TGF-β 信号通路 | 腹泻、恶心、呕吐、体重减轻、肝毒性 | [98-101] |

阿奇霉素是一种大环内酯类抗生素，可降低 BOS 患者的气道中性粒细胞增多和 IL-8 信使 RNA 的表达，从而改善 NRAD 表型中的 $FEV_1$[56]。2014 年，ISHLT 发布了对在诊断为 BOS 的患者中至少使用 3 个月的阿奇霉素的建议[57]。阿奇霉素的随机对照试验（RCT）对治疗已发生的 BOS 与预防 BOS 显示出不同的结果。与安慰剂组相比，对于发生的 BOS，服用阿奇霉素的患者的 $FEV_1$ 平均升高 0.3 L，较基线增加 10%[58]。相较于安慰剂组患者，移植后早期开始使用阿奇霉素并在前 2 年服用阿奇霉素的受者的 $FEV_1$ 更好，BOS 患病率较低（12.5% *vs.* 44.2%），2 年无 BOS 生存率更高[59]。与安慰剂组相比，

## 第12章 慢性移植肺功能障碍

移植前和移植后1个月使用阿奇霉素对3个月的$FEV_1$或无CLAD生存期无影响[60]。一项比较阿奇霉素预防CLAD前后的结果的单中心研究报告称,其改善了CLAD的生存率,但没有降低CLAD的风险或发展至CLAD经历的时间[61]。阿奇霉素作为CLAD的预防方式已经在世界各地的肺移植中心中采用,其中包括我们的中心在内。

孟鲁司特是一种白三烯受体拮抗剂,可减少气道嗜酸性炎症,用于治疗哮喘。有关闭塞性毛细支气管炎的潜在益处的报道,随着造血干细胞移植后的移植物抗宿主病的发生,促使孟鲁司特被用于纤维增殖性BOS的研究[62]。一项开放标签试验研究表明,每天10 mg孟鲁司特能减轻6个月内$FEV_1$的衰减。随后对30例已经服用阿奇霉素的BOS患者进行为期1年的随机对照试验,发现其肺功能和生存率没有差异[63]。虽然总体上是阴性试验,但事后分析建议加入孟鲁司特能使早期1期BOS患者术后$FEV_1$维持稳定[63]。

ECP是通过暴露于紫外线A光诱导白细胞中补骨脂素介导的DNA交联,从而导致淋巴细胞、NK细胞和T细胞的凋亡[64]。ECP最初在20世纪80年代用于治疗皮肤T细胞淋巴瘤,随后是其他T细胞介导的疾病,包括克罗恩病、GVDH和实质器官移植排斥反应。ECP是一种免疫调节疗法,而非免疫抑制疗法,其发生感染性并发症的风险较低[65]。虽然其免疫调节机制尚不清楚,但增强调节性T(Treg)细胞反应已被提出[66-68]。在BOS中,ECP诱导的外周血Treg细胞的增加或稳定与$FEV_1$的稳定相关,而Treg反应的缺失与$FEV_1$的进行性下降相关[67]。ECP还与抑制性细胞因子IL-4和IL-10的增加,促炎细胞因子IL-1b、IL-2、IFN-γ、IL-17、IP-1和MCP-1的减少,以及BOS患者中DSA的清除有关[69]。

尽管在非随机研究中,ECP与CLAD中$FEV_1$下降率降低[65,67,69-72]以及生存率增加[65]相关,但临床反应是可变的[65]。尚不明确这种变异性是否反映了独立于ECP的CLAD的病程进展。移植后3年以上的BOS的晚期发展,$FEV_1$的快速下降,在更晚期的BOS阶段开始使用ECP,以及RAS表型与更差的反应相关[65,73]。目前,ECP主要推荐用于BOS,治疗时间由$FEV_1$反应指导[74]。一项随机多中心试验对ECP治疗难治性和新诊断的BOS的疗效和耐受性进行了评估(临床试验注册号NCT02181257)。

mTOR抑制剂(哺乳动物雷帕霉素靶蛋白抑制剂),西罗莫司和依维莫司,可防止B细胞和T细胞增殖[75],减少NK细胞、间充质细胞和成纤维细胞的增殖,并与Treg细胞的增殖有关。这些作用形成了mTOR抑制作为BOS的潜在治疗方法的假说[76]。虽然mTOR抑制剂通常被用于减轻其他免疫抑制剂的不良事件——肾毒性、白细胞减少、胃肠道不良反应——但关于它们对CLAD进展的影响的证据有限。4项EVER LUNG随

### 肺移植：胸外科临床问题

机试验显示，与三联免疫抑制相比，经以依维莫司为基础的四联低 CNI 免疫抑制治疗后 1 年肾功能更优，但 CLAD 的发展没有差异[77]。一项多中心随机对照试验（RCT）显示，在稳定期肺移植受者（接受泼尼松 + 环孢素治疗）中，依维莫司相较于硫唑嘌呤可降低 12 个月时闭塞性细支气管炎综合征（BOS）的发生率，但 24 个月时两组元显著差异[78]。依维莫司停用的不良事件主要是感染和肾脏损害。一项针对 CLAD 的依维莫司的回顾性研究发现，6 个月时 BOS 的 $FEV_1$ 有所改善，但 RAS 患者的 $FEV_1$ 迅速下降[79]。mTOR 抑制剂对 CLAD 进展的长期影响需要在 RCT 研究中进一步评估，特别是由于其广泛作用，包括增强天然免疫系统的激活（如巨噬细胞和树突状细胞）可导致炎症不良事件[75]，如肺炎。

吸入环孢霉素是一种钙调神经磷酸酶抑制剂，可以在 T 细胞受体激活时，通过阻止 IL-2 和其他细胞因子的转录来降低 T 细胞效应。全身使用环孢霉素的副作用限制了异位移植所需的浓度，引出局部用药的概念——更高的局部药物浓度引起的全身不良反应更少。动物研究发现，雾化后的肺环孢霉素浓度高于全身途径[80]。对伴有难治性排斥反应的肺受者进行的小型单中心研究显示，吸入环孢霉素能使肺中的组织学 ACR 和 $FEV_1$ 以剂量依赖的方式得到改善[81]。在一项对 21 例 BOS 患者进行的随机试验中，每天 2 次吸入脂质体环孢霉素可使 $FEV_1$ 和 FVC 达到稳定，而标准护理组持续下降[82]。接受环孢素治疗的患者中位无再移植生存期为 4.1 年，显著优于标准护理组的 2.7 年[82]。最近有一项评估吸入脂质体环孢霉素治疗 BOS 的疗效分析的大型随机对照试验完成（ClinicalTrials.gov NCT03657342）。

阿仑单抗是一种单克隆抗体，可与 B 细胞、T 细胞、NK 细胞、树突状细胞和巨噬细胞的细胞膜中的 CD52 结合[83]。阿仑单抗的诱导与改善肺移植相关生存率和无 BOS 时间相关[84]。尽管阿仑单抗对难治性 ACR 有所改善，但其作为逆转已发生的 BOS 的使用与 $FEV_1$ 的短暂增加有关，特别是 1 期 BOS，但并不能改善长期预后[85-87]。此外，由此产生的严重和长期的淋巴细胞减少及其引起的显著的感染风险增加。

ATG 是一种抗 T 细胞免疫球蛋白，来源于马和兔子，可以消耗循环中的淋巴细胞。其可以用于 ACR 的诱导和治疗[88]。在一项对 71 例接受 ATG 治疗的 CLAD 患者进行的单中心研究中，有 23% 的患者 $FEV_1$ 有所改善或保持稳定，40% 的患者 $FEV_1$ 下降减弱，37% 出现 $FEV_1$ 下降恶化[89]。CLAD 表型与反应无关。感染性并发症很常见——有 1/3 的患者培养呈阳性，4% 的患者因感染住院。尽管其他因素的影响尚不清楚，但反应与更好的无再移植生存率相关。

## 第12章 慢性移植肺功能障碍

全淋巴细胞照射包括对所有主要的膈上和膈下血管周围淋巴结、脾脏和胸腺的靶向照射，导致其功能衰竭、功能受损以及T细胞异常成熟，从而产生强大的免疫抑制[90]。在包括超过150例BOS患者的若干回顾性病例系列中，将反应定义为$FEV_1$的稳定或其下降的衰减，主要发生在快速进展的BOS患者中，在36%~100%的患者中得到报告[91]。造成这种可变性的原因尚不清楚[91,92]。无再移植生存率在全淋巴放射治疗后可变[91]。一种8 Gy分10次照射的方案已被广泛使用。尽管减少了抗增殖药物的使用和严重感染，但骨髓抑制仍使多达1/3的患者早期停止全淋巴细胞照射。

吡非尼酮是一种抑制人肺成纤维细胞增殖和分化成肌成纤维细胞的小分子[93]药物。吡非尼酮可减缓IPF患者的FVC值下降，改善无进展生存期[94]。它的抗纤维化作用提出了吡非尼酮是否也能减缓CLAD的进展的问题[95]。在该病例系列中观察到RAS患者在开始使用吡非尼酮后，能够缓解FVC的衰减和$FEV_1$的下降[95-97]。尽管如此，也有报道称仍有一半的患者出现了不良反应，主要是厌食症和恶心，需要减少吡非尼酮剂量并增加20%的CNI剂量需求[97]。一项评估吡非尼酮在限制性慢性肺同种异体移植物功能障碍（CLAD）患者中52周用药安全性和耐受性的前瞻性开放标签研究正在进行中（临床试验注册号NCT03359863）。尽管目前吡非尼酮治疗CLAD的证据只是轶事，但2项随机、安慰剂对照研究有望提供可靠的数据：最近完成的吡非尼酮治疗BOS的欧洲试验（EPOS；临床试验注册号NCT02262299）和一项正在进行的试验，通过参数反应映射（parametric response mapping，PRM）评估吡非尼酮对CLAD的作用，这是一种新兴的成像诊断方法（临床试验注册号NCT03473340）。

尼达尼布是一种多重酪氨酸激酶抑制剂，可抑制人肺成纤维细胞中的肌成纤维细胞分化[98]。尼达尼布可以减缓IPF[99]、硬皮病相关间质性肺病[100]和进行性纤维性间质性肺病[101]患者的FVC下降。与吡非尼酮类似，其抗纤维化作用可减缓CLAD的进展。一项多中心随机试验，评估6个月的尼达尼布对BOS患者$FEV_1$变化的影响正在进行中（临床试验注册号NCT03283007）。IPF单肺移植后继续使用尼达尼布以保留固有的肺功能的研究也在进行中（临床试验注册号NCT03562416）。

再移植是目前唯一可以延长CLAD的生存期的治疗方法。然而，在所有时间点上，再移植后的生存率都低于初次肺移植[102]。有多中心研究报告称，再移植后RAS的生存率明显低于BOS[103]。虽然导致该差异的原因尚不明确，但研究观察到，与因闭塞性细支气管炎综合征（BOS）接受再移植的患者相比，因RAS再移植的患者具有更高的术后死亡率和更早的CLAD复发。

## 12.4 争 议

对 CLAD 定义本身就是不确定的[6,10]，因此，其发病率和无 CLAD 生存率的估计也不确定。人们对 CLAD 的自然史仍然知之甚少。早期的生物标志物异常可能会阐明其机制并细化风险分层。

虽然肺功能下降一直是 CLAD 诊断的主要预后因素和基石，但影像学异常，特别是 RAS 样磨玻璃影，可能先于功能改变并能够预测生存[104,105]。利用 CT 表现作为替代肺活量测定诊断 RAS[106]。此外，随着新的图像分析方法的出现，常规 CT 扫描的预后效用正在扩大，比如 PRM[107]。

除了用于评估感染和 ACR 的用途，支气管镜逐渐成为 CLAD 生物标志物预测的来源。气道刷分析可显示检测同种异体排斥基因通路、CLAD 发病过程中的路径、微生物组的改变，以及其他细胞和表观遗传学的变化[25,49,108]。

## 12.5 总 结

CLAD 是一种肺移植后肺功能进行性下降的综合征，目前尚无治愈方法。需要更好地定义 CLAD 的内型和预后生物标志物来了解其病理生物学和开发有效的疗法。虽然单中心研究可以提出假设，但还需要大型多中心的 RCT 来评估当前和未来 CLAD 的疗效。

### 声明

A.Venado：参与了由 Genentech 资助的限制性慢性肺移植功能障碍（PIRCLAD）研究（担任首席研究员）。J.Kukreja：参与了 Lung Bioengineering（数据安全监测委员会）；Transmedics（研究）。John Greenland：担任 Atara Biotherapeutics、Theravance Biopharma、Boehringer Ingelheim 的科学顾问委员会成员；研究资金来自 Theravance Biopharma。

## 参考文献

1. Cooper JD, Billingham M, Egan T, et al. A working formulation for the standardization of nomenclature and for clinical staging of chronic dysfunction in lung allografts. International Society for Heart and Lung Transplantation. J Heart Lung Transpl 1993;12(5):713–716.

2. Dugger DT, Fung M, Hays SR, et al. Chronic lung allograft dysfunction small airways reveal a lymphocytic inflammation gene signature. Am J Transpl 2021;21(1):362–371.

3. Estenne M, Maurer JR, Boehler A, et al. Bronchiolitis obliterans syndrome 2001: an update of the diagnostic criteria. J Heart Lung Transpl 2002; 21(3):297–310.

4. Hachem RR, Chakinala MM, Yusen RD, et al. The predictive value of bronchiolitis obliterans syndrome stage 0-p. Am J Respir Crit Care Med 2004;169(4):468–472.

5. Glanville AR. Bronchoscopic monitoring after lung transplantation. Semin Respir Crit Care Med 2010;31(2):208–221.

6. Sato M, Waddell TK, Wagnetz U, et al. Restrictive allograft syndrome (RAS): a novel form of chronic lung allograft dysfunction. J Heart Lung Transpl 2011;30(7):735–742.

7. Verleden GM, Raghu G, Meyer KC, et al. A new classification system for chronic lung allograft dysfunction. J Heart Lung Transplant 2014;33(2):127–133.

8. Verleden GM, Glanville AR, Lease ED, et al. Chronic lung allograft dysfunction: definition, diagnostic criteria, and approaches to treatment-A consensus report from the Pulmonary Council of the ISHLT. J Heart Lung Transpl 2019;38(5):493–503.

9. Glanville AR, Verleden GM, Todd JL, et al. Chronic lung allograft dysfunction: definition and update of restrictive allograft syndrome-A consensus report from the Pulmonary Council of the ISHLT. J Heart Lung Transpl 2019;38(5):483–492.

10. Verleden GM, Vos R, Verleden SE, et al. Survival determinants in lung transplant patients with chronic allograft dysfunction. Transplantation 2011;92(6):703–708.

11. Todd JL, Jain R, Pavlisko EN, et al. Impact of forced vital capacity loss on survival after the onset of chronic lung allograft dysfunction. Am J Respir Crit Care Med 2014;189(2):159–166.

12. Van Herck A, Verleden SE, Sacreas A, et al. Validation of a post-transplant chronic lung allograft dysfunction classification system. J Heart Lung Transpl 2019;38(2):166–173.

13. Tazelaar HD, Yousem SA. The pathology of combined heart-lung transplantation: an autopsy study. Hum Pathol 1988;19(12):1403–1416.

14. Burke CM, Theodore J, Dawkins KD, et al. Posttransplant obliterative bronchiolitis and other late lung sequelae in human heart-lung transplantation. Chest 1984;86(6):824–829.

15. Greenland JR, Jones K, Singer JP. Bronchiolitis. In: Broaddus VC, Ernst JD, King TE, et al, editors. Murray & Nadel's textbook of respiratory medicine, vol. 1, 7th edition. Philadelphia, PA: Elsevier; 2021. p. 994–1004.

16. Chua F, Desai SR, Nicholson AG, et al. Pleuroparenchymal fibroelastosis. A review of clinical, radiological, and pathological characteristics. Ann Am Thorac Soc 2019;16(11):1351–1359.

17. Verleden SE, Von der Thusen J, Roux A, et al. When tissue is the issue a histological review of chronic lung allograft dysfunction. Am J Transpl 2020;20(10):2644–2651.

18. Belperio JA, Weigt SS, Fishbein MC, et al. Chronic lung allograft rejection: mechanisms and therapy. Proc Am Thorac Soc 2009;6(1):108–121.

19. Higuchi T, Maruyama T, Jaramillo A, et al. Induction of obliterative airway disease in murine tracheal allografts by CD81 CTLs recognizing a single minor histocompatibility antigen. J Immunol 2005;174(4):

1871–1878.

20. Glanville AR, Aboyoun CL, Havryk A, et al. Severity of lymphocytic bronchiolitis predicts long-term outcome after lung transplantation. Am J Respir Crit Care Med 2008;177(9):1033–1040.
21. Verleden SE, Scheers H, Nawrot TS, et al. Lymphocytic bronchiolitis after lung transplantation is associated with daily changes in air pollution. Am J Transpl 2012;12(7):1831–1838.
22. Greenland JR, Jones KD, Hays SR, et al. Association of large-airway lymphocytic bronchitis with bronchiolitis obliterans syndrome. Am J Respir Crit Care Med 2013;187(4):417–423.
23. Levy L, Huszti E, Tikkanen J, et al. The impact of first untreated subclinical minimal acute rejection on risk for chronic lung allograft dysfunction or death after lung transplantation. Am J Transpl 2019;20(1): 241–249.
24. Khalifah AP, Hachem RR, Chakinala MM, et al. Minimal acute rejection after lung transplantation: a risk for bronchiolitis obliterans syndrome. Am J Transpl 2005;5(8):2022–2030.
25. Iasella CJ, Hoji A, Popescu I, et al. Type-1 immunity and endogenous immune regulators predominate in the airway transcriptome during chronic lung allograft dysfunction. Am J Transpl 2021;21(6): 2145–2160.
26. Lemaitre PH, Vokaer B, Charbonnier LM, et al. Cyclosporine A drives a Th17and Th2-mediated posttransplant obliterative airway disease. Am J Transpl 2013;13(3):611–620.
27. Vos R, Verleden SE, Ruttens D, et al. Azithromycin and the treatment of lymphocytic airway inflammation after lung transplantation. Am J Transpl 2014;14(12):2736–2748.
28. Vanaudenaerde BM, Wuyts WA, Geudens N, et al. Macrolides inhibit IL17-induced IL8 and 8-isoprostane release from human airway smooth muscle cells. Am J Transpl 2007;7(1):76–82.
29. Tikkanen JM, Singer LG, Kim SJ, et al. De Novo DQ donor-specific antibodies are associated with chronic lung allograft dysfunction after lung transplantation. Am J Respir Crit Care Med 2016; 194(5):596–606.
30. Levine DJ, Glanville AR, Aboyoun C, et al. Antibody-mediated rejection of the lung: a consensus report of the International Society for Heart and Lung Transplantation. J Heart Lung Transpl 2016; 35(4):397–406.
31. Roux A, Le Lan I, Holifanjaniaina S, et al. Antibody-mediated rejection in lung transplantation: clinical outcomes and donor-specific antibody characteristics. Am J Transpl 2016;16(4):1216–1228.
32. Valenzuela NM, Reed EF. Antibodies in transplantation: the effects of HLA and non-HLA antibody binding and mechanisms of injury. Methods Mol Biol 2013;1034:41–70.
33. Calabrese DR, Lanier LL, Greenland JR. Natural killer cells in lung transplantation. Thorax 2019; 74(4):397–404.
34. Paul P, Pedini P, Lyonnet L, et al. FCGR3A and FCGR2A genotypes differentially impact allograft rejection and patients' survival after lung transplant. Front Immunol 2019;10:1208.
35. Reznik SI, Jaramillo A, Zhang L, et al. Anti-HLA antibody binding to hla class I molecules induces proliferation of airway epithelial cells: a potential mechanism for bronchiolitis obliterans syndrome. J Thorac Cardiovasc Surg 2000;119(1):39–45.
36. Hachem RR, Yusen RD, Meyers BF, et al. Anti-human leukocyte antigen antibodies and preemptive antibody-directed therapy after lung transplantation. J Heart Lung Transpl 2010;29(9):973–980.
37. Islam AK, Sinha N, DeVos JM, et al. Early clearance vs persistence of de novo donor-specific antibodies following lung transplantation. Clin Transpl 2017;31(8):10.
38. Ius F, Sommer W, Tudorache I, et al. Preemptive treatment with therapeutic plasma exchange and rituximab

for early donor-specific antibodies after lung transplantation. J Heart Lung Transpl 2015; 34(1):50–58.

39. Hachem RR, Tiriveedhi V, Patterson GA, et al. Antibodies to K-alpha 1 tubulin and collagen V are associated with chronic rejection after lung transplantation. Am J Transpl 2012;12(8):2164–2171.

40. Kastelijn EA, van Moorsel CH, Ruven HJ, et al. Genetic polymorphisms and bronchiolitis obliterans syndrome after lung transplantation: promising results and recommendations for the future. Transplantation 2012;93(2):127–135.

41. Calabrese DR, Wang P, Chong T, et al. Dectin-1 genetic deficiency predicts chronic lung allograft dysfunction and death. JCI Insight 2019;4(22):e133083.

42. Calabrese DR, Aminian E, Mallavia B, et al. Natural killer cells activated through NKG2D mediate lung ischemia-reperfusion injury. J Clin Invest 2021; 131(3):e137047.

43. Greenland JR, Sun H, Calabrese D, et al. HLA mismatching favoring host-versus-graft NK cell activity via KIR3DL1 is associated with improved outcomes following lung transplantation. Am J Transpl 2017; 17(8):2192–2199.

44. Calabrese DR, Chong T, Wang A, et al. NKG2C natural killer cells in bronchoalveolar lavage are associated with cytomegalovirus viremia and poor outcomes in lung allograft recipients. Transplantation 2019;103(3):493–501.

45. Weigt SS, Copeland CAF, Derhovanessian A, et al. Colonization with small conidia Aspergillus species is associated with bronchiolitis obliterans syndrome: a two-center validation study. Am J Transpl 2013;13(4):919–927.

46. Suzuki Y, Cantu E, Christie JD. Primary graft dysfunction. Semin Respir Crit Care Med 2013; 34(3):305–319.

47. Nawrot TS, Vos R, Jacobs L, et al. The impact of traffic air pollution on bronchiolitis obliterans syndrome and mortality after lung transplantation. Thorax 2011;66(9):748–754.

48. Biswas Roy S, Elnahas S, Serrone R, et al. Early fundoplication is associated with slower decline in lung function after lung transplantation in patients with gastroesophageal reflux disease. J Thorac Cardiovasc Surg 2018;155(6):2762–2771. e1.

49. Dugger DT, Fung M, Zlock L, et al. Cystic fibrosis lung transplant recipients have suppressed airway interferon responses during pseudomonas infection. Cell Rep Med 2020,1(4):100055.

50. Khalifah AP, Hachem RR, Chakinala MM, et al. Respiratory viral infections are a distinct risk for bronchiolitis obliterans syndrome and death. Am J Respir Crit Care Med 2004;170(2):181–187.

51. Kelly FL, Kennedy VE, Jain R, et al. Epithelial clara cell injury occurs in bronchiolitis obliterans syndrome after human lung transplantation. Am J Transpl 2012;12(11):3076–3084.

52. Liu Z, Liao F, Scozzi D, et al. An obligatory role for club cells in preventing obliterative bronchiolitis in lung transplants. JCI Insight 2019;5(9):e124732.

53. Naikawadi RP, Disayabutr S, Mallavia B, et al. Telomere dysfunction in alveolar epithelial cells causes lung remodeling and fibrosis. JCI Insight 2016; 1(14):e86704.

54. Faust HE, Golden JA, Rajalingam R, et al. Short lung transplant donor telomere length is associated with decreased CLAD-free survival. Thorax 2017; 72(11):1052–1054.

55. Peng T, Frank DB, Kadzik RS, et al. Hedgehog actively maintains adult lung quiescence and regulates repair

and regeneration. Nature 2015; 526(7574):578–582.

56. Verleden GM, Vanaudenaerde BM, Dupont LJ, et al. Azithromycin reduces airway neutrophilia and interleukin-8 in patients with bronchiolitis obliterans syndrome. Am J Respir Crit Care Med 2006; 174(5):566–567.

57. Meyer KC, Raghu G, Verleden GM, et al. An international ISHLT/ATS/ERS clinical practice guideline: diagnosis and management of bronchiolitis obliterans syndrome. Eur Respir J 2014;44(6): 1479–1503.

58. Corris PA, Ryan VA, Small T, et al. A randomised controlled trial of azithromycin therapy in bronchiolitis obliterans syndrome (BOS) post lung transplantation. Thorax 2015;70(5):442–450.

59. Vos R, Vanaudenaerde BM, Verleden SE, et al. A randomised controlled trial of azithromycin to prevent chronic rejection after lung transplantation. Eur Respir J 2011;37(1):164–172.

60. Van Herck A, Frick AE, Schaevers V, et al. Azithromycin and early allograft function after lung transplantation: a randomized, controlled trial. J Heart Lung Transpl 2019;38(3):252–259.

61. Li D, Duan Q, Weinkauf J, et al. Azithromycin prophylaxis after lung transplantation is associated with improved overall survival. J Heart Lung Transpl 2020;39(12):1426–1434.

62. Verleden GM, Verleden SE, Vos R, et al. Montelukast for bronchiolitis obliterans syndrome after lung transplantation: a pilot study. Transpl Int 2011;24(7):651–656.

63. Ruttens D, Verleden SE, Demeyer H, et al. Montelukast for bronchiolitis obliterans syndrome after lung transplantation: a randomized controlled trial. PLoS One 2018;13(4):e0193564.

64. Knobler R, Arenberger P, Arun A, et al. European dermatology forum updated guidelines on the use of extracorporeal photopheresis 2020-part 1. J Eur Acad Dermatol Venereol 2020;34(12): 2693–2716.

65. Jaksch P, Scheed A, Keplinger M, et al. A prospective interventional study on the use of extracorporeal photopheresis in patients with bronchiolitis obliterans syndrome after lung transplantation. J Heart Lung Transpl 2012;31(9):950–957.

66. Lamioni A, Parisi F, Isacchi G, et al. The immunological effects of extracorporeal photopheresis unraveled:induction of tolerogenic dendritic cells in vitro and regulatory T cells in vivo. Transplantation 2005;79(7):846–850.

67. Meloni F, Cascina A, Miserere S, et al. Peripheral CD4(1)CD25(1) TREG cell counts and the response to extracorporeal photopheresis in lung transplant recipients. Transpl Proc 2007;39(1): 213–217.

68. Maeda A, Schwarz A, Kernebeck K, et al. Intravenous infusion of syngeneic apoptotic cells by photopheresis induces antigen-specific regulatory T cells. J Immunol 2005;174(10):5968–5976.

69. Baskaran G, Tiriveedhi V, Ramachandran S, et al. Efficacy of extracorporeal photopheresis in clearance of antibodies to donor-specific and lung-specific antigens in lung transplant recipients. J Heart Lung Transpl 2014;33(9):950–956.

70. Morrell MR, Despotis GJ, Lublin DM, et al. The efficacy of photopheresis for bronchiolitis obliterans syndrome after lung transplantation. J Heart Lung Transpl 2010;29(4):424–431.

71. Vazirani J, Routledge D, Snell GI, et al. Outcomes following extracorporeal photopheresis for chronic lung allograft dysfunction following lung transplantation: a single-center experience. Transpl Proc 2021;53(1):296–302.

72. Hage CA, Klesney-Tait J, Wille K, et al. Extracorporeal photopheresis to attenuate decline in lung function

due to refractory obstructive allograft dysfunction. Transfus Med 2021.

73. Greer M, Dierich M, De Wall C, et al. Phenotyping established chronic lung allograft dysfunction predicts extracorporeal photopheresis response in lung transplant patients. Am J Transpl 2013;13(4): 911–918.
74. Knobler R, Arenberger P, Arun A, et al. European dermatology forum: updated guidelines on the use of extracorporeal photopheresis 2020 Part 2. J Eur Acad Dermatol Venereol 2021;35(1):27–49.
75. Säemann MD, Haidinger M, Hecking M, et al. The multifunctional role of mTOR in innate immunity: implications for transplant immunity. Am J Transpl 2009;9(12):2655–2661.
76. de Pablo A, Santos F, Solé A, et al. Recommendations on the use of everolimus in lung transplantation. Transpl Rev (Orlando) 2013;27(1):9–16.
77. Gottlieb J, Neurohr C, Muller-Quernheim J, et al. A randomized trial of everolimus-based quadruple therapy vs standard triple therapy early after lung transplantation. Am J Transpl 2019;19(6):1759–1769.
78. Snell GI, Valentine VG, Vitulo P, et al. Everolimus versus azathioprine in maintenance lung transplant recipients: an international, randomized, doubleblind clinical trial. Am J Transpl 2006;6(1):169–177.
79. Patrucco F, Allara E, Boffini M, et al. Twelve-month effects of everolimus on renal and lung function in lung transplantation: differences in chronic lung allograft dysfunction phenotypes. Ther AdvChronic Dis 2021;12. 2040622321993441.
80. Mitruka SN, Won A, McCurry KR, et al. In the lung aerosol cyclosporine provides a regional concentration advantage over intramuscular cyclosporine. J Heart Lung Transpl 2000;19(10):969–975.
81. Iacono AT, Smaldone GC, Keenan RJ, et al. Doserelated reversal of acute lung rejection by aerosolized cyclosporine. Am J Respir Crit Care Med 1997;155(5):1690–1698.
82. Iacono A, Wijesinha M, Rajagopal K, et al. A randomised single-centre trial of inhaled liposomal cyclosporine for bronchiolitis obliterans syndrome post-lung transplantation. ERJ Open Res 2019; 5(4):00167-2019–02019.
83. Zhao Y, Su H, Shen X, et al. The immunological function of CD52 and its targeting in organ transplantation. Inflamm Res 2017;66(7):571–578.
84. Furuya Y, Jayarajan SN, Taghavi S, et al. The impact of alemtuzumab and basiliximab induction on patient survival and time to bronchiolitis obliterans syndrome in double lung transplantation recipients. Am J Transpl 2016;16(8):2334–2341.
85. Ensor CR, Rihtarchik LC, Morrell MR, et al. Rescue alemtuzumab for refractory acute cellular rejection and bronchiolitis obliterans syndrome after lung transplantation. Clin Transpl 2017;31(4):10.
86. Reams BD, Musselwhite LW, Zaas DW, et al. Alemtuzumab in the treatment of refractory acute rejection and bronchiolitis obliterans syndrome after human lung transplantation. Am J Transpl 2007; 7(12):2802–2808.
87. Moniodis A, Townsend K, Rabin A, et al. Comparison of extracorporeal photopheresis and alemtuzumab for the treatment of chronic lung allograft dysfunction. J Heart Lung Transpl 2018;37(3):340–348.
88. Ippoliti G, Lucioni M, Leonardi G, et al. Immunomodulation with rabbit anti-thymocyte globulin in solid organ transplantation. World J Transpl 2015;5(4): 261–266.
89. Kotecha S, Paul E, Ivulich S, et al. Outcomes following ATG therapy for chronic lung allograft dysfunction. Transpl Direct 2021;7(4):e681.
90. Tochner Z, Slavin S. Immune modulation by ionized irradiation. Curr Opin Immunol 1988;1(2):261–268.
91. Lebeer M, Kaes J, Lambrech M, et al. Total lymphoid irradiation in progressive bronchiolitis obliterans

syndrome after lung transplantation: a single-center experience and review of literature. Transpl Int 2020;33(2):216–228.

92. Fisher AJ, Rutherford RM, Bozzino J, et al. The safety and efficacy of total lymphoid irradiation in progressive bronchiolitis obliterans syndrome after lung transplantation. Am J Transpl 2005;5(3): 537–543.

93. Conte E, Gili E, Fagone E, et al. Effect of pirfenidone on proliferation, TGF-beta-induced myofibroblast differentiation and fibrogenic activity of primary human lung fibroblasts. Eur J Pharm Sci 2014;58:13–19.

94. King TE Jr, Bradford WZ, Castro-Bernardini S, et al. A phase 3 trial of pirfenidone in patients with idiopathic pulmonary fibrosis. N Engl J Med 2014; 370(22):2083–2092.

95. Vos R, Verleden SE, Ruttens D, et al. Pirfenidone: a potential new therapy for restrictive allograft syndrome? Am J Transpl 2013;13(11):3035–40.

96. Bennett D, Lanzarone N, Fossi A, et al. Pirfenidone in chronic lung allograft dysfunction: a single cohort study. Panminerva Med 2020;62(3):143–149.

97. Vos R, Wuyts WA, Gheysens O, et al. Pirfenidone in restrictive allograft syndrome after lung transplantation: a case series. Am J Transpl 2018;18(12): 3045–3059.

98. Rangarajan S, Kurundkar A, Kurundkar D, et al. Novel mechanisms for the antifibrotic action of nintedanib. Am J Respir Cell Mol Biol 2016;54(1): 51–59.

99. Richeldi L, du Bois RM, Raghu G, et al. Efficacy and safety of nintedanib in idiopathic pulmonary fibrosis. N Engl J Med2014;370(22):2071–2082.

100. Distler O, Highland KB, Gahlemann M, et al. Nintedanib for systemic sclerosis-associated interstitial lung disease. N Engl J Med 2019;380(26):2518–2528.

101. Flaherty KR, Wells AU, Cottin V, et al. Nintedanib in progressive fibrosing interstitial lung diseases. N Engl J Med 2019;381(18):1718–1727.

102. Yusen RD, Edwards LB, Kucheryavaya AY, et al. The registry of the International Society for Heart and Lung Transplantation: thirty-first adult lung and heart-lung transplant report–2014; focus theme: retransplantation. J Heart Lung Transpl 2014;33(10):1009–1024.

103. Verleden SE, Todd JL, Sato M, et al. Impact of CLAD phenotype on survival after lung retransplantation: a multicenter study. Am J Transpl 2015; 15(8):2223–2230.

104. Levy L, Huszti E, Renaud-Picard B, et al. Risk assessment of chronic lung allograft dysfunction phenotypes: validation and proposed refinement of the 2019 International Society for Heart and Lung Transplantation classification system. J Heart Lung Transpl 2020;39(8):761–770.

105. Dettmer S, Shin HO, Vogel-Claussen J, et al. CT at onset of chronic lung allograft dysfunction in lung transplant patients predicts development of the restrictive phenotype and survival. Eur J Radiol 2017;94:78–84.

106. Suhling H, Dettmer S, Greer M, et al. Phenotyping chronic lung allograft dysfunction using body plethysmography and computed tomography. Am J Transpl 2016.

107. Belloli EA, Degtiar I, Wang X, et al. Parametric response mapping as an imaging biomarker in lung transplant recipients. Am J Respir Crit Care Med 2017;195(7):942–952.

108. Dugger DT, Calabrese DR, Gao Y, et al. Lung allograft epithelium DNA methylation age is associated with graft chronologic age and primary graft dysfunction. Front Immunol 2021;12:704172.

# 第 13 章 非同种异体肺移植的并发症

Tany Thaniyavarn, Harpreet Singh Grewal, Hilary J. Goldberg, Selim M. Arcasoy  著

扶志敏  译

周建平  校

【关键词】
- 肺移植  • 非同种异体移植物  • 并发症  • 免疫抑制

【要点】
- 非同种异体移植物并发症对肺移植术后短期和长期预后有重要的影响。
- 慢性免疫抑制可导致现有医学合并症的恶化，或可能导致新的医学合并症的发展。
- 非同种异体移植物并发症的管理需要密切监测和多学科团队协作。

## 13.1 引　言

钙调磷酸酶抑制剂（CNI）是现代免疫抑制治疗的基石，能够提高肺移植（LTx）受者的长期存活率。根据国际心肺移植学会（ISHLT）登记处的数据，2019年，移植后1年生存下来的经历双肺和单肺移植（single lung transplantation，SLT）受者的中位生存时间分别为10.2年和6.5年[1]。长期使用CNI及其他免疫抑制剂，特别是皮质类固醇，可能会加剧原有的慢性疾病或导致新的慢性疾病，如糖尿病、高血压、高脂血症、心血管疾病等（表13-1）。此外，在长期免疫抑制的背景下，发生恶性肿瘤的风险也会增加。由于移植受者普遍存在多药的联合治疗，因此，应对药物相互作用、药物吸收和此人群中的不良反应重点关注。本章将关注肺移植后最常见的医学疾病及其影响，包括糖尿病、高血压、高脂血症、急性肾损伤（AKI）、慢性肾病（chronic kidney disease，CKD）和恶性肿瘤。

表 13-1　肺移植后的非同种异体移植并发症

| 器官系统 | 并发症 | 器官系统 | 并发症 |
| --- | --- | --- | --- |
| 心血管* | 房性心律失常<br>冠状动脉疾病<br>急性心包炎<br>高血压* | 恶性肿瘤* | 皮肤癌<br>移植后淋巴细胞增生性疾病<br>支气管癌<br>其他实体及血液恶性肿瘤 |
| 肾脏* | 急性肾损伤*<br>慢性肾脏疾病* | 胃、食管、肠道和肝脏 | 胃食管反流病<br>胃轻瘫<br>肠梗阻<br>肠壁囊样积气症<br>肠缺血和穿孔<br>囊性纤维化的远端肠梗阻综合征<br>胆囊炎<br>憩室炎<br>胰腺炎<br>肝结节性再生增生 |
| 神经系统 | 震颤<br>癫痫发作<br>认知功能障碍<br>后部可逆性脑病综合征<br>卒中<br>进行性多灶性白质脑病 | 代谢* | 糖尿病*<br>血脂异常*<br>低镁血症<br>高钾血症<br>肥胖 |
| 肌肉骨骼 | 危重性肌病<br>横纹肌溶解<br>缺血性坏死<br>骨质疏松症<br>衰弱 | 其他 | 高氨血症<br>移植物抗宿主病<br>低丙球蛋白血症<br>药物的相互作用 |
| 血液系统 | 静脉血栓栓塞<br>血细胞减少<br>免疫性溶血<br>血栓性微血管病 | | |

注：*表示将在本文中讨论的并发症

# 13.2 糖尿病

## 13.2.1 流行病学和风险因素

在肺移植受者中，术后糖尿病（posttransplant diabetes mellitus，PTDM）的患病率在第一年为 20%~43%，33%~60% 的受者在 5 年内将发展为 PTDM[1,2]。对 PTDM 诊断的一个注意事项是区分短暂性高血糖和 PTDM。术后初期及皮质类固醇治疗排斥反应后常见短暂性高血糖，但其也是 PTDM 的一个风险因素。因此，2013 年国际术后糖尿病共识会议[3]和 2014 年美国糖尿病协会（American Diabetes Association，ADA）[4]提出护理标准建议，在患者处于稳定状态且免疫抑制治疗减至维持水平时，在门诊环境中再斟酌进行 PTDM 的诊断。诊断标准应与非移植情况下的标准相同。在术后第 1 年，特别是术后初期，应谨慎参考血红蛋白 A1C，因为贫血可能会降低测试的敏感性。PTDM 诊断的金标准仍然是口服葡萄糖耐量测试。PTDM 的风险因素包括传统因素和移植相关的因素，如表 13-2 所述。

表 13-2 移植后糖尿病的危险因素

| 传统风险因素 | 移植相关的危险因素 |
| --- | --- |
| · 45 岁及以上 | |
| · 非裔美国人、西班牙裔美国人、印度裔美国人、亚裔美国人或太平洋岛民 | |
| · 糖尿病家族史及遗传危险因素 | · CNIs（他克莫司＞环孢素） |
| · 妊娠糖尿病史 | · 移植后短暂性高血糖 |
| · 糖尿病前期 | · 频繁的排斥反应 |
| · 多囊卵巢综合征 | · 低镁血症 |
| · 低 HDL 和（或）高三酰甘油 | · 丙型肝炎（可能的危险因素） |
| · 肥胖 | · CMV 感染（可能的危险因素） |
| · 久坐的生活方式 | |
| · 吸烟 | |
| · 西方饮食 | |

注：CMV，巨细胞病毒；CNIs，钙调磷酸酶抑制剂；HDL，高密度脂蛋白胆固醇。数据来自参考文献[3,4,73-75]

### 13.2.2 预防

应强调生活方式的改变（健康饮食、每周至少 150 分钟的中等强度体育活动，以及使用经认证的技术辅助糖尿病预防计划）在移植前后都非常重要。早期发现 PTDM 对于管理至关重要，应对有已知风险因素的患者特别关注，尤其那些术后出现高血糖的患者。尽管与普通人群相比，血红蛋白 A1C 的敏感性可能较低，但 ADA 仍推荐使用空腹血糖测试与血红蛋白 A1C 水平联合筛查 PTDM[4]。

### 13.2.3 管理

不论 PTDM 风险如何，都应采用对受者和移植物最佳的免疫抑制方案[3,4]。与环孢素相比，他克莫司与 PTDM 的发生相关性更高[5]。然而，基于他克莫司的方案能够降低排斥的风险[1]。因此，不应仅因为代谢并发症的风险会增加就轻易替换他克莫司。

在急性病期和高剂量皮质类固醇治疗阶段，如术后早期和治疗排斥反应期间，胰岛素是治疗高血糖最可靠的方法。术后高血糖 3 周内开始使用基础胰岛素治疗，可能可以防止 PTDM 的发展 [6]。ADA（2021）推荐对持续高血糖（≥ 180 mg/dL）开展胰岛素治疗，目标血糖范围为 140~180 mg/dL [4]。当患者免疫抑制状态稳定时，应强调调整生活方式，也可以使用口服降糖药（oral hypoglycemic agent，OHA）。然而，关于 OHA 在肺移植受者中的有效性缺乏证据。在小型研究中成功使用了二甲双胍、噻唑烷二酮和二肽基肽酶 -4（dipeptidyl peptidase 4，DPP-4）抑制剂 [7,8]。除了噻唑烷二酮可能导致 CNI 和 mTOR 抑制剂水平下降外，其他 OHA 与 CNI 或 mTOR 抑制剂之间没有重大的药物相互作用。因此，选择合适的 OHA 应基于其不良反应的特点。例如，二甲双胍的使用可能因肾功能不全和肠胃不良反应在术后患者中受限。已知噻唑烷二酮会导致液体潴留，可能限制其使用。DPP-4 抑制剂是理想的选择，因为其不良反应最小。对于有动脉粥样硬化心血管疾病（atherosclerotic cardiovascular disease，ASCVD）或高 ASCVD 风险的患者（年龄 ≥ 55 岁，冠状动脉、颈动脉或下肢动脉狭窄 > 50%，或左心室肥厚），已确诊肾病或心力衰竭，ADA 推荐使用对心血管有益的钠葡萄糖共转运体 2 抑制剂或胰高血糖素样肽 1 受体激动剂作为治疗方案的一部分 [4]。然而，这 2 类药物可能增加 CNI 和 mTOR 抑制剂的肾毒性，因此，在移植受者人群中应谨慎使用。鉴于移植受者中低镁血症的高发病率及其对 PTDM 的影响，补充镁剂可能有益 [9]。可能需要较高剂量的镁（可能引起腹泻）以维持正常或接受正常的血清镁水平。某些镁制剂，如甘氨酸镁或乳酸镁，可能因其肠胃不良反应较少而最为合适。

## 13.3 高血压

### 13.3.1 流行病学和风险因素

50%~80% 的肺移植受者在移植后 1~5 年被诊断为高血压 [10]。高血压的风险因素包括但不限于高龄、肥胖、高血压家族史、非裔美国人种族、高钠饮食和缺乏体力活动。已知环孢素和皮质类固醇会导致高血压。

### 13.3.2 预防

美国心脏协会 / 美国心脏病学院（American Heart Association/American College of

# 第13章 非同种异体肺移植的并发症

Cardiology, AHA/ACC）建议对于超重或肥胖者的减重，应采取有益于心血管的健康饮食，增加体力活动，限制钠摄入，以饮食形式补充钾，并且减少酒精摄入[11]。然而，移植受者有几个重要的特征。鉴于CNI和皮质类固醇引起的高血压中有显著的水钠潴留，应优先考虑限制钠摄入。许多中心要求移植前停止饮酒，然而，应对可能已恢复饮酒的受者进行特殊关注，临床医生需在移植后询问饮酒情况。通常不需要对由CNI抑制剂、甲氧苄啶-磺胺甲噁唑使用和肾功能损害引起的移植受者高钾血症补充钾。

### 13.3.3 管理

在移植患者中诊断高血压的方法与普通人群相似。然而，关于肺移植受者的血压（blood pressure，BP）治疗目标及特定药物使用没有明确依据。在肾移植受者中使用的目标BP低于130/80 mmHg，因其与延长移植物存活期相关[11,12]。肺移植受者中高血压的药物管理取决于高血压发展的时机、药物不良反应和药物的相互作用。

在肺移植后的初期阶段，液体超负荷、房性心律失常和AKI会影响药物选择。液体超负荷可能导致BP升高，应强调使用利尿剂或噻嗪类利尿剂进行液体优化。在肺移植后的即刻阶段，30%~50%的受者会出现房性心律失常，常用β受体阻滞剂进行管理，通常也有助于控制BP[13,14]。最后，在这一阶段有52.5%的患者会发生AKI，因此，应避免使用血管紧张素转换酶抑制剂（angiotensin-converting enzyme inhibitors，ACEI）和血管紧张素受体阻滞剂（angiotensin receptor blockers，ARB）。此外，ACEI可能会通过抑制红细胞生成素的产生而导致贫血。尽管在糖尿病人群中应用ACEI和ARB对心血管有益，但其对肾移植受者患者生存的影响尚不明确[15,16]。

二氢吡啶类CCB（如氨氯地平）比非二氢吡啶类CCB具有更强的血管扩张效应，常用于移植后高血压的治疗，可抵消CNI的血管收缩效应[17]。然而，由CYP3A4调节的CCB与常用的移植药物（如CNI、他汀类药物和唑类药物）之间的药物相互作用可能会导致每种药物的毒性增加。已有报道称此类组合可导致横纹肌溶解症[18]，因此应考虑调整CCB剂量。二氢吡啶类CCB，尤其是非二氢吡啶类CCB，会导致CNI水平升高。因此，使用时应密切监测CNI浓度。相反，这种组合可能对快速代谢者有用，以减少达到目标水平所需的CNI剂量。其他抗高血压药物，如α1受体阻滞剂，在移植后受者中也能安全使用，但不应将其作为一线药物。

## 13.4 高脂血症

### 13.4.1 流行病学和风险因素

高脂血症是肺移植后另一种常见的合并症,其在移植后1年和5年分别为26.7%和58.2%[10]。高脂血症的风险因素与糖尿病和高血压的相似。应将即使在总胆固醇水平未升高的情况下也可能发生的血脂异常(即异脂血症)与高脂血症区分开来。其包括其他脂质异常,如高密度脂蛋白(high-density lipoprotein,HDL)胆固醇偏低、极低密度脂蛋白(very low-density lipoprotein,VLDL)升高、载脂蛋白B偏高、小而密低密度脂蛋白(low-density lipoprotein,LDL)升高等。在Reed及其同事的研究中,发现89%的慢性阻塞性肺疾病患者在肺移植后HDL下降[19]。然而,肺移植受者中其他血脂异常的发生率尚未知。

### 13.4.2 预防

高脂血症通常伴随其他与移植相关的合并症,特别是糖尿病和高血压。预防或改善这些合并症,调整生活方式可能对血脂水平产生积极影响。

### 13.4.3 管理

对于40~75岁的患者,高脂血症的治疗取决于10年ASCVD风险,该风险是使用ASCVD风险评估器计算的[20]。然而,肺移植存活时间在实质器官移植中最短,双肺移植受者的中位存活时间为10.2年[1]。心血管疾病导致的死亡在移植后10年以上的患者中占6.8%[1]。因此,治疗高脂血症以预防ASCVD在肺移植接受者中的益处仍有争议。另一方面,有证据表明,高脂血症与肺移植后肾功能快速下降有关[21]。在肾移植受者中,低HDL与心血管事件和全因死亡率增加有关[22]。对于20~39岁的患者,如果家族史中有ASCVD的早发病例且LDL ≥ 160 mg/dL,建议给予他汀类药物治疗。对于75岁以上的患者,他汀类药物治疗的益处尚不清楚,应进行综合判断[23]。然而,如果患者已经开始使用他汀类药物且能够耐受,继续治疗是合理的。移植后患者的目标脂质水平尚未建立,通常使用AHA/ACC对普通人群的指南建议[23]。

关于高甘油三酯血症,AHA/ACC建议对ASCVD风险 ≥ 7.5%的患者开始他汀类药物治疗,同时处理高甘油三酯血症的风险因素和继发因素。尽管使用他汀类药物并处理其继发因素，但仍有空腹甘油三酯≥500 mg/dL，特别是≥1000 mg/dL 的患者，应开始实行极低脂肪饮食、避免精制碳水化合物和酒精、ω-3 脂肪酸的摄入。如果必要，可以使用贝特类药物以预防胰腺炎。

用于治疗高脂血症的药物通常会与其他常用的移植后药物产生药物相互作用或干扰其吸收。他汀类药物是最常用的抗高脂血症药物，与他克莫司合用似乎是安全的，但与环孢素联用时需要减少剂量[24]。除了免疫抑制药物外，当他汀类药物与其他药物（特别是唑类药物和CCB）联用时，需要酌情调整剂量。高 ASCVD 风险或糖尿病患者需要使用高强度他汀类治疗，使用高剂量阿托伐他汀或瑞舒伐他汀。然而，如果患者正在使用环孢素，则该组合可能存在药物相互作用，在这种情况下，可能需要使用其他降脂药物。一般认为蛋白酶转化酶亚型 9 抑制剂作为治疗高脂血症的最新药物非常安全，无需对移植患者进行剂量调整[25]。

## 13.5 急性肾损伤

### 13.5.1 流行病学和风险因素

肺移植后 AKI 是一种常见的并发症，其定义不一，既包括血清肌酐翻倍，也使用了 AKI 的分类系统。肺移植文献中最常用的分类系统包括急性肾损伤网络（acute kidney injury network，AKIN）、RIFLE（风险、损伤、衰竭、肾功能丧失和终末期肾病）和 KDIGO（肾脏病：改善全球结果）标准[14,26,27]。AKI 的发生率高达 80%，在不同研究间差异很大[14,28,29]。尽管 AKI 的定义存在异质性，但在肺移植受者中报告的 AKI 结果和风险因素一致[28-35]。与 AKI 发展相关的风险因素包括移植时疾病的严重程度、血流动力学失代偿、心肺支持的使用、手术类型（单侧与双侧）及手术持续时间（方框 13-1）[28,30-32,36,37]。移植后即刻 AKI 与住院时间延长、CKD 风险增加、机械通气持续时间及死亡率增加有关[31,34,35]。5%~8% 的受者需要肾脏替代治疗，与不需要肾脏替代治疗的受者相比，该群体的 30 天内死亡风险几乎增加了 10 倍，1 年死亡风险增加了 5 倍以上[37]。重要的是，Lertjitabanjong 及其同事的 Meta 分析显示，研究期间的年份并不影响肺移植后 AKI 的发生率[14]。

> **方框 13-1　移植后 AKI 的危险因素**
>
> - 高肺源分配评分
> - 移植前肺动脉平均压 > 35 mmHg
> - 移植前全身性高血压
> - 体外膜肺氧合支持
> - 机械通气桥接移植
> - 移植术后延长机械通气时间
> - 术中体外循环支持
> - 术中、术后低血压
> - 移植后全身性感染
> - 使用 CNI
> - 除 COPD 以外的肺移植适应证
> - 双侧肺移植和再次肺移植
>
> 数据来源于参考文献[28,30-32,36,37]

### 13.5.2 预防和管理

上述数据突显了在移植前阶段识别 AKI 发展风险患者的重要性。为制定旨在减少肺移植后 AKI 风险同时确保预防二次损伤的策略提供可能。从长远来看，在基线肾功能障碍的患者中评估移植候选资格，然后在该高风险人群中定期评估肾功能十分重要[28,31,37,38]。肾小球滤过率（glomerular filtration rate，GFR）方程无法准确评估这些患者的肾脏储备功能，并且也可能会高估营养不良或肌肉萎缩的患者的肾功能[39]。应在早期申请肾脏科专科介入以准确诊断和对肾功能障碍进行分级，并在选定的候选者中考虑肾脏移植[40]。考虑适当改良手术方法，以避免或最小化有发展成肾衰竭风险的患者在手术中使用体外循环的可能。在手术过程中与麻醉和灌注团队进行多学科合作，以最小化灌注压的波动，有利于受者的预后。适当补液和血流动力学复苏策略以缓解血流动力学紊乱在所有护理阶段是必需的。使用依赖于诱导治疗的替代免疫抑制方案，可以在极易早期出现肾功能障碍的患者中延迟启动 CNI 治疗。药剂师管理可确保适当药物选择和剂量使用[29]。与多学科团队合作平衡体液状态和肾脏保护管理策略也十分有益。密切监测尿量至关重要，因为其可能是肾功能障碍的最早迹象，对其进行相应的干预措施可以改善死亡率（方框 13-2）[41]。

> **方框 13-2　急性肾损伤**
>
> - AKI 与住院时间延长、CKD 的风险、机械通气时间以及死亡风险相关。
> - 移植后 AKI 最常见的病因是肾脏低灌注和急性肾小管坏死的肾前状态。
> - 识别可改变的风险因素，并采取措施以降低风险，可以帮助降低移植后 AKI 的发生率及减少不良后果。

## 13.6 慢性肾病

### 13.6.1 流行病学和风险因素

与 AKI 一样，CKD 是肺移植后公认的并发症。根据 KDIGO 指南，CKD 被定义为影像学上的结构异常或肾功能下降超过 3 个月，包括 5 个阶段。根据最新的移植受者科学登记数据库（SRTR）报告，CKD 患者中血肌酐水平超过 2.5 mg/dL、需要长期透析或肾移植的比例在 1 年时为 6.2%，到 5 年时增加到 17.3%[35]。AKI 仍然是 CKD 发展最重要的风险因素[14,42]。肺移植后第 1 个月内 GFR 的早期下降可以预测 CKD 的发生[42]。此外，报告中还提到肾功能损失过程是双相的，即在移植后的前 6 个月内快速损失，之后缓慢下降[43]。根据 SRTR 报告，以血清肌酐翻倍作为 CKD 的标志，在移植后 1 年和 5 年的发生率分别为 34% 和 53%[26,27]。术前高血压、移植后高血压的发展（特别是舒张压超过 90 mmHg），以及环孢素的使用是 CKD 和终末期肾病的风险因素[27,44,45]。

### 13.6.2 预防和管理

CKD 预防的基石在于 AKI 的预防和评估可改变的风险因素。高血压是导致 CKD 的重要因素，应使用前一节描述的适当管理措施。应考虑避免使用肾毒性药物（即非甾体抗炎药），在可行的情况下调整治疗性 CNI 水平，必要时转向替代免疫抑制策略（如西罗莫司），同时平衡每种策略的不良效应和排斥风险[46,47]。Canales 及其同事报告，移植后存活超过 6 年的受者在不到 1 年和超过 6 年时的 GFR 相似。这一关联表明，肺移植后早期的肾脏损伤可能对肾功能有长期影响[27,47,48]。让肾病医生参与这些患者的管理可能会有帮助，对于选定的晚期 CKD 患者，可以考虑进行肾移植（方框 13-3）。

> **方框 13-3　慢性肾脏病**
> - 移植后 AKI 是 CKD 的重要危险因素。
> - 术前全身性高血压，移植后舒张压＞ 90 mmHg 和环孢素的使用增加了患 CKD 的风险。
> - 积极地预防术后 AKI 对肾功能有长期的积极影响。

## 13.7 恶性肿瘤

### 13.7.1 流行病学和风险因素

恶性肿瘤是继细支气管炎闭塞性综合征之后，肺移植受者在存活超过 5 年后第二大常见死因，约占死亡总数的 17%。与普通人群相比，移植受者恶性肿瘤的发生率更高[1,49]。在所有实质器官移植中，肺移植受者的癌症风险最高，可能与其免疫抑制治疗的强度有关[50]。移植后恶性肿瘤的风险因素包括一般风险因素和特定于移植的风险因素，如表 13-3 所示。在肺移植受者中报告了各种类型的恶性肿瘤。我们将重点关注该人群中最常见的恶性肿瘤，包括皮肤鳞状细胞癌（SCC）、移植后淋巴增殖性疾病（PTLD）和肺癌[49,50]。

肺移植后癌症发展的机制包括新感染和致癌病毒的再激活、紫外线照射造成的突变负担、免疫抑制的直接效应以及罕见的供者来源的恶性肿瘤。移植后恶性肿瘤最重要的风险是诱导和慢性免疫抑制治疗对抗肿瘤和抗病毒 T 细胞免疫监测的损害[51]。

### 表 13-3　移植后恶性肿瘤的风险因素

| 一般风险因素 | 移植相关风险因素 |
| --- | --- |
| • 高龄<br>• 遗传易感性<br>• 恶性肿瘤家族史<br>• 恶性肿瘤个人史<br>• 移植前烟草暴露<br>• 饮酒<br>• 日照等环境因素 | • 使用 T 细胞消耗剂 [ 莫罗单抗（不再使用）、阿仑单抗和 ATG]，而不是非 T 细胞消耗剂，如巴利昔单抗和达利珠单抗<br>• 免疫抑制剂（mTOR 抑制剂除外，可能有保护作用）、持续时间和峰度<br>• 皮肤癌<br>　◦ 硫唑嘌呤，而不是霉酚酸酯<br>　◦ 伏立康唑使用<br>• PTLD<br>　◦ EBV D+/R-<br>　◦ 白种人<br>　◦ 年龄 < 40 岁<br>　◦ CMV D+/R-<br>　◦ 任何移植前恶性肿瘤<br>　◦ 受者基因型 *HLA Bw22*、*B18* 或 *B21*<br>　◦ 较少 HLA 匹配<br>• 肺癌<br>　◦ 单肺移植（IPF 和 COPD 中原生肺恶性肿瘤）<br>• 供体恶性肿瘤转移 |

注：ATG，抗胸腺细胞球蛋白；EBV D+/R-，EB 病毒（Epstein-Barr virus）供本血清反应阳性 / 受体血清反应阴性；CMV D+/R-，巨细胞病毒供体血清阳性 / 受体血清阴性；COPD，慢性阻塞性肺疾病；HLA，人类白细胞抗原；IPF，特发性肺纤维化；mTOR，哺乳动物雷帕霉素靶蛋白；PTLD，移植后淋巴细胞增生性疾病
数据来自参考文献 [49,50,52,58-60]

### 13.7.2 皮肤癌

皮肤癌虽然通常不致命，但却是实质器官移植后最常见的恶性肿瘤，包括肺移植后。皮肤癌症的累积发病率在肺移植术后 5 年为 31%，10 年为 47%[52]（图 13-1）。SCC 和基底细胞癌（BCC）占所有皮肤癌的 95%[53,54]。皮肤鳞状细胞癌和基底细胞癌主要累及阳光照射的部位。BCC 倾向于面部和上半身，SCC 倾向于手臂、上身和面部[54]。黑色素瘤通常是色素性病变，可以通过 ABCDE（不对称、边界、颜色、直径和进化）技术进行评估[55]。在这些皮肤癌中，SCC 的发病率最高，侵袭性最强。与普通人群相比，肺移植受者的皮肤鳞状细胞癌往往分化较差且具有侵袭性[56]。在一项随访 2 年的转移性 SCC 研究中，1/3 的移植受者已经死亡，2/3 患有转移性疾病。相比之下，80% 的非免疫受损患者在 2 年时间内没有疾病发生，也没有观察到死亡[57]。肺移植受者复发和转移疾病的风险在皮肤 SCC 治疗后 1.5 年分别高达 14% 和 8%[56]。

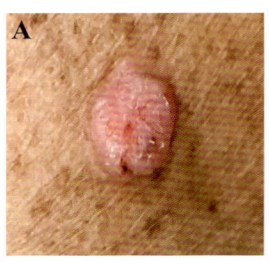 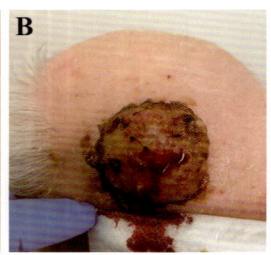 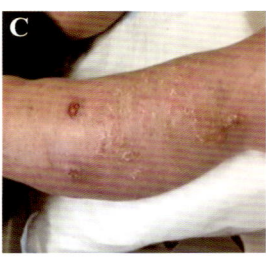 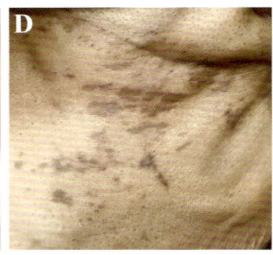

图 13-1　皮肤恶性肿瘤的例子

注：（A）手臂皮肤鳞状细胞癌；（B）头皮鳞状细胞癌快速生长后大出血；（C）脂膜炎并发多发性溃疡和出血的多灶多形性真皮肉瘤结节；（D）卡波西肉瘤累及胸壁和肺移植切口部位

### 13.7.3　移植后淋巴增生障碍

PTLD 会影响 1.8%~9.4% 的肺移植受者，在 EBV 血清阴性受者（EBV R-）接受血清阳性供体（EBV D+）的肺移植时，其发生率可能高达 20%~30%[50,58,59]。大多数 PTLD 发生在移植后的第一年，最常见于 EBV D+/R- 血清状态的患者。6.2% 的 EBV D+/R- 血清状态患者发展为 PTLD，60.8% 的患者在移植后的第一年内发展为 PTLD[58]。这些早期的 PTLD 大多来源于受者的 B 细胞，与 EBV（Epstein-Barr 病毒）相关，涉及肺移植器官，并对减少免疫抑制反应良好[50,60]。发生在肺移植后 1 年以上的晚期 PTLD 可能来源于其他细胞，如 T 细胞和 NK 细胞，更可能是 EBV 阴性的，且在诊断时可能是肺外的以及已经扩散的[50]。

### 13.7.4　肺癌

肺移植后的肺癌可能在异体移植肺（作为供者传播或新生恶性肿瘤）、原生肺中发展，或者如果为了这个指征进行肺移植时，则可能代表受者原发肺癌的复发。在被摘除的肺中，肺癌也可能是在移植肺中偶然发现的。与普通人群相比，肺移植受者中肺癌的发生率增加了 4.8 倍。SLT 的受者肺癌发生率是正常人群的 13 倍，大多数发生在原生的右肺，可能是因为右肺体积更大的缘故[50,61]。诊断的中位时间为移植后 3.9 年[61]。

### 13.7.5　预防和筛查

移植前的癌症筛查是强制性的，特别是在有风险因素的人群中。ISHLT 对候选者选择的共识指南推荐，对于大多数类型的既存恶性肿瘤，在进行移植前应至少有 5 年无病间隔[62]。然而，尽管满足此要求，也应考虑癌症复发的风险，而候选资格应基于多学科

# 第13章 非同种异体肺移植的并发症

决策。另外，对于某些恶性肿瘤，如局限性前列腺癌或非黑色素瘤皮肤癌，2年无病间隔时间结合预测癌症复发低风险的患者可能是合理的。除了在囊性纤维化（CF）人群中进行结直肠癌筛查外，没有专门针对肺移植后癌症筛查的指南。通常使用恶性肿瘤的一般筛查指南进行筛查（表 13-4）。表 13-4 总结了在肺移植前后期通常实施的恶性肿瘤筛查建议。许多移植中心每年进行 1 次胸部 CT 扫描以常规评估移植肺，也可作为肺癌筛查，特别是在进行 SLT 的患者中。

表 13-4 癌症筛查建议[a]

| 癌症 | 条件 | 筛查建议 |
| --- | --- | --- |
| 乳腺癌 | 女性，50~74 岁 | 每 2 年做 1 次乳房 X 线检查 |
| 宫颈癌 | < 21 岁 | 不用筛查 |
| | 21~29 岁 | 每 3 年做 1 次宫颈细胞学检查 |
| | 30~65 岁 | 每 3 年做 1 次宫颈细胞学检查或每 5 年做 1 次 hrHPV 检测或每 5 年做 1 次 hrHPV 宫颈细胞学检查 |
| | > 65 岁 | 不用筛查 |
| 结直肠癌 | 年龄 < 60 岁有 CRC 或晚期息肉的直系亲属或任何年龄有 2 个以上有 CRC 或晚期息肉的直系亲属 | 40 岁或在最年轻的患病亲属患病之前进行 10 年的时间结肠镜检查，以较早者为准 |
| | 45~49 岁 | 可能建议进行结肠镜检查 |
| | 50~75 岁 | 每 10 年做 1 次结肠镜检查[b] |
| | CF 移植前 | 结肠镜检查从 40 岁开始<br>每 5 年重新筛查 1 次<br>所有腺瘤性息肉每 3 年复查 1 次 |
| | CF 移植后 | 年龄 ≥ 30 岁，术后 2 年内进行结肠镜检查，过去 5 年内结肠镜检查均为阴性<br>每 5 年复查 1 次<br>所有需要重新筛查的腺瘤性息肉每 3 年复查 1 次 |

注：CF，囊性纤维化；CRC，结直肠癌；hrHPV，高危人类乳头瘤病毒
[a] 本表不包括特殊情况，如患有易患恶性肿瘤的遗传疾病的患者。某些恶性肿瘤如前列腺癌、肝癌、卵巢癌或胰腺癌筛查不推荐在普通人群中进行
[b] 结肠镜检查在检测结直肠癌和息肉以及切除病灶方面灵敏度最高。因此，与其他筛查方式相比，在器官移植前后进行结肠镜检查是首选
参考文献 [76-79] 中的数据

应常规进行移植前的教育和筛查。对于皮肤癌的风险评估，最近的德尔菲小组推荐使用基于证据的风险分层工具对候选者进行风险分层，并由皮肤科医生对移植患者进行全身检查[63]。一个基于证据的皮肤癌筛查工具示例是皮肤和紫外线肿瘤移植风险评估计算器（Skin and Ultraviolet Neoplasia Transplant Risk Assessment Calculator，SUNTRAC）。其已被开发用于基于种族、年龄、性别、既往皮肤癌史和器官移植类型对患者进行风险分层。SUNTRAC 工具将患者分为低风险到非常高风险的 4 个等级。该类风险分层可能会帮助临床医生根据每个患者皮肤癌发展的风险制定皮肤癌筛查计划[64]。

应建议患者使用防晒系数≥30的防晒霜，穿着足够覆盖身体的衣物，戴帽子和太阳镜，使其有常规的自我检查意识，并至少 1 年看一次皮肤科医生[53,54]。EBV D+/R- 血清状态的 PTLD 患者应密切进行 EBV 病毒载量监测。可能的情况下，应考虑使用低强度免疫抑制剂，尤其是在有 EBV 病毒血症的人中。更昔洛韦预防性治疗可以将 PTLD 风险降低至 83%[65]。

## 13.7.6 评估与治疗

### 13.7.6.1 皮肤癌

在确诊为皮肤癌的患者中，通常会采取降低免疫抑制强度的方法，但应始终与移植物排斥反应的风险相权衡。在癌前或早期非侵袭性皮肤癌中，可用切除术或破坏性技术进行治疗，如莫氏手术。其他治疗方法包括局部治疗和全身治疗。应采用多学科方法，在必要时尽早让皮肤科、肿瘤学和外科专家参与，并进行密切监测，以确保最佳结果。应对患者是否有复发或转移性疾病进行监测（图 13-2）。

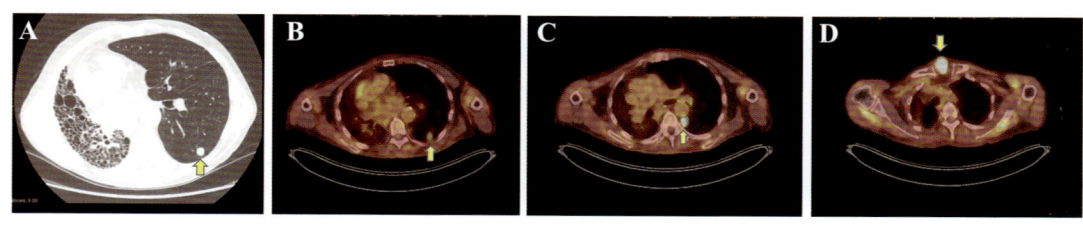

图 13-2 转移性皮肤 SCC

注：（A）胸部 CT 扫描，同种异体移植物左下叶有圆形肺结节；（B）PET 扫描显示结节 FDG 亲和力；（C）另一个 FDG 常见的肺结节，紧临降主动脉；（D）胸骨上方区域的一个体积大的明显的 FDG 皮下 SCC 肿块

### 13.7.6.2 移植后淋巴增生性疾病

PTLD 有多种表现。非特异性全身症状包括发热、疲劳和体重减轻。在胸腔内的 PTLD 可能会观察到单个或多个肺结节、肿块或肺叶实变以及胸腔积液。其他体征和症状取决于受累器官（图 13-3）[54]。例如，肺部受累时出现新发咳嗽，胃肠道 PTLD 时表现为便秘伴腹痛，中枢神经系统疾病时出现意识改变或局灶性神经学体征，或者膀胱 PTLD 时出现尿毒症（图 13-4）[54,66]。PTLD 的一般管理方法包括谨慎降低免疫抑制（通常是停用细胞周期抑制剂）、使用利妥昔单抗的抗 B 细胞疗法、化疗和放疗[67,68]。PTLD 的有效治疗需要移植和肿瘤团队的密切合作[54]。

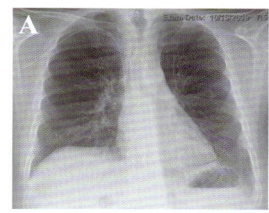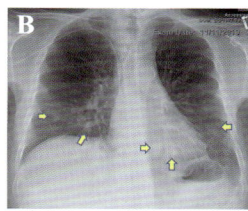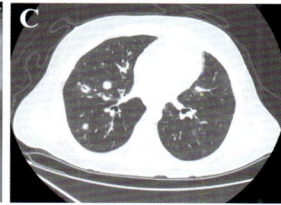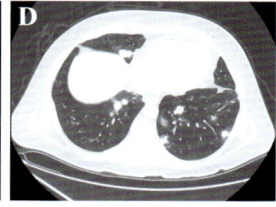

图 13-3　肺移植第一年内的胸腔 B 细胞 PTLD

注：（A）基线胸部 X 线检查，无肺结节；（B）基线胸部 X 线检查 4 周后观察到轻微的双侧肺结节性混浊（黄色箭头）；（C，D）胸部 CT 扫描显示双侧不同形状和大小的肺结节

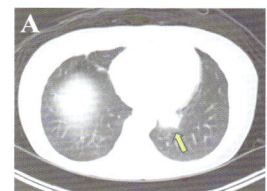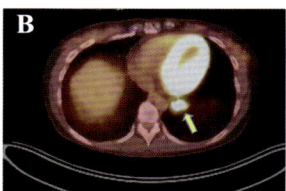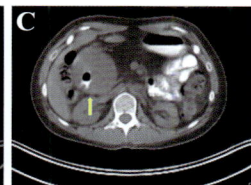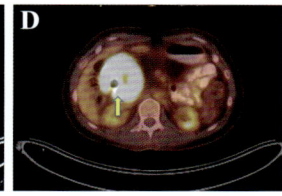

图 13-4　肺移植后 8 年 T 细胞 PTLD 合并肺和胃肠道受累导致十二指肠梗阻

注：（A）胸部 CT 扫描显示左下叶心旁肺肿块；（B）PET 扫描显示该肿块的 FDG 亲和力；（C）腹部 CT 扫描显示十二指肠第二部分周围的软组织肿块；（D）十二指肠肿块在 PET 扫描上显示出强烈的 FDG 亲和力

### 13.7.6.3 肺癌

广义来说，肺癌分为小细胞肺癌和非小细胞肺癌。这 2 种类型都可能出现全身症状（如厌食、乏力和体重减轻），或出现肺部症状（包括新发咳嗽、呼吸困难、胸痛），或罕见的咯血。其也可能表现为无症状，常规胸部 X 线片中偶然发现肺结节或淋巴结肿大（图 13-5）[54]。在免疫抑制的影响下，肺癌通常进展迅速，这种快速进展有时可能会与感染[69,70]相似。移植患者肺癌的诊断和分期策略与非移植人群相同，但可能会由于移

**肺移植：胸外科临床问题**

植时的淋巴结切除而受到限制[54]。尽可能尝试根治性切除。化疗的选择受到受者并发症的限制，在免疫检查点抑制剂的情况下，排斥反应的风险增加[54]。与 PTLD 和皮肤癌一样，肺癌患者通常会减少免疫抑制，尽管其益处并不清楚[50,54]。

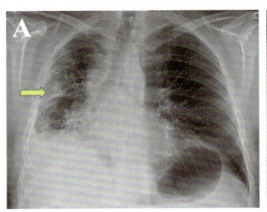 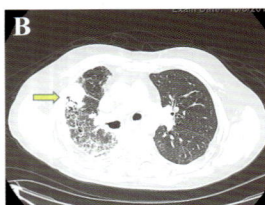 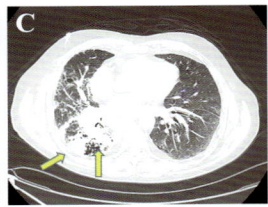 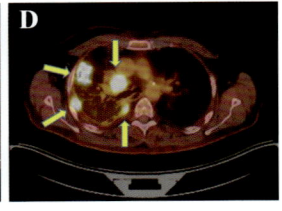

图 13-5　原生肺中的非小细胞支气管肺癌

注：（A）胸部 X 线片显示，纤维化的原生肺出现一个新的外围不透明的三角形；（B）胸部 CT 扫描证实周围肿块病变；（C）在同一胸部 CT 上，右下叶中央和外周可见其他肿块；（D）PET 扫描显示多发性高代谢性肺部病变和纵隔腺病

## 13.8　总　结

总体而言，肺移植后患者的排斥和感染是主要的问题，但很可能还有许多医疗并发症，并需要多学科合作进行科学细致的管理。长期暴露于免疫抑制剂环境中可能会加剧现有疾病，导致新的急性和慢性疾病的发展，并增加恶性肿瘤发生的风险。这些并发症会对（肺移植患者的）短期和长期预后产生负面影响，且这种影响独立于移植肺的健康状况。

【临床护理要点】

- 肺移植后糖尿病的诊断应在患者处于稳定状态且正在接受维持性免疫抑制治疗阶段时[3,4]进行。
- 糖化血红蛋白 A1C 在诊断肺移植后糖尿病方面的敏感性降低，尤其是在移植后第一年[3,4]。
- 胰岛素是肺移植后高血糖的主要治疗方法，早期开始治疗可以预防真性的糖尿病的发展[4,6]。
- 口服降糖药仅在患者接受稳定维持性免疫抑制治疗时使用[4]。
- 抗高血压药物对于移植后的患者通常是安全的。药物的选择主要取决于其他临床情况。例如，在液体超负荷的情况下使用利尿剂，在房性心律失常的情况下使用β受体阻滞剂，或使用二氢吡啶类钙通道阻滞剂来缓解CNI的血管收缩效应[13,17]。

- 钙通道阻滞剂，尤其是非二氢吡啶类，可能会增加CNI的水平，其使用需要密切监测并进行CNI剂量调整。
- 肺移植后患者的高脂血症管理基于ASCVD风险，与一般人群类似，使用AHA/ACC推荐的相同的指南，但应特别注意避免药物相互作用[23]。
- 可以依赖诱导治疗延迟开始肺移植受者CNI治疗，尤其是在肺移植后发生AKI的情况下[28,46]。
- 进行药物管理以确保适当的围手术期和移植后药物剂量[29]。
- 密切监测尿量至关重要，因为其是肾功能不全的最早迹象，并可以提醒医疗团队尽早修改管理策略[28,37,41,71]。
- 肺移植术后早期的肾脏损伤可能会影响长期肾功能[27,47,48]。
- 恶性肿瘤是存活超过5年的肺移植受者中，继细支气管炎闭塞性综合征之后的第二大常见死因[1]。
- 皮肤癌，特别是鳞状细胞癌，是肺移植后受者中最常见的癌症[52]。
- 大多数移植后淋巴增生性疾病在移植后第一年内发生，在接受EBV血清阳性供者肺器官的EBV血清阴性患者中更为常见[58]。
- 建议囊性纤维化患者在40岁开始结肠镜检查（移植前），并在30岁前（且不晚于术后2年）进行结肠镜筛查（移植术后）[72]。
- 在移植护理的所有阶段，应常规使用基于证据的指南和工具（如SUNTRAC计算器）进行恶性肿瘤风险、预防策略和恶性肿瘤筛查的教育[53,54,62,63]。

## 声明

作者没有与此项目有关的任何商业、金融利益或资金冲突。

## 参考文献

1. Chambers DC, Cherikh WS, Harhay MO. The international thoracic organ transplant registry of the international society for heart and lung transplantation: thirty-sixth adult lung and heartlung transplantation report – 2019; focus theme: donor and recipient size match. J Heart Lung Transplant 2019;38(10):1042–1055.
2. Hackman KL, Snell GI, Back LA. Prevalence and predictors of diabetes after lung transplantation: a prospective, longitudinal study. Diabetes Care 2014;37(11):2919–2925.
3. Sharif A, Hecking M, Vries APJ. Proceedings from an international consensus meeting on posttransplantation diabetes mellitus: recommendations and future directions. Am J Transplant 2014;14(9):1992–2000.
4. Classification and Diagnosis of Diabetes. Standards of Medical Care in Diabetes—2021. Diabetes Care 2021;44:S15–33.
5. Vincenti F, Friman S, Scheuermann E. Results of an international, randomized trial comparing glucose metabolism disorders and outcome with cyclosporine versus tacrolimus. Am J Transplant 2007;7(6). 1606-1514.
6. Hecking M, Haidinger M, Döller D. Early basal insulin therapy decreases new-onset diabetes after renal transplantation. J Am Soc Nephrol 2012;23(4): 739–749.
7. Kurian B, Joshi R, Helmuth A. Effectiveness and long-term safety of thiazolidinediones and metformin in renal transplant recipients. Endocr Pract 2008; 14(8):979–984.
8. Halden TAS, Åsberg A, Vik K. Short-term efficacy and safety of sitagliptin treatment in long-term stable renal recipients with new-onset diabetes after transplantation. Nephrol Dial Transplant 2014;29(4): 926–33.
9. Peled Y, Ram E, Lavee J. Hypomagnesemia is associated with new-onset diabetes mellitus following heart transplantation. Cardiovasc Diabetol 2019; 18(1):132.
10. Yusen RD, Edwards LB, Dipchand AI. The registry of the international society for heart and lung transplantation: thirty-third adult lung and heart-lung transplant report – 2016; focus theme: primary diagnostic indications for transplant. J Heart Lung Transplant 2016;35(10):1170–1184.
11. Whelton PK, Carey RM, Aronow WS. ACC/AHA/AAPA/ABC/ACPM/AGS/APhA/ASH/ASPC/NMA/PCNA guideline for the prevention, detection, evaluation, and management of high blood pressure in adults: executive summary: a report of the american college of cardiology/american heart association task force onclinical practice guidelines. Hypertension 2017;71(6):1269–1324.
12. Weir MR, Burgess ED, Cooper JE. Assessment and management of hypertension in transplant patients. J Am Soc Nephrol 2015;26. Published online June.
13. Fan J, K Z, S L. Incidence, risk factors and prognosis of postoperative atrial arrhythmias after lung transplantation: a systematic review and meta-analysis. Interact Cardiovasc Thorac Surg 2016;23(5): 790–799.
14. Lertjitbanjong P, Thongprayoon C, Cheungpasitporn W, et al. Acute kidney injury after lung transplantation: a systematic review and meta-analysis. J Clin Monit 2019;8(10):1713. https://doi.org/10.3390/jcm8101713.
15. Heinze G, Mitterbauer C, Regele H. Angiotensin-converting enzyme inhibitor or angiotensin II type 1 receptor antagonist therapy is associated with prolonged patient and graft survival after renal transplantation. J Am Soc Nephrol 2006;17(3): 889–899.
16. Opelz G, Zeier M, Laux G. No improvement of patient or graft survival in transplant recipients treated with

angiotensin-converting enzyme inhibitors or angiotensin II type 1 receptor blockers: a collaborative transplant study report. J Am Soc Nephrol 2006; 17(11):3257–3262.

17. Grzésk G, Wiciński M, Malinowski B. Calcium blockers inhibit cyclosporine A-induced hyperreactivity of vascular smooth muscle cells. Mol Med Rep 2012;5(6):1469–1474.

18. Khan S, Khan I, Novak M. The concomitant use of atorvastatin and amlodipine leading to rhabdomyolysis. Cureus 2018;10(1):e2020.

19. Reed RM, Hashmi S, Eberlein M, et al. Impact of lung transplantation on serum lipids in COPD. Respir Med 2011;105(12):1961–1968.

20. Estimator ASCVDR. ; 2021. Available at: https://tools.acc.org/ldl/ascvd_risk_estimator/index.html/calulate/estimator/.

21. Stephany BR, Alao B, Budev M. Hyperlipidemia is associated with accelerated chronic kidney disease progression after lung transplantation. Am J Transplant 2007;7(11):2553–2560.

22. Barn K, Laftavi M, Pierce D. Low levels of highdensity lipoprotein cholesterol: an independent risk factor for late adverse cardiovascular events in renal transplant recipients. Transpl Int 2010;23(6):574–579.

23. Grundy SM, Stone NJ, Bailey AL. AHA/ACC/AACVPR/AAPA/ABC/ACPM/ADA/AGS/APhA/ASPC/NLA/PCNA guideline on the management of blood cholesterol: executive summary. Circulation 2018; 139(25):1082–1143.

24. Migliozzi DR, Asal NJ. Clinical controversy in transplantation: tacrolimus versus cyclosporine in statin drug interactions. Ann Pharmacother 2020;54(2): 171–177.

25. Uyanik-Uenal K, Stoegerer-Lanzenberger M, Auersperg K. Treatment of Therapy-resistant hyperlipidemia after heart transplant with PCSK9-inhibitors. J Heart Lung Transplant 2019;38(4):S213–214.

26. Hingorani S. Chronic kidney disease after liver, cardiac, lung, heart–lung, and hematopoietic stem cell transplant. Pediatr Nephrol 2008;23(6):879–888.

27. Ishani A, Erturk S, Hertz MI, et al. Predictors of renal function following lung or heart-lung transplantation. Kidney Int 2002;61(6):2228–2234.

28. Puttarajappa CM, Bernardo JF, Kellum JA. Renal complications following lung transplantation and heart transplantation. Crit Care Clin 2019;35(1):61–73.

29. Du WW, Wang XX, Zhang D, et al. Retrospective analysis on incidence and risk factors of early onset acute kidney injury after lung transplantation and its association with mortality. Ren Fail 2021;43(1): 535–542.

30. Xue J, Wang L, Chen CM, et al. Acute kidney injury influences mortality in lung transplantation. Ren Fail 2014;36(4):541–545.

31. Rocha PN, Rocha AT, Palmer SM, et al. Acute renal failure after lung transplantation: incidence, predictors and impact on perioperative morbidity and mortality. Am J Transplant 2005;5(6):1469–1476.

32. Jacques F, El-Hamamsy I, Fortier A, et al. Acute renal failure following lung transplantation: risk factors, mortality, and long-term consequences. Eur J Cardio-Thoracic Surg 2011. https://doi.org/10.1016/j.ejcts.2011.04.034.

33. Logan AT, Casale JP, Doligalski CT. Early acute kidney injury in lung transplantation is associated with significant mortality. The J Heart Lung Transplant 2016;35(4):S235.

34. Fidalgo P, Ahmed M, Meyer SR, et al. Incidence and outcomes of acute kidney injury following orthotopic

lung transplantation: a population-based cohort study. Nephrol Dial Transplant 2014;29(9):1702–1709. https://doi.org/10.1093/ndt/gfu226.

35. Valapour M, Lehr CJ, Skeans MA, et al. OPTN/SRTR 2019 Annual data report: lung. Am J Transplant 2021;21(S2):441–520.
36. Atchade E, Barour S, Tran-Dinh A, et al. Acute kidney injury after lung transplantation: perioperative risk factors and outcome. Transplant Proc 2020; 52(3):967–976.
37. Banga A, Mohanka M, Mullins J, et al. Characteristics and outcomes among patients with need for early dialysis after lung transplantation surgery. Clin Transplant 2017;31(11):e13106. https://doi.org/10.1111/ctr.13106.
38. Osho AA, Castleberry AW, Snyder LD, et al. Assessment of different threshold preoperative glomerular filtration rates as markers of outcomes in lung transplantation. The Ann Thorac Surg 2014;98(1):283–290.
39. Barraclough K, Menahem S, Bailey M, et al. Predictors of decline in renal function after lung transplantation. J Heart Lung Transplant 2006;25(12):1431–1435.
40. Yerokun BA, Mulvihill MS, Osho AA, et al. Simultaneous or sequential lung-kidney transplantation confer superior survival in renal-failure patients undergoing lung transplantation: a national analysis. J Heart Lung Transplant 2017;36(4):S95.
41. Jin K, Murugan R, Sileanu FE, et al. Intensive monitoring of urine output is associated with increased detection of acute kidney injury and improved outcomes. Chest 2017;152(5):972–979.
42. Wehbe E, Brock R, Budev M, et al. Short-term and long-term outcomes of acute kidney injury after lung transplantation. J Heart Lung Transplant 2012; 31(3):244–251.
43. Pattison JM, Petersen J, Kuo P, et al. The incidence of renal failure in one hundred consecutive heart-lung transplant recipients. Am J Kidney Dis 1995; 26(4):643–648.
44. Kunst H, Thompson D, Hodson M. Hypertension as a marker for later development of end-stage renal failure after lung and heart-lung transplantation: a cohort study. J Heart Lung Transplant 2004;23(10): 1182–1188.
45. Esposito C, De Mauri A, Vitulo P, et al. Risk factors for chronic renal dysfunction in lung transplant recipients. Transplantation 2007;84(12):1701–1703.
46. Naesens M, Kuypers DRJ, Sarwal M. Calcineurin inhibitor nephrotoxicity. Clin J Am Soc Nephrol 2009; 4(2):481–508.
47. Ivulich S, Westall G, Dooley M, et al. The evolution of lung transplant immunosuppression. Drugs 2018; 78(10):965–982.
48. Canales M, Youssef P, Spong R, et al. Predictors of chronic kidney disease in long-term survivors of lung and heart-lung transplantation. Am J Transplant 2006;6(9):2157–2163.
49. Engels EA, Pfeiffer RM, Fraumeni JF. Spectrum of cancer risk among U. S. solid organ transplant recipients: The transplant cancer match study. J Am Med Assoc 2011;306(17):1891–1901.
50. Shtraichman O, Ahya VN. Malignancy after lung transplantation. Ann Transl Med 2020;8(6):416. https://doi.org/10.21037/atm. 2020. 02. 126.
51. Cangemi M, Montico B, Faè DA. Dissecting the multiplicity of immune effects of immunosuppressive drugs to better predict the risk of de novo malignancies in solid organ transplant patients. Front Oncol 2019;9. Published online March.

52. Rashtak S, Dierkhising RA, Kremers WK. Incidence and risk factors for skin cancer following lung transplantation. J Am Acad Dermatol 2015;72(1):92–98.
53. Tejwani V, Deshwal H, Ho B, et al. Cutaneous complications in recipients of lung transplants. Chest 2019;155(1):178–193.
54. Benvenuto L, Aversa M, Arcasoy SM. Malignancy following lung transplantation. In: Reference module in biomedical sciences. Elsevier; 2021. https://doi.org/10.1016/B978-0-08-102723-3.00120-7. B9780081027233001000.
55. Abbasi NR, Shaw HM, Rigel DS, et al. Early diagnosis of cutaneous melanoma: revisiting the ABCD criteria. J Am Med Assoc 2004;292(22):2771–2776.
56. Mittal A, Colegio OR. Skin cancers in organ transplant recipients. Am J Transplant 2017;17(10): 2509–2530.
57. Carucci JA, Martinez JC, Zeitouni NC, et al. InTransit metastasis from primary cutaneous squamous cell carcinoma in organ transplant recipients and nonimmunosuppressed patients: clinical characteristics, management, and outcome in a series of 21 patients. Dermatol Surg 2004;30(4p2):651–655.
58. Courtwright AM, Burkett P, Divo M. Posttransplant lymphoproliferative disorders in epstein-barr virus donor positive/recipient negative lung transplant recipients. Ann Thorac Surg 2018;105(2):441–447.
59. Cheng J, Moore CA, Iasella CJ. Systematic review and meta-analysis of post-transplant lymphoproliferative disorder in lung transplant recipients. Clin Transplant 2018;32(5):e13235.
60. Neuringer IP. posttransplant lymphoproliferative disease after lung transplantation. Clin Dev Immunol 2013;2013:1–11.
61. Triplette M, Crothers K, Mahale P. Risk of lung cancer in lung transplant recipients in the United States. Am J Transplant 2019;19(5):1478–1490.
62. Weill D, Benden C, Corris PA, et al. A consensus document for the selection of lung transplant candidates: 2014—an update from the pulmonary transplantation council of the international society for heart and lung Transplantation. J Heart Lung Transplant 2015;34(1):1–15.
63. Crow LD, Jambusaria-Pahlajani A, Chung CL, et al. Initial skin cancer screening for solid organ transplant recipients in the United States: Delphi method development of expert consensus guidelines. Transpl Int 2019;32(12):1268–1276.
64. Jambusaria-Pahlajani A, Crow LD, Lowenstein S, et al. Predicting skin cancer in organ transplant recipients: development of the SUNTRAC screening tool using data from a multicenter cohort study. Transpl Int 2019;32(12):1259–1267.
65. Funch DP, Walker AM, Schneider G. Ganciclovir and acyclovir reduce the risk of post-transplant lymphoproliferative disorder in renal transplant recipients. Am J Transplant 2005;5(12):2894–2900.
66. Grewal HS, Lane C, Highland KB, et al. Post-transplant lymphoproliferative disorder of the bladder in a lung transplant recipient. Oxford Med Case Rep 2018;2018(3).
67. Trappe R, Oertel S, Leblond V, et al. Sequential treatment with rituximab followed by CHOP chemotherapy in adult B-cell post-transplant lymphoproliferative disorder (PTLD): the prospective international multicentre phase 2 PTLD-1 trial. Lancet Oncol 2012;13(2):196–206.
68. Choquet S. Efficacy and safety of rituximab in B-cell post-transplantation lymphoproliferative disorders: results of a prospective multicenter phase 2 study. Blood 2006;107(8):3053–3057.

69. Arcasoy SM, Hersh C, Christie JD, et al. Bronchogenic carcinoma complicating lung transplantation. J Heart Lung Transplant 2001;20(10): 1044–1053.
70. Grewal AS, Padera RF, Boukedes S, et al. Prevalence and outcome of lung cancer in lung transplant recipients. Respir Med 2015;109(3):427–433.
71. Ollech JE, Kramer MR, Peled N. Post-transplant diabetes mellitus in lung transplant recipients: incidence and risk factors. Eur J Cardiothorac Surg 2008;33(5):844–848.
72. Maldonado F, Tapia G, Ardiles L. Early hyperglycemia: a risk factor for posttransplant diabetes mellitus among renal transplant recipients. Transplant Proc 2009;41(6):2664–2667.
73. Hjelmesæth J, Sagedal S, Hartmann A. Asymptomatic cytomegalovirus infection is associated with increased risk of new-onset diabetes mellitus and impaired insulin release after renal transplantation. Diabetologia 2004;47(9):1550–1556.
74. Shaukat A, Kahi CJ, Burke CA. ACG clinical guidelines: colorectal cancer screening 2021. Am J Gastroenterol 2021;116(3):458–479.
75. Siu AL, USPST Force. Screening for breast cancer:u. s. preventive service task force recommendation statement. Ann Intern Med 2016;164(4):279–296.
76. Curry SJ, Krist AH, Owens DK. Screening for cervical cancer: us preventive service task force recommendation statement. J Am Med Assoc 2018; 320(7):674–686.
77. Bibbins-Domingo K, Grossman DC, Curry SJ. Screening for colorectal cancer: us preventive services task force recommendation statement. J Am Med Assoc 2016;315(23):2564–2575.
78. Bennett D, Fossi A, Marchetti L, et al. Postoperative acute kidney injury in lung transplant recipients. Interact Cardiovasc Thorac Surg 2019;28(6): 929–935.
79. Hadjiliadis D, Khoruts A, Zauber AG, et al. Cystic fibrosis colorectal cancer screening consensus recommendations. Gastroenterology 2018;154(3):736–745. e14.

# 第 14 章 肺再移植

Eriberto Michel, Matthew Galen Hartwig, Wiebke Sommer 著

杨燕华 译

周建平 校

【关键词】
- 肺移植 • 再移植 • 重做肺移植 • 慢性同种异体肺移植物功能障碍

【要点】
- 急性移植物衰竭、慢性同种异体肺移植物功能障碍和气道并发症是肺再移植的适应证。
- 仔细筛选受者和供者对于获得满意的患者治疗结果至关重要。
- 微创手术技术前景广阔，但进行安全手术操作才是最终和最重要的目标。
- 随着时间的推移，肺再移植的结果有所改善，某些受者的结果与第一次肺移植相当。

## 14.1 背　景

随着 Hardy 及其同事于 1963 年在密西西比大学进行了第一例人类肺移植（LTx）手术，并在 20 世纪 80 年代进行了首次成功的系列手术，肺移植在患有终末期肺病患者中的临床应用不断发展和扩大。遗憾的是，急性移植物衰竭和慢性肺同种异体移植物功能障碍（CLAD）仍然很常见，移植物衰竭是长期生存最重要的限制。再移植肺是治疗不可逆的同种异体肺移植物衰竭的唯一方法。再移植最初的报道令人沮丧，因为其显示接受早期再移植的患者生存率较低，并且在术后几年内同种异体移植肺功能下降[1,2]。幸运的是，更多的近期的报道显示结果有所改善，从而导致肺再移植的需求不断增加[3]（图14-1）。

# 肺移植：胸外科临床问题

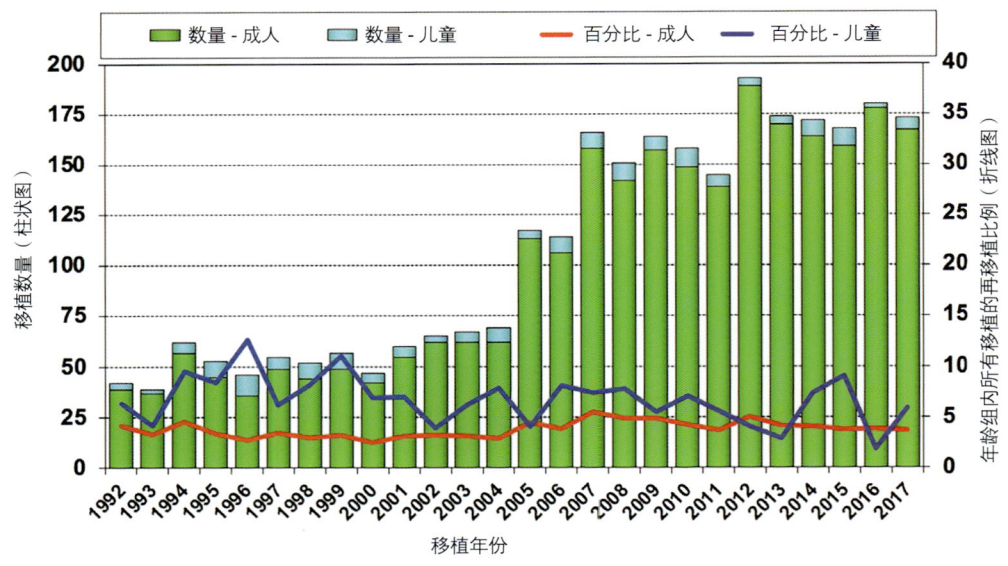

**图 14-1** 按年份和年龄组划分的成人和儿童肺再移植情况

注：来自国际心肺移植协会。国际胸腔器官移植（TTX）登记数据幻灯片。2019 年幻灯片：肺移植总体统计数据。https://ishlt.org/research-data/registries/ttx-registry/ttx-registry-slides

CLAD 是晚期死亡和再移植指征的最常见原因，约 40% 的首次肺同种异体移植物会在 5 年内出现这种情况[4]。尽管 CLAD 很常见，但肺移植的中位生存率仍维持在 6 年左右，在当今时代肺再移植仅占所有肺移植的 4%，多年来该比例没有明显变化[5]。患有 CLAD 的受者数量与最终接受再次肺移植的受者数量之间的差距可能反映了受者、医疗保健系统、临床结果和伦理等综合因素。

## 14.2 肺再移植的指征

导致原发性肺移植受者同种异体移植物衰竭的主要情况有 3 种：继发于原发性移植物功能不全（PGD）的急性移植物衰竭、CLAD 和术后气道并发症[6,7]。

### 14.2.1 急性移植物衰竭

由于广泛的缺血 / 再灌注损伤，首次肺移植后可能会发生 PGD。超急性同种异体移植排斥尽管不常见，但可导致早期急性同种异体移植物衰竭。急性同种异体移植物功能障碍通常是自限性的，不会导致移植物衰竭。因此，许多中心避免紧急再移植，将其保留为特殊情况下的挽救生命的措施。

然而，无论病因如何，早期肺再移植的结果始终较差，其 1 年生存率低于 50%[7-10]。严重急性移植物衰竭的治疗，通常本质上是支持性治疗，即延长机械通气、镇静和（或）体外膜肺氧合（ECMO）支持。早期再移植受者由于长期机械通气、镇静、瘫痪和 ICU 相关操作、与免疫抑制和血流动力学不稳定相关的肾功能衰竭以及其他终末器官损伤（如缺血性胆管病、肠缺血等）而面临感染并发症的风险更高。这些众多因素进一步增加了后续干预的风险，从而增加了并发症发生的风险。同样地，在临床实践中往往难以判断早期移植物衰竭是否已不可逆，从而导致再次移植的决定被延迟，直至出现多器官系统衰竭。因此，除特殊情况外，许多中心都会避免因急性移植物衰竭而进行紧急再移植。

### 14.2.2 慢性同种异体肺移植物功能障碍

大多数接受肺再移植的受者都患有首次同种异体移植物的慢性排斥反应。CLAD 可进一步分为阻塞性同种异体移植功能障碍［闭塞性细支气管炎综合征（BOS）］和限制性表型（rCLAD）［限制性同种异体移植综合征（RAS）］。CLAD 的表型对病程以及肺再移植后的预后具有重大影响，在决定是否进行再移植时应予以考虑。

CLAD 的特点是 $FEV_1$ 从移植后基线值持续下降（≥ 20%），基线值定义为术后 2 次最佳测量值的平均值。BOS 影响大约 70% 的 CLAD 患者出现由小气道纤维闭塞引起的进行性气流阻塞。BOS 在放射影像学中通常不显示肺部浸润，并且病程差异很大[11,12]（图 14-2）。在经验丰富的中心，肺再移植后的 BOS 预后已被证明与初次肺移植相似[7,12]。

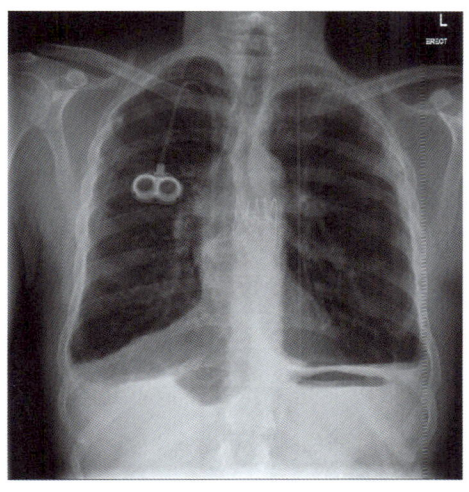

**图 14-2** 双侧肺移植后患有闭塞性细支气管炎综合征的患者的胸部 X 线检查
注：胸部 X 线检查未显示明显的肺野浸润和膈肌扁平，提示肺过度充气

RAS 表现为持续的放射学浸润和胸膜增厚、FEV$_1$、FVC 下降以及总肺容量下降（图 14-3）。在疾病发展过程中，可能会出现间质网状阴影和牵拉性支气管扩张[13]。RAS 的肺部组织学通常显示肺胸膜实质弹力纤维增生和肺泡间隔结构中有胶原沉积[14]。RAS 通常显示出更快的疾病进展，发病后的中位生存期是 BOS 患者的一半[15]。同样，在肺再移植病例中，RAS 的生存率也不如 BOS[12]。

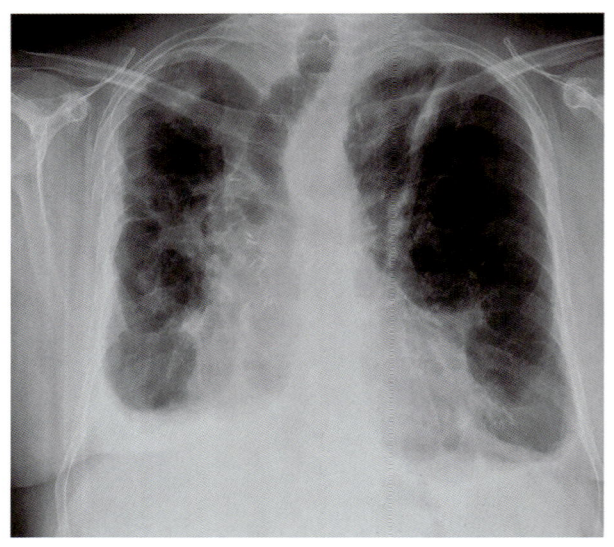

图 14-3　双侧肺移植后出现限制性同种异体移植综合征 (rCLAD) 的患者的胸部 X 线检查
注：胸部 X 线检查显示典型的胸膜增厚、间质网状阴影和气管移位

多项报告表明，少数患者会发展为混合型 CLAD，同时具有阻塞性和限制性的特点，伴或不伴放射学表现，如肺实质浸润和(或)胸膜增厚[16]。由于缺乏可靠的药物治疗，对于纯表型和混合表型的患者，肺再移植仍然是晚期 CLAD 的唯一选择[12]。

### 14.2.3 气道并发症

肺移植后支气管吻合术的并发症并不常见，但如果并发症严重导致支气管镜和传统手术治疗失败时，可能需要再次移植。严重气道并发症（包括狭窄和裂开）的总体发生率在不同中心之间存在 1.5%~13% 的差异[7,17,18]。总体而言，严重气道并发症的发生率随着时间的推移而下降，其原因很可能是手术技术的改进和支气管内治疗选择。最近的报道显示，因支气管并发症导致的肺再移植数量大幅减少，显示出良好的中长期效果[7,17]。

## 14.3 肺再移植患者的评估和选择

肺再移植患者的选择对于获得可接受的结果至关重要，并且必须考虑围术期死亡的风险。此外，还应考虑供体器官稀缺的伦理困境，在评估肺再移植患者时需要多学科团队有更广泛的视角。

一般来说，再移植患者的选择应采用与初次肺移植相同的标准[19]。因此，恶性肿瘤、严重晚期非肺部疾病和不受控制的感染通常是再移植肺的禁忌证。应特别注意患者对既往药物治疗的总体依从性。再移植前的总体临床状态是一个重要的考虑因素，因为与在医院等待的患者相比，在家中等待再移植的患者无论有或没有机械支持，都明显有更好的结果[12]。CLAD 表型是肺再移植术后生存率相关的决定因素，RAS 和 BOS 患者的生存率不同。与 BOS 受者相比，在 RAS 患者中，BMI 较低对生存有负面影响[12]。相反，在大型 SRTR 登记分析中，需要再移植的肥胖患者（BMI > 29.9）的术后生存率较低[20]。初次移植后第一年内的早期再移植以及急性排斥反应和 PGD 的诊断与术后生存率较差有关[5,6,21-23]。同样，需要术前机械通气和（或）体外生命支持桥接进行再移植的患者的生存率甚至更差[3,6,7,24]。

虽然一项登记研究（UNOS）显示，对需要 ECMO 桥接肺再移植的受者，随着时间的推移，用于桥接目的的体外支持的使用总体增加，但与无需 ECMO 桥接再移植相比，ECMO 桥接再移植后的 90 天和 1 年生存率显著较低。术前高血清胆红素、ICU 住院、机械通气和 PGD 均与 ECMO 队列中死亡率较高相关。因此，采用体外生命支持桥接策略的再移植与死亡率显著增加相关，必须极其谨慎地考虑[20]。此外，年龄（特别是 65 岁以上）以及终末器官功能障碍［如慢性肾功能衰竭（GFR < 50~60 mL/min）］已被确定为术后死亡率和 1 年生存率降低的其他重要独立危险因素[25,26]。由于普遍使用钙调神经磷酸酶抑制作为标准维持免疫疗法，肾功能在再移植环境中几乎都是受损的。肺再移植手术类型（单侧 vs. 双侧）也已在多篇出版物中进行了分析，结果不一[6,10,21,22,27,28]。最后，多次肺再移植的结果特别差[22,23]。

## 14.4 肺再移植的免疫学方面

初次肺移植对受者来说是一次免疫事件，导致同种异体反应性记忆 T 细胞的存在，该细胞可能在抗原再暴露时转化为效应 T 细胞，并具有引发同种异体移植排斥反应的能力[29]。

### 14.4.1 供体选择

在存在预先形成的人类白细胞抗原（HLA）抗体的情况下选择供体，需要对供体进行 HLA 分型以及循环 HLA 抗体分型以识别潜在的供体特异性[30,31]。使用供体 HLA 进行虚拟交叉配型分型和受者的 HLA 抗体分型可以预测供体 - 受者的兼容性。因此，在选择致敏受者的供体时，必须充分了解供体完整的 HLA 分型，以避免交叉配型阳性移植。在受者体内缺乏循环 HLA 抗体的情况下，选择与第一个肺捐献者的 HLA 类型不同的供体可能不会影响术后结果。因此，在供体 - 受者匹配期间无需避免此类供体[32]。

### 14.4.2 免疫敏感的受者

已知先前存在的循环 HLA 抗体会通过与不匹配的 HLA 结合而引起超急性排斥反应，从而导致术后早期或甚至在手术台上突然出现移植物衰竭，并伴有出血性肺水肿和严重的实质浸润[33,34]。因此，检测移植前现有的 HLA 抗体对于初次移植和再移植至关重要。目前的诊断标准是使用固相测定进行定期血清筛查，该测定使用单一抗原珠来确定抗体的类型。建议在再移植前常规进行重新检测，尤其是在输血等免疫事件之后[35]。选择供体时，其 HLA 谱应避免受者中预先形成供体特异性抗体。免疫敏感的受者在移植后发生严重 PGD、急性细胞排斥反应（ACR）和抗体介导的排斥反应（AMR）的风险较高，会对生存率产生负面影响[36-39]。术前脱敏方案包括治疗性血浆置换、静脉注射免疫球蛋白（IVIG）和 B 细胞耗竭剂（如利妥昔单抗和硼替佐米）。然而，接受治疗和未接受治疗的免疫敏感受者的术后结果并没有显著差异[40]。

### 14.4.3 再移植后新生的供体特异性抗体

移植后，12%~40% 的受者会产生新生供体特异性 HLA 抗体（donor-specific HLA antibodies，DSA），而再移植是新生 DSA 的独立危险因素[41-43]。因此，建议肺再移植后定期监测受者新生 DSA，特别是术后第一年内，以改善移植效果[42-44]。鉴于肺移植后持久性 DSA 对无 CLAD 生存的负面影响，多个中心已发表他们对免疫敏感患者进行围术期治疗的方案，以实现与没有 DSA 的受者相似的无 CLAD 生存[41-43,45,46]。在没有 DSA 的情况下，肺再移植不会带来更高的急性同种异体移植排斥反应或发生 CLAD 的风险[3,5,7]。

## 14.5 手术技术

再次胸腔移植手术是一项重大技术。粘连性疾病表现为致密的胸膜增厚、血管与胸壁粘连（图 14-4）、大量出血和潜在的肾功能不全，这仅仅是导致这项困难而艰巨的手术的其中几个因素。进行肺再移植时必须考虑到几个关键问题。

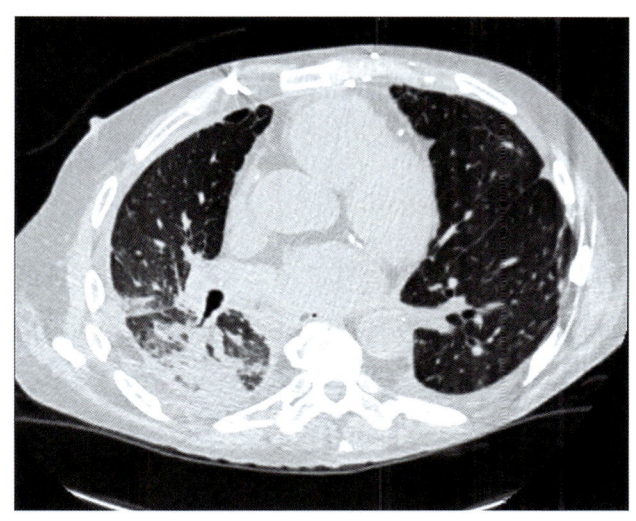

图 14-4　接受双侧胸膜固定术的肺再移植候选者的计算机断层扫描显示胸膜增厚

### 14.5.1 蛤壳术式与侧开胸术

考虑到与再移植相关的技术挑战，历来许多中心首选双侧经胸胸廓切开术（蛤壳术式）大切口，其提供了进入双侧胸膜腔、肺门和前纵隔的良好通道。然而，蛤壳术式切口可能会导致疼痛、恢复时间延长以及潜在的伤口并发症。这些限制促使一些中心采用替代方法。

Bhama 及其同事报道了他们使用保留胸骨的方法进行双侧肺再移植的早期经验。在这项小样本的回顾性研究中，结果显示术后疗效没有显著差异，并且有减少术后机械通气时间和住院时间的趋势[47]。在更大的系列中，汉诺威研究小组报道了他们在肺再移植的微创方案方面的经验，其中包括支持双侧肺移植、避免同种异体移植物缩小、保留胸骨的前胸廓微创切开术、避免体外循环、避免使用肝素和预防性凝血因子输注。结果显示微创方案可减少术后透析、机械通气、气管切开术的需要以及 ICU 住院时间，并显示出较高的住院、30 天和 1 年生存率[7]。尽管微创肺再移植因各种原因很有吸引力，但最

**肺移植：胸外科临床问题**

终手术的安全性和暴露性仍然是最重要的。在再次移植手术之前进行首次手术或干预手术（例如，针对反复积液的胸膜固定术或针对滞留肺的剥脱术）可以在再次移植的方法和实施中发挥相当大的作用。第一次移植后的任何胸膜操作都会使再次移植手术在技术上更加困难，并且更有可能需要大量输血。通常采用关闭主动脉插管部位上方的心包上部的方法以避免灾难性的再出血。为了避免心包积液或心包缩窄（这是一种罕见但严重的并发症），一般不会完全关闭心包。对于肺门，在肺动脉（PA）和支气管吻合口之间放置软组织（通常是胸腺脂肪）可以促进再移植时的解剖分离。关闭支气管周围软组织也可能有助于在再移植解剖过程中分离支气管和PA。

### 14.5.2 单侧与双侧原位肺再移植

在过去的30年里，双侧原发性肺移植已成为几乎所有适应证的趋势[5]。化脓性肺病和严重特发性肺动脉高压一直是首次受者双侧移植的经典绝对适应证。尽管同样的原则也适用于再移植，但双肺或单肺再移植的适应证尚不清楚。在对2005—2013年间联合器官共享网络登记处的审查中，Shum及其同事确定了410例接受肺再移植的患者。他们观察到，无论初次移植或再移植类型如何，再移植受者之间的生存率都没有显著差异，由此得出结论，无论以前的移植类型如何，都应该选择单肺再移植，以最大限度地利用有限的器官资源[28]。在另一项UNOS研究中，Kon及其同事回顾了325例在单肺移植后接受肺再移植的患者的结果。研究发现，与对侧和双侧肺再移植相比，同侧单肺再移植的早期和中期死亡风险增加。事实上，对侧和双侧肺再移植的30天和1年生存率与初次肺移植相当[48]。这些发现并不令人意外，因为决定进行同侧再移植表明人们倾向于避免进行对侧再移植手术，而这些理由无法从国家登记册中获取。杜克大学研究小组此前曾发表过对具有较高手术风险的间质性肺病患者进行分期双侧移植的经验[49]。其包括65岁以上的患者、患有严重冠状动脉疾病的患者以及表现出功能状态下降的患者。接受单肺移植的患者经过一段时间的恢复后进行重新评估，因原发肺疾病再次列入移植清单，随后进行对侧单肺移植。研究发现，这些患者有类似的短期生存率和1年肺功能测试结果，且肾损伤发生率降低。先前因原发性肺疾病进行单肺移植后的对侧单肺移植（即"分期双侧肺移植"）不应被误解为因同种异体移植物衰竭而进行的再移植。

我们的做法是对之前接受过双侧移植的患者优先选择双侧再移植。对于之前接受过单侧肺移植的患者来说，答案更加微妙。例如，对于那些由于对侧胸腔环境"恶劣"而接受单侧肺移植（而非双侧）的患者，我们将选择进行同侧单肺再次移植。对于因身体虚弱、慢性病急性发作，但对侧胸腔解剖结构良好的患者，我们则会进行对侧单肺再次移植。我们很少对之前接受过单肺移植的患者进行双侧肺再移植，然而，根据受者的微生物环境和其他因素的考虑，这可能是必要的。要求对每个病例都仔细评估和审查，以最大限度地提高成功的机会。

### 14.5.3 体外循环

随着时间的推移，体外循环在肺移植中的应用不断发展。在肺移植手术中，体外循环（CPB）最初是维持术中血流动力学和呼吸功能的主要手段。然而，CPB 的使用与更高的输血需求以及与更高的 PGD 率（与全身炎症反应增加有关）相关。虽然许多项目选择"非体外循环"进行肺移植，但现在越来越多的中心常规使用术中 ECMO，事实证明这种方法安全有效，可减少 PGD、输血需求和术后终末器官功能障碍[50,51]。此外，如果患者需要术后支持，ECMO 可以轻松地重新配置并在 ICU 中继续使用[51]。

目前关于肺再次移植术中体外循环支持的使用的数据较少。Wallinder 及其同事的研究报道了初次移植和再次移植手术中使用体外循环的比例相似。然而，其大部分病例都是在没有循环支持的情况下进行的[21]。由于体外循环通常需要全身抗凝，因此需要将出血风险增加的缺点与心肺支持的必要性进行权衡。在再次移植手术中，由于解剖过程中误伤肺动脉或肺静脉的风险更高，可能需要 CPB 形式的机械支持。否则，在胸膜剥离过程中避免使用机械支持通常会更具优势，能够尽量减少血管粘连引起的出血。

### 14.5.4 血液学管理

围手术期血液学管理在肺再移植中至关重要。考虑到这种高难度手术的技术挑战，肺再移植需要更高的输血要求也就不足为奇了[52,53]。由于输血率的增加与较高的 PGD 发生率和较低的生存率相关，努力减少患者的输血势在必行[52-56]。然而，关于输血对肺移植结果影响的高质量数据仍然缺乏。在一项关于肺移植中输血和结果的系统性回顾中，Klapper 及其同事强调了移植计划需要制定围手术期血液学管理的算法方法[57]。

Smith 及其同事的研究表明，实施床旁旋转式血栓弹性测量（rotational thromboelastometry，ROTEM）和规范化出血管理方案，可以显著减少输注红细胞悬浮液、新鲜冰冻血浆和血小板的需求[58]。减少围术期输血需求的另一个有前景的方法是使用重组和浓缩的凝血因子制剂[59]。这些治疗还能避免传统产品带来的容量负荷。

## 14.6 术后管理和其他重要考虑因素

初次移植和再次移植的术后管理实际上是相同的，但也有一些重要的区别。

### 14.6.1 保持胸腔开放

在一些高难度的肺移植手术中，包括并不罕见的再次移植手术、部分关闭手术切口或"保持胸腔开放"并使用临时无菌敷料都是重要的辅助手段。尽管我们的目标是最终闭合手术切口，但由于术中更容易出血、供体-受体尺寸不匹配以及需要继续体外支持的 PGD，因此在某些情况下，手术结束后暂时保持胸腔开放可能更安全。对于需要持续应用中心静脉插管进行静脉-动脉体外膜肺氧合（ECMO），或存在严重凝血障碍性出血需要持续抢救的情况，我们的做法不是"过度填塞"胸腔，而是优先实现止血目标。我们使用定制的 Esmarch 绷带和 Ioban 敷料制作临时敷料，将其缝合固定在适当的位置。然后重新打开胸腔，每 24~48 小时更换一次敷料，直到出血得到控制，或者可以逐渐撤离体外循环支持并且适合进行最终的切口闭合为止。

### 14.6.2 供体-受体尺寸匹配

另一个重要的考虑因素是由于瘢痕组织而导致的再次手术中胸腔相对固定的特性。应特别注意尺寸匹配，强调避免尺寸过大。固定而僵硬的胸腔结构会限制生理活动，加上供体肺尺寸过大以及肺移植过程中和术后立即出现的总体顺应性降低，常常导致严重的呼吸困难。另一种情况下，暂时保持胸腔开放可能是有益的，同时增加一个临时的"支撑"，可以增加胸腔的尺寸。因为患者需要长时间卧床休息，重症监护和护理团队必须努力监测敷料的完整性，并密切关注压疮的情况。

## 14.7 长期结果

### 14.7.1 生存率

历史上，与初次肺移植相比，再移植的结果较差，第 1 年内死亡率最高。1992—2017 年的登记数据显示，肺再移植受者的 1 年生存率为 69.8%，而同一时间范围内的初次移植的 1 年生存率为 89.9%。同样，再移植的 5 年生存率为 41.9%，而初次移植的 5

年生存率为 56.4%[60]。

然而，当考虑再移植的基础诊断时，在经验丰富的中心，患有 CLAD 的受者表现出与初次移植相似的生存率，1 年生存率大于 85%[7,10,61]。相比之下，在初次肺移植早期出现严重 PGD 的受者，接受第二次肺移植的预后明显更差，多项文献报道了 1 年生存率为 38%～44%[7,25,27]。

CLAD 的表型也会影响术后生存率。再移植后 RAS 患者的 1 年生存率显著低于 BOS 患者，分别为 59% 和 84%[12]。据报道，肺再移植后第一年内的主要死亡原因没有显著差异，移植物衰竭和感染并发症是患者死亡的主要原因[62]。术后第一年之后，慢性同种异体移植排斥反应是死亡的主要原因，与初次移植后的患者类似[62]。

### 14.7.2 肺再移植后慢性同种异体肺功能障碍

慢性排斥反应发生在再移植肺后的第 1 年，其中大多数在术后第 3～5 年之间被诊断为 CLAD。当代肺再移植队列的无 CLAD 生存期中位数为 59～63 个月，与初次肺移植相似[7,62]。然而，CLAD 的表型也会影响术后无 CLAD 生存率。RAS 患者会在再移植后更早更频繁地出现慢性同种异体移植功能障碍。一项多中心研究报告显示，RAS 患者再移植后 3 年的无 CLAD 生存率为 51%，而同一时间点 BOS 患者的无 CLAD 生存率为 69%[12]。

## 14.8 总　结

肺再移植仍然是不可逆同种异体肺移植物衰竭的标准治疗方法。尽管早期经验显示结果接近令人望而却步，但随着患者选择、手术技术、术中和围术期管理的改善，以及使用 ECMO 和指导输血管理的血栓弹性图等安全辅助手段，肺再移植已成为对患者和医疗项目而言可行且重要的治疗方法。

> 【临床护理要点】
> 
> - 急性移植物衰竭、慢性肺移植物功能障碍和气道并发症是肺再移植的最重要适应证。
> - 慎重选择患者和供者对于达到满意的预后至关重要。
> - 微创手术技术在改善患者预后方面具有很大的潜力。
> - 初次肺移植和肺再移植的术后管理类似。

## 声明

EM：没有声明。

WS：没有声明。

MGH：直觉外科（咨询和研究）、Paragonix（咨询和研究）、BiomedInnovations（咨询和研究）、Mallinckrodt（研究）。

## 参考文献

1. Miller JD, Patterson GA. Retransplantation following isolated lung transplantation. Semin Thorac Cardiovasc Surg 1992;4(2):122–125.
2. Novick RJ, Schafers HJ, Stitt L, et al. Seventy-two pulmonary retransplantations for obliterative bronchiolitis: predictors of survival. Ann Thorac Surg 1995;60(1):111–116.
3. Halloran K, Aversa M, Tinckam K, et al. Comprehensive outcomes after lung retransplantation: a single center review. Clin Transplant 2018;32(6):e13281.
4. Yusen RD, Edwards LB, Kucheryavaya AY, et al. The registry of the international society for heart and lung transplantation: thirty-second official adult lung and heart-lung transplantation report–2015; focus theme:early graft failure. J Heart Lung Transplant 2015;34(10):1264–1277.
5. Yusen RD, Edwards LB, Kucheryavaya AY, et al. The registry of the International Society for Heart and Lung Transplantation: thirty-first adult lung and heart-lung transplant report–2014; focus theme: re-transplantation. J Heart Lung Transplant 2014; 33(10):1009–1024.
6. Kawut SM, Lederer DJ, Keshavjee S, et al. Outcomes after lung retransplantation in the modern era. Am J Respir Crit Care Med 2008;177(1):114–120.
7. Sommer W, Ius F, Kuhn C, et al. Technique and out comes of less invasive lung retransplantation. Transplantation 2018;102(3):530–537.
8. Harringer W, Wiebe K, Struber M, et al. Lung transplantation–10-year experience. Eur J Cardiothorac Surg 1999;16(5):546–554.
9. Wekerle T, Klepetko W, Wisser W, et al. Lung retransplantation: institutional report on a series of twenty patients. J Heart Lung Transplant 1996;15(2):182–189.
10. Osho AA, Castleberry AW, Snyder LD, et al. Differential outcomes with early and late repeat transplantation in the era of the lung allocation score. Ann Thorac Surg 2014;98(6):1914–20 [discussion 1911–1920].
11. Godinas L, Van Raemdonck D, Ceulemans LJ, et al. Lung retransplantation: walking a thin line between hope and false expectations. J Thorac Dis 2019; 11(11):E200–203.
12. Verleden SE, Todd JL, Sato M, et al. Impact of CLAD phenotype on survival after lung retransplantation: a multicenter study. Am J Transplant 2015;15(8): 2223–2230.
13. Sato M, Hwang DM, Waddell TK, et al. Progression pattern of restrictive allograft syndrome after lung transplantation. J Heart Lung Transplant 2013; 32(1):23–30.

14. Ofek E, Sato M, Saito T, et al. Restrictive allograft syndrome post lung transplantation is characterized by pleuroparenchymal fibroelastosis. Mod Pathol 2013;26(3):350–356.
15. Sato M, Hirayama S, Matsuda Y, et al. Stromal activation and formation of lymphoid-like stroma in chronic lung allograft dysfunction. Transplantation 2011;91(12):1398–1405.
16. Yoshiyasu N, Sato M. Chronic lung allograft dysfunction post-lung transplantation: the era of bronchiolitis obliterans syndrome and restrictive allograft syndrome. World J Transpl 2020;10(5):104–116.
17. Schweiger T, Nenekidis I, Stadler JE, et al. Single running suture technique is associated with low rate of bronchial complications after lung transplantation. J Thorac Cardiovasc Surg 2020;160(4): 1099–1108. e3.
18. Moreno P, Alvarez A, Algar FJ, et al. Incidence, management and clinical outcomes of patients with airway complications following lung transplantation. Eur J Cardiothorac Surg 2008;34(6):1198–1205.
19. Orens JB, Estenne M, Arcasoy S, et al. International guidelines for the selection of lung transplant candidates: 2006 update–a consensus report from the Pulmonary Scientific Council of the International Society for Heart and Lung Transplantation. J Heart Lung Transplant 2006;25(7):745–755.
20. Hayanga JW, Aboagye JK, Hayanga HK, et al. Extracorporeal membrane oxygenation as a bridge to lung re-transplantation: Is there a role? J Heart Lung Transplant 2016;35(7):901–905.
21. Wallinder A, Danielsson C, Magnusson J, et al. Outcomes and long-term survival after pulmonary re-transplantation: a single-center experience. Ann Thorac Surg 2019;108(4):1037–1044.
22. Thomas M, Belli EV, Rawal B, et al. Survival after lung retransplantation in the united states in the current era (2004 to 2013): better or worse? Ann ThoracSurg 2015;100(2):452–457.
23. Dubey GK, Hossain A, Dobrescu C, et al. Repeat lung retransplantation and death risk. J Heart Lung Transplant 2020;39(8):841–845.
24. Collaud S, Benden C, Ganter C, et al. Extracorporeal life support as bridge to lung retransplantation: a multicenter pooled data analysis. Ann Thorac Surg 2016;102(5):1680–1686.
25. Ren D, Kaleekal TS, Graviss EA, et al. Retransplantation outcomes at a large lung transplantation program. Transpl Direct 2018;4(11):e404.
26. Osho AA, Castleberry AW, Snyder LD, et al. Determining eligibility for lung transplantation: a nationwide assessment of the cutoff glomerular filtrationrate. J Heart Lung Transplant 2015;34(4):571–579.
27. Hall DJ, Belli EV, Gregg JA, et al. Two decades of lung retransplantation: a single-center experience. Ann Thorac Surg 2017;103(4):1076–1083.
28. Schumer EM, Rice JD, Kistler AM, et al. Single versus double lung retransplantation does not affect survival based on previous transplant type. Ann Thorac Surg 2017;103(1):236–240.
29. Abou-Daya KI, Tieu R, Zhao D, et al. Resident memory T cells form during persistent antigen exposure leading to allograft rejection. Sci Immunol 2021; 6(57):eabc8122.
30. Bosanquet JP, Witt CA, Bemiss BC, et al. The impact of pre-transplant allosensitization on outcomes after lung transplantation. J Heart Lung Transplant 2015; 34(11):1415–1422.
31. Hulbert AL, Pavlisko EN, Palmer SM. Current challenges and opportunities in the management of antibody-mediated rejection in lung transplantation. Curr Opin Organ Transpl 2018;23(3):308–315.
32. Sommer W, Hallensleben M, Ius F, et al. Repeated human leukocyte antigen mismatches in lung re-transplantation. Transpl Immunol 2017;40:1–7.

33. Frost AE, Jammal CT, Cagle PT. Hyperacute rejection following lung transplantation. Chest 1996; 110(2):559–562.

34. Kulkarni HS, Bemiss BC, Hachem RR. Antibody-mediated rejection in lung transplantation. Curr Transpl Rep 2015;2(4):316–323.

35. Levine DJ, Glanville AR, Aboyoun C, et al. Antibody-mediated rejection of the lung: a consensus report of the International Society for Heart and Lung Transplantation. J Heart Lung Transplant 2016; 35(4):397–406.

36. Hadjiliadis D, Chaparro C, Reinsmoen NL, et al. Pretransplant panel reactive antibody in lung transplant recipients is associated with significantly worse post-transplant survival in a multicenter study. J Heart Lung Transplant 2005;24(7 Suppl):S249–254.

37. Brugiere O, Suberbielle C, Thabut G, et al. Lung transplantation in patients with pretransplantation donor-specific antibodies detected by Luminex assay. Transplantation 2013;95(5):761–765.

38. Kim M, Townsend KR, Wood IG, et al. Impact of pretransplant anti-HLA antibodies on outcomes in lung transplant candidates. Am J Respir Crit Care Med 2014;189(10):1234–1239.

39. Lau CL, Palmer SM, Posther KE, et al. Influence of panel-reactive antibodies on posttransplant outcomes in lung transplant recipients. Ann Thorac Surg 2000;69(5):1520–1524.

40. Snyder LD, Gray AL, Reynolds JM, et al. Antibody desensitization therapy in highly sensitized lung transplant candidates. Am J Transplant 2014;14(4): 849–856.

41. Verleden SE, Vanaudenaerde BM, Emonds MP, et al. Donor-specific and -nonspecific HLA antibodies and outcome post lung transplantation. Eur Respir J 2017;50(5):1701248.

42. Ius F, Sommer W, Tudorache I, et al. Early donors-pecific antibodies in lung transplantation: risk factors and impact on survival. J Heart Lung Transplant 2014;33(12):1255–1263.

43. Ius F, Muller C, Sommer W, et al. Six-year experience with treatment of early donor-specific anti-HLA antibodies in pediatric lung transplantation using a human immunoglobulin-based protocol. Pediatr Pulmonol 2020;55(3):754–764.

44. Hachem RR. Donor-specific antibodies in lung transplantation. Curr Opin Organ Transpl 2020;25(6): 563–567.

45. Tinckam KJ, Keshavjee S, Chaparro C, et al. Survival in sensitized lung transplant recipients with perioperative desensitization. Am J Transplant 2015;15(2):417–426.

46. Courtwright AM, Cao S, Wood I, et al. Clinical outcomes of lung transplantation in the presence of donor-specific antibodies. Ann Am Thorac Soc 2019;16(9):1131–1137.

47. Bhama JK, Bansal A, Shigemura N, et al. Sternal-sparing approach for reoperative bilateral lung transplantation. Interact Cardiovasc Thorac Surg 2013;17(5):835–837.

48. Kon ZN, Bittle GJ, Pasrija C, et al. The optimal procedure for re-transplantation after single lung transplantation. Ann Thorac Surg 2017;104(1):170–175.

49. Hartwig MG, Ganapathi AM, Osho AA, et al. Staging of bilateral lung transplantation for high-risk patients with interstitial lung disease: one lung at a time. Am J Transplant 2016;16(11):3270–3277.

50. Ius F, Kuehn C, Tudorache I, et al. Lung transplantation on cardiopulmonary support: venoarterial extracorporeal membrane oxygenation outperformed cardiopulmonary bypass. J Thorac Cardiovasc Surg 2012;144(6):1510–1516.

51. Hoetzenecker K, Schwarz S, Muckenhuber M, et al. Intraoperative extracorporeal membrane oxygenation and the possibility of postoperative prolongation improve survival in bilateral lung transplantation. J Thorac Cardiovasc Surg 2018;155(5):2193–2206. e3.
52. Grande B, Oechslin P, Schlaepfer M, et al. Predictors of blood loss in lung transplant surgery-a single center retrospective cohort analysis. J Thorac Dis 2019;11(11):4755–4761.
53. Cernak V, Oude Lansink-Hartgring A, van den Heuvel ER, et al. Incidence of massive transfusion and overall transfusion requirements during lung transplantation over a 25-year period. J Cardiothorac Vasc Anesth 2019;33(9):2478–2486.
54. Ong LP, Thompson E, Sachdeva A, et al. Allogeneic blood transfusion in bilateral lung transplantation: impact on early function and mortality. Eur J Cardiothorac Surg 2016;49(2):668–674 [discussion 674].
55. Hayes D Jr, Higgins RS, Kilic A, et al. Extracorporeal membrane oxygenation and retransplantation in lung transplantation: an analysis of the UNOS registry. Lung 2014;192(4):571–576.
56. Diamond JM, Lee JC, Kawut SM, et al. Clinical risk factors for primary graft dysfunction after lung transplantation. Am J Respir Crit Care Med 2013;187(5):527–534.
57. Klapper JA, Hicks AC, Ledbetter L, et al. Blood product transfusion and lung transplant outcomes: a systematic review. Clin Transplant 2021;35(10): e14404.
58. Smith I, Pearse BL, Faulke DJ, et al. Targeted bleeding management reduces the requirements for blood component therapy in lung transplant recipients. J Cardiothorac Vasc Anesth 2017;31(2): 426–433.
59. Bhaskar B, Zeigenfuss M, Choudhary J, et al. Use of recombinant activated Factor VII for refractory after lung transplant bleeding as an effective strategy to restrict blood transfusion and associated complications. Transfusion 2013;53(4):798–804.
60. Chambers DC, Cherikh WS, Harhay MO, et al. The International Thoracic Organ Transplant Registry of the International Society for Heart and Lung Transplantation: thirty-sixth adult lung and heart-lung transplantation report-2019; Focus theme: donor and recipient size match. J Heart Lung Transplant 2019;38(10):1042–1055.
61. Biswas Roy S, Panchanathan R, Walia R, et al. Lung retransplantation for chronic rejection: a single-center experience. Ann Thorac Surg 2018;105(1): 221–227.
62. Lund LH, Edwards LB, Kucheryavaya AY, et al. The registry of the International Society for Heart and Lung Transplantation: thirty-first official adult heart transplant report–2014; focus theme: retransplantation. J Heart Lung Transplant 2014;33(10): 996–1008.